Clinical Pharmacology for Nurses

For Churchill Livingstone:

Commissioning Editor: Ninette Premdas
Project Manager: Gail Murray
Project Development Manager: Dinah Thom

Clinical Pharmacology for Nurses

John Trounce MD FRCP
Professor Emeritus of Clinical Pharmacology, United Medical and Dental Schools,
and Physician Emeritus, Guy's Hospital, London, UK

Nursing Adviser

Dinah Gould BSc MPhil PhD RGN RNT
Professor of Nursing, Faculty of Health, South Bank University, London, UK

SIXTEENTH EDITION

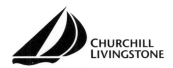
CHURCHILL
LIVINGSTONE

EDINBURGH LONDON NEW YORK PHILADELPHIA ST LOUIS SYDNEY TORONTO 2000

CHURCHILL LIVINGSTONE
An imprint of Harcourt Publishers Limited

© E&S Livingstone Ltd 1958, 1961, 1964, 1967, 1970
© Longman Group Limited 1973, 1977, 1979, 1981, 1983,
1985, 1988, 1990, 1994
© Pearson Professional Limited 1997
© Harcourt Publishers Limited 2000

First edition 1958
Second edition 1961
Third edition 1964
Fourth edition 1967
Fifth edition 1970
Sixth edition 1973
Seventh edition 1977
Eighth edition 1979
Ninth edition 1981

Tenth edition 1983
Eleventh edition 1985
Twelfth edition 1988
Thirteenth edition 1990
Fourteenth edition 1994
Fifteenth edition 1997
Sixteenth edition 2000

ISBN 0 443 06244 7
  Reprinted 2000
  Reprinted 2002

International Edition ISBN 0 443 06249 8
  Reprinted 2000
  Reprinted 2001
  Reprinted 2002

British Library Cataloguing in Publication Data
A catalogue record for this book is available from the British
Library

Library of Congress Cataloging in Publication Data
A catalog record for this book is available from the Library
of Congress.

Note
Medical knowledge is constantly changing. As new
information becomes available, changes in treatment,
procedures, equipment and the use of drugs become
necessary. The editors and contributors and the publishers
have, as far as it is possible, taken care to ensure that the
information given in this text is accurate and up to date, but
mistakes may have occurred. However, readers are strongly
advised to confirm that the information, especially with
regard to drug usage, complies with latest legislation
and standards of practice.

The
publisher's
policy is to use
**paper manufactured
from sustainable forests**

Printed in China by RDC Group Limited
W/03/04

Contents

Contributors

Chapter 11. Anaesthetics

M.B. Barnett MB BS FRC Anaes
Consultant Anaesthetist,
Guy's Hospital, London, UK

Chapter 25. Drugs and the eye

D.M. Watson TD FRCS FRCOphth
Consulting Ophthalmic Surgeon Emeritus
Guy's and St Thomas' Hospitals, London, UK

Contribution to Chapter 26. The local application of drugs

Lynette Stone CBE BA RGN RM (NSW) DMS
Nursing and Business Development Manager,
Dermatological and Dental Group,
Guy's Hospital, London, UK

Chapter 3. Nurses and the pharmaceutical service and Chapter 29. Herbal medicines

Anne Joshua MSc MRPharm S
Consultant Pharmacist

Preface to the Sixteenth Edition

This edition introduces some important new drugs and their use in the management of disease. The text has been revised and seven new illustrations have been added.

An understanding of pharmacology and its application to patient care is an integral part of pre- and post-registration nursing education, with the current trend towards extending nurse prescribing. In addition to the actions and uses of drugs in treatment, some account is given of their role in prevention, where this is relevant.

Nurses are frequently responsible for the application of drugs to the skin and the eye and these parts have been written by specialists who give precise instruction of techniques used.

A short section on homeopathy follows the chapter on herbal medicines, as these complementary therapies are now widely practised.

Nurses should be familiar with the regulation and control of drugs, adverse reactions and monitoring, the introduction and licensing of new drugs, clinical trials, ethics committees and the economic aspects of medicine, not only because of their increasing involvement with prescribing but also because there is much public discussion and media coverage of these subjects. The lists for further reading have been revised and updated.

We bid farewell to Roger Horne, with our thanks for all the help he has given us over many editions. His section is now covered by Anne Joshua.

Finally, we would like to thank the staff of Churchill Livingstone, yet again, for their unfailing assistance in the preparation of this book.

London 1999

J.R.T.
D.J.G.

Acknowledgements

We would like to thank the following for permission to reproduce their illustrations:

Allen and Hanbury Ltd—Figure 4.8

Becton Dickinson—Figures 2.1, 2.2, 2.3

The European Resuscitation Council 1997 who hold the copyright for Figure 11.2

MTP Press—Figures 4.6, 6.2, 6.3, 8.2, 15.1 from *Commonsense Use of Medicines* by J. Fry, J. Trounce and M. Godfrey

Prentice Hall International—Figures 14.12, 14.14 from *Nursing Care of Women* by Dinah Gould

Graseby Medical for permission to use their name in the illustration, Figure 9.3

Professor D'Arcy and the Oxford University Press for Tables 29.1, 29.2

Edward Arnold and Professor Ritter for Figure 21.3 from *A Textbook of Clinical Pharmacology*

The BMJ Publishing Group and Professor Eastell for Figure 14.7

HMSO for Figure 17.2 from *Immunisation against Infectious Disease*

and the following for their help and advice:

Dr Virginia Murray, The National Poisons Information Service, New Cross Hospital, London

Stephanie Barnes and Susanna Gilmour-White, Department of Clinical Pharmacology, St Thomas' Hospital, and the Drug Information Unit, Guy's Hospital, London

Dr Camilla Davies, Department of Anaesthetics, Guy's Hospital, London

Theo King

Louise Farrow.

Nomenclature

In 1998 the recommended International Non-proprietary Name (rINN) replaced the British Approved Name (BAN) for drugs. There are several drugs, widely used in the UK, for which the INN differs from the BAN. For main headings in the text and in the index, where this occurs, the BAN will be shown in parentheses after the rINN for drugs where it is considered that confusion could occur. For example:

Epinephrine (adrenaline)

1

Introduction

Pharmacology may be defined as the study of drugs. This includes their origin, chemical structure, preparation, administration, actions, metabolism and excretion. The application of the action of drugs and other measures in the treatment of disease is called therapeutics.

Drugs have been used in treating disease for thousands of years. The writings of most of the ancient civilizations contain directions for the preparation and administration of drugs. Nearly all the remedies described had little, if any, effect, but it is of interest that among the bizarre prescriptions containing such ingredients as fat of the hippopotamus and pig bile, can be found drugs which are still used today. The ancient Egyptians were familiar with the purging effect of castor oil, the Arabians used both opium and senna, and in more recent times the effects of digitalis on oedema were known to country people with no medical training. Nevertheless, the use of drugs in the treatment of disease remained entirely empirical and usually misdirected until the nineteenth century. This period saw the emergence of rational physiology and pathology and on this foundation it was possible to study the effect of drugs and their use in disease.

At first, investigation was confined to observation of the effect on the whole animal or human patient. With the rise of experimental physiology it became possible to investigate the action of drugs on isolated organs and thus obtain a much clearer picture of their effects and potential uses as therapeutic agents. These investigations have

1

brought into use such drugs as adrenaline and ergometrine.

While this work was progressing the chemical structure of many drugs was being unravelled and it thus proved practicable to relate the function of drugs to their chemical composition. This was an important advance for it meant that by slightly altering the structure of a drug it might be possible to enhance its useful action and remove any troublesome side-effects. This led to the introduction of many synthetic substances which have proved invaluable in the treatment of disease.

Although extensive experiments in animals led to many useful advances, it is now realized that there are important differences between the pharmacology of drugs in animals and humans. Even in the relatively early stages of introducing a new drug, investigation of its action requires studies in humans. This has led to the emergence of clinical pharmacology which is essentially the study of drug actions in humans.

At the present time the frontiers of pharmacology are still being extended, and much work is now concerned with the actual effect of the drug on the complex chemical reactions which are continually occurring within the living cell. Much of this work is difficult, expensive and time consuming, but it is by such a methodical approach, occasionally illuminated by a flash of empirical genius, that pharmacology will advance and the therapeutic armoury of the nurse and doctor be enlarged.

THE USE OF DRUGS

In the management of any patient a therapeutic plan should be formulated to decide the realistic objectives of treatment. This plan will frequently include the use of drugs, but before giving any drug to a patient certain factors should be considered:

1. Is the drug appropriate, not only for the disorder being treated, but also for that individual, taking into account age, state of health and general circumstances?

2. How has the patient responded to drugs in the past? A careful drug history is essential.

3. Does the patient understand the implications of treatment? A full explanation is necessary, including the objectives of treatment, the action of the drug (simplified, if necessary) and the possibility of adverse effects.

4. Has the correct therapy been chosen? Choosing the correct therapy for a patient has always been to some extent based on evidence derived from previous experience, investigation and research. However, this evidence may be biased by prejudice, false impressions and ignorance. To improve this situation there is a move to practise medicine (including the choice of drugs) on the basis of the current best evidence available; this is called *evidence based medicine*.

Patient care is now seen as a team activity and nurses will play their part in several capacities. They are increasingly involved in the drug aspects of treatment, as prescribers, in administering drugs and in noting therapeutic and adverse effects. It is therefore important that they have an understanding of the underlying principles and mechanisms involved in addition to their knowledge of the use of drugs.

ABSORPTION, METABOLISM AND ELIMINATION OF DRUGS (PHARMACOKINETICS)

The study of the way in which the body handles drugs from administration to elimination is called pharmacokinetics. Although this is a complex subject, some understanding of the principles is useful in that it is concerned with the dosage, distribution and duration of action of the drug.

Drugs may be given to a patient in various ways; they may be injected, absorbed from the gastrointestinal tract after oral or rectal administration, applied locally or inhaled.

The term *bioavailability* is used to denote that proportion of the administered dose of a drug which reaches the circulation. If it is given intravenously then the bioavailability is obviously 100%; if it is swallowed then only a proportion may reach the circulation.

Oral administration is the commonest and easiest way to give a drug and the bioavailability by this route depends on several factors.

1. *Absorption.* Most drugs are absorbed by diffusion through the wall of the intestine into the bloodstream, a process aided by the very large surface area of the gut wall. A few drugs are absorbed by active transport processes. The rate and extent of absorption will depend on the physical properties of the drug which determine how easily it will pass through the wall of the gut, and on the formulation of the drug by the manufacturer.

Absorption may be complete or incomplete and may be modified by the rate at which the stomach empties, the presence or absence of food in the stomach and, sometimes, interactions with other drugs or diseases of the gastrointestinal tract (p. 9).

2. *First pass effect.* When absorbed from the gastrointestinal tract drugs have to pass via the portal vein to the liver before reaching the general circulation (Fig. 1.1). This may be important as many drugs are metabolized (broken down) as they pass through the liver so that only a proportion of the amount absorbed actually reaches the circulation and thus their bioavailability is reduced. This removal of the drug as it passes through the liver is called the first pass effect. Drugs which show a very large first pass effect are almost inactive if swallowed, examples being lignocaine and glyceryl trinitrate, and these have to be injected or, if absorbed from the oral mucosa, can be chewed or sucked, thus bypassing the liver.

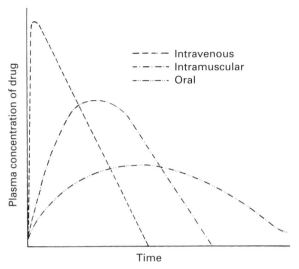

Figure 1.2 The effect of the route of administration of a drug on the plasma concentrations after a single dose.

After absorption, drugs enter the bloodstream and are carried round the body. They may be in simple solution in the plasma, but many are poorly soluble and are partially bound to plasma proteins which act as carriers. *It is important to realize that the fraction of a drug which is bound to protein is inactive and only the free unbound portion has any pharmacological action.*

The concentration of a drug in the bloodstream is a good index of whether the correct dose is being given to produce a satisfactory therapeutic effect. Therefore, the nurse should know something of the factors which govern the blood concentration.

1. *The dose.* It is obvious that the larger the dose, the higher the concentration achieved.

2. *The route of administration.* Intravenous injection produces a rapid rise in blood concentration whereas oral administration gives a slower rise and a lower peak concentration. Intramuscular injection rates lie between the two (Fig. 1.2).

3. *The distribution of the drug.* This is another important factor in determining the plasma concentration and also its activity and therapeutic usefulness (Fig. 1.3). Some drugs are confined to the bloodstream and this obviously limits their effect; for instance, an antibiotic which would

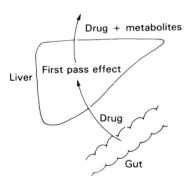

Figure 1.1 First pass metabolism of a drug.

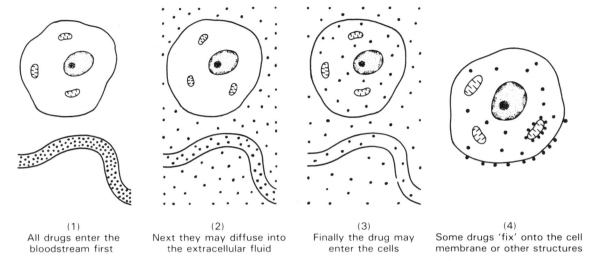

(1)	(2)	(3)	(4)
All drugs enter the bloodstream first	Next they may diffuse into the extracellular fluid	Finally the drug may enter the cells	Some drugs 'fix' onto the cell membrane or other structures

Figure 1.3 Distribution of drugs in the body.

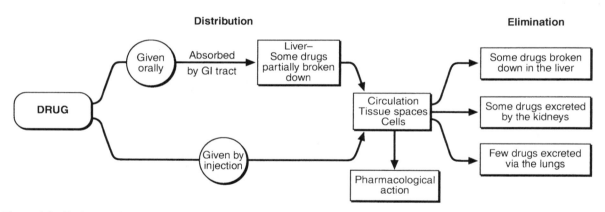

Figure 1.4 Pathways of systemically-acting drugs.

not enter the tissues would be useless in treating most infections.

Other drugs diffuse out of the circulation into the tissue spaces and some enter the cells and spread through the total water of the body. A few drugs are actually concentrated in cells.

The average volume of the distribution space for an adult is:

Plasma	3 litres
Extracellular space	15 litres
Total body water	36 litres

It can be seen, therefore, that the more widely a drug diffuses, the lower will be the concentration produced by a given dose.

4. *The rate of elimination.* The faster the body breaks down or excretes a drug, the more rapidly the blood level falls.

Drugs are usually eliminated in one or two ways (Fig. 1.4):

a. They may be broken down or combined with some other chemical so that they are no longer pharmacologically active. This usually occurs in the liver and is brought about by substances called enzymes. Enzymes have the property of promoting certain chemical reactions, and some of these are concerned with the inactivation of drugs. Therefore, if the liver cells are damaged by disease or the circulation to the liver is reduced, as in cardiac failure, the inactivation process may be slower than normal. The activity of the liver enzymes can be increased or decreased by drugs and this has important implications in treating patients (see Drug Interactions. p. 298).

There are also *genetically determined differences* in the rate at which some drugs can be broken down by the body (see p. 7). Suxamethonium normally produces a transient paralysis of voluntary muscle as it is broken down by an enzyme, but in certain families this enzyme is lacking or abnormal and suxamethonium causes a prolonged paralysis.

With certain types of drug, if given repeatedly, the breakdown process becomes more effective. Therefore, larger and larger doses are required to produce the same effect and this is known as *drug tolerance.*

b. Drugs or their breakdown products may be excreted through the kidneys and, if these are damaged by disease, excretion will be delayed and accumulation can occur. By the age of 80 years, kidney function is reduced to about half that of young adults, so with some drugs reduced dosage is required in the elderly. Rarely, drugs are excreted through the lungs and this route is important in the case of volatile anaesthetics.

The speed of elimination is the main factor in deciding the duration of action of a drug and is referred to as the *plasma half-life* ($t_{\frac{1}{2}}$) of that drug. This figure is obtained experimentally by giving a single dose, usually intravenously, and measuring the plasma concentration at intervals. The time taken for this concentration to halve is the plasma or biological half-life (Fig. 1.5).

Prodrugs are drugs which have been modified so that they are well absorbed or distributed but are pharmacologically inactive. In the body they are changed to the active form: for example, enalapril to the active form enalaprilat and levodopa to dopamine.

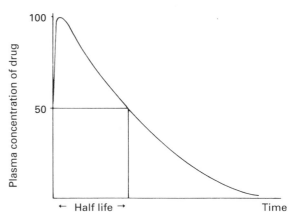

Figure 1.5 Plasma levels and half-life of a drug after a single intravenous injection.

FACTORS INFLUENCING THE DOSAGE REGIME

Several factors must be considered when a drug is given to a patient. *The time it takes to act* is largely determined by the route of administration. For the most rapid effect, the drug is usually given intravenously. *The blood level and therapeutic effectiveness* depend on the dose, distribution within the body and to some degree on the mode of administration and speed of elimination.

Rapidly excreted drugs with short half-lives will require frequent administration or even continuous infusion to maintain a fairly constant concentration in the body, whereas those that are eliminated slowly can be given once or twice daily. With repeated dosing, the concentration in the plasma climbs until a more or less steady level is obtained. This is termed *steady state* (Fig. 1.6). The time taken to reach steady state is approximately five times the half-life of the drug. For example, the half-life of digoxin is 36 hours, so steady state for digoxin given regularly will be reached in $36 \times 5 = 180$ hours.

It can be seen that the shorter the half-life (i.e. the quicker the elimination) of a drug, the more rapidly it will reach steady state. To hasten the achievement of steady state and full therapeutic effect with more slowly excreted drugs, a large *loading dose* may be given followed by smaller maintenance doses (see Fig. 1.6).

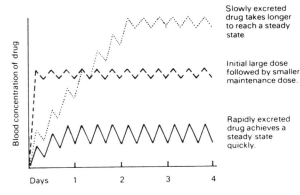

Slowly excreted drug takes longer to reach a steady state.

Initial large dose followed by smaller maintenance dose.

Rapidly excreted drug achieves a steady state quickly.

Figure 1.6 Steady state concentrations of drugs.

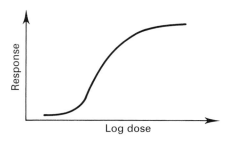

Figure 1.7 Dose/response curve.

DOSE RESPONSE

In general the response to a drug is related to the dose; an increased dose leads to a greater response. If the log of the dose is plotted against the response (Fig. 1.7), most drugs show a sigmoid curve.

With the majority of drugs, when used therapeutically, the dose/response is on the steep part of the curve, i.e. increased dose → increased effect. However, with some drugs, for example the analgesic buprenorphine, the dose/response is towards the upper end of the curve so that increasing the dose beyond a certain level does not enhance the therapeutic effect of the drug.

FACTORS WHICH MAY MODIFY DRUG RESPONSE

There are a number of variables that can influence drug response. It is true that the pharmacological action of a drug rarely differs between subjects, but the intensity and duration of that action often differs considerably.

This may occur for two main reasons:

1. Because the concentration of the drug within the body, and thus its intensity of action, is subject to interindividual variation.
2. Because the sensitivity and responsiveness of receptor mechanisms involved in drug action may differ between subjects.

Although many of these interindividual differences in drug response are not large enough to be of practical importance, with some drugs, particularly if there is only a narrow margin between toxicity and therapeutic effect, such variations in response may represent the difference between success and disaster and therefore some knowledge of the factors involved is useful to the nurse and they are discussed in the following sections.

Size of the patient

This can be expressed either in terms of body weight or body surface area. It is obvious that when a drug, after absorption, is distributed throughout the body, the larger that body (and thus the volume of distribution) the lower will be the concentration of a given dose of a drug and the less intense will be its actions.

To correct for variations due to differences in weight the dose may be expressed as:

Dose per kilogram weight of the patient.

Example: For a patient weighing 60 kg and a dose of 10 mg/kg.

$$\text{Dose} = 60 \times 10 = 600 \text{ mg}$$

Even greater accuracy can be achieved by relating the dose to the surface area of the patient, this being derived from the patient's height and weight. The dose is then expressed as:

Dose per square metre of body surface area.

This removes as far as possible variations in response due to differences in patient size.

Age of the patient

There are considerable variations in response related to age, due to difference in patient size and to other factors and these are considered in Chapter 22 page 287.

Genetic factors

There are a number of inherited variations in drug response largely related to differences in drug elimination. Many drugs are broken down by enzymes (usually in the liver) and this terminates their actions. It is now believed that there can be considerable interperson differences in the activity of these enzymes.

With certain drugs it is possible to distinguish between two populations of people: one group with a highly active enzyme system which is able to break down the drug rapidly and the other with a less active system and relatively slower breakdown of the drug. This type of genetic variation, where two populations can exist which differ in the metabolism of a drug, is known as *genetic polymorphism*.

Example

A number of important drugs including isoniazid (p. 232) and hydralazine (p. 68) are inactivated by acetylation, a process involving enzyme action. In the UK 40% of the population are fast acetylators (with highly active acetylator enzymes) and 60% are slow acetylators. This is an inherited characteristic and the ratio of fast/slow acetylators varies in different parts of the world—100% of Inuit are rapid acetylators whereas 80% of Egyptians are slow acetylators. Differences in acetylator status do not usually matter in the UK, except when high doses of the drugs are being used when there is a slightly increased risk of toxic effects in subjects who are slow acetylators. In the less developed world where, for reasons of expense, very minimal doses may be necessary—for example, isoniazid in the treatment of tuberculosis—those who are rapid acetylators may suffer some falling-off of therapeutic efficacy.

Another example of genetic polymorphism is deficiency in the enzyme glucose-6-phosphate dehydrogenase (G6PD). This involves largely Africans and Indians, affecting about 100 million people. It is due to an abnormal enzyme in the red blood cells and results in the breakdown of these cells when exposed to certain substances:

- Quinine
- Sulfonamides
- Broad beans
- Chloroquine
- Chloramphenicol.

There are many other examples of inherited differences in response to drugs and some are still being discovered.

Nutritional factors

Frank malnutrition can modify responses to drugs. Loss of body mass is one factor involved and reduction of enzyme activity, which can occur as a result of a lack of protein, may result in the slowed breakdown of drugs. Malnutrition as such is not usual in the UK, but prolonged illness, perhaps associated with sepsis and fever, can produce very much the same result. Under these circumstances the response to a drug may be greater than expected.

Example

Warfarin (see p. 80) is an anticoagulant which is broken down in the liver by enzymes. Its effect on coagulation is often greater in patients who have suffered a long illness and are in a poor nutritional state and they may require a smaller than usual dose.

Even without malnutrition diet can affect drug response. Vegetarians and heavy smokers both show several differences in enzyme activity which could modify drug response, although the changes are usually too small to cause serious problems.

Race and drug response

The increasing movement of populations means that the nurse may be looking after patients of several ethnic groups and it is becoming apparent that with some drugs different races may show differing sensitivities. For instance, it has been shown that in America the β blocker propranolol is less effective in lowering blood pressure in black than in white subjects. These differences could be due to:

1. Genetic differences in drug metabolizing enzymes leading to variations in the blood levels achieved.
2. Different lifestyles (e.g. diet) which could also alter the metabolizing enzymes.
3. Differences in the actual response to the drug.

At present very little is known about the problem and with many drugs it is probably unimportant, but it provides an interesting field for further research.

Intercurrent illness

This may both *modify drug elimination* and *affect receptor sensitivity* and is an important cause of altered response to a drug.

Most drugs are either broken down by the liver or excreted by the kidneys, so disease of these organs with diminished function can lead to accumulation of the drug with a more intense and prolonged action which can reach dangerous proportions.

Example

Morphine when given to a patient with cirrhosis of the liver has a more marked and prolonged effect than normal, and dangerous depression of respiration can develop.

Normally, morphine is broken down in the liver; in cirrhosis distortion of the normal anatomy, so that blood bypasses the liver, and loss of liver cells both result in decreased enzyme activity, and thus accumulation of morphine.

It is not always necessary for there to be liver damage for drug metabolism to be altered. In heart failure the blood flow through the liver is reduced and this alone may be sufficient to reduce appreciably the breakdown of drugs.

Example

Lidocaine (p. 63) is used to treat cardiac arrhythmias, particularly after myocardial infarction; it is broken down by the liver. If it is given to patients with heart failure (a not uncommon occurrence) then its elimination is slowed and toxicity will result if the dose is not reduced.

Kidney function may also modify drug response.

Example

Gentamicin (see p. 228) is excreted by the kidneys and when renal function is reduced serious accumulation occurs with normal dosage. This is why careful monitoring of blood levels with subsequent modification of doses is required when gentamicin is given, particularly in renal disease.

Receptor sensitivity may also be affected by disease.

Example

In chronic respiratory disease, because the respiratory centre is chronically short of oxygen, it becomes very sensitive to the depressing effect of morphine and normal doses can result in severe respiratory depression.

Drug interactions

One drug can modify the response to another drug in a number of different ways. This is discussed on page 298.

Other factors including psychological ones may also be important in drug response. Expectation of a successful outcome may appear to improve the results of treatment: for example, analgesics are more effective if ignorance and fear are dispelled.

Thus the response of a patient to a particular drug should be looked at as shown in Figure 1.8.

Choosing and adjusting the dose

Most drugs are given in doses which have been found by experience to be satisfactory, although

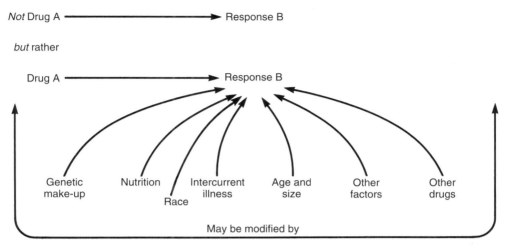

Not Drug A ⟶ Response B

but rather

Drug A ⟶ Response B

May be modified by

Genetic make-up • Nutrition • Race • Intercurrent illness • Age and size • Other factors • Other drugs

Figure 1.8 Response of a patient to a particular drug.

the dose may be modified by the factors discussed above. As a result, formularies usually give a range of doses. In the light of the clinical response some alterations may be needed (e.g. the dose of hypotensive drugs is adjusted until a satisfactory fall in blood pressure is achieved).

Therapeutic monitoring

With a few drugs there may be considerable interperson variation in plasma concentration, and when this must be kept within a narrow range to avoid toxicity whilst achieving a satisfactory therapeutic effect, it is necessary to measure the plasma concentration at regular intervals and adjust the dose as needed. The correct sampling time depends on the drug being used but it is important that it is adhered to if the result is to provide meaningful information. The drugs which usually require this are:

- Gentamicin and other aminoglycoside antibiotics
- Lithium
- Phenytoin
- Cyclosporin.

Other drugs which may require monitoring of plasma concentrations are:

- Theophylline
- Methotrexate
- Carbamazepine
- Digoxin.

THE ADMINISTRATION OF DRUGS

Drugs are given in many ways and as this is often the duty of nurses the methods are considered in detail in Figure 1.9 and in Chapter 2.

Orally

The easiest and most usual way to give drugs is by mouth and there are many formulations for this purpose.

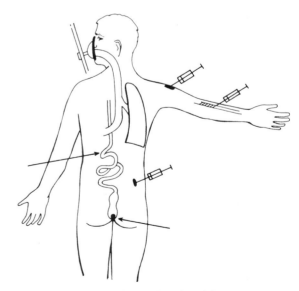

Figure 1.9 Methods of administration of drugs.

Tablets are prepared by mixing a drug with a base which binds it together. They are usually coated and may be coloured.

Capsules are made of gelatin or some similar substance and contain a drug which is liberated when the wall of the capsule is digested in the stomach or intestine.

The actual formulation of tablets and capsules is very important and determines how satisfactorily the drug is released. This governs its absorption and bioavailability. A great deal of care is taken in the manufacture of tablets to ensure the maximum bioavailability. It is also possible, by coating the tablets, by modifying the capsule or by binding the drug to some inert substance, to slow down the release of the active ingredient and thus prolong its absorption and effect. These may be called sustained-release or *retard* preparations.

Mixtures are liquids which contain several ingredients dissolved or diffused in water or some other solvent.

An *emulsion* is a mixture of two liquids in which one is dispersed through the other in a finely divided state.

A *linctus* is a liquid which contains some sweet syrupy substance used for its soothing effect on coughs.

When liquid drugs are prescribed they are accompanied by the British Standard oral syringe which measures up to 5 ml and is marked with 0.5 ml divisions. This should be used to draw up the fluid to achieve the exact dose. For doses of 5 ml or more, the standard 5 ml plastic spoon can be used. The syringe is issued with a manufacturer's information leaflet advising on use and storage, but verbal explanations are still valuable, especially as liquid medicines are usually given to children and frequently administered by anxious parents. Families appreciate practical demonstrations of the use of the syringe provided by the nurse.

The absorption of drugs given by mouth is affected by several factors other than drug formulation:

1. **Food.** If a drug is taken with or after a meal it is absorbed more slowly. This is due to delayed emptying of the stomach where little absorption occurs and because certain drugs become temporarily bound to food. When a rapid effect is required it should be given on an empty stomach. Drugs which may irritate the stomach should be given with food.

2. **Rate of gastric emptying and drug interactions.** Gastric emptying may be affected by drugs and this may modify absorption. For instance, atropine-like drugs delay gastric emptying, whereas metoclopramide, which is often used for nausea, actually increases the speed of gastric emptying and thus the rate of absorption. If drugs are given together they may bind to each other and prevent absorption, although this is a rare occurrence and, in practice, several different types of drug are often given at the same time.

By injection

Injections may be given *intravenously, intramuscularly, subcutaneously, intradermally* or into various body cavities such as the pleura or peritoneum, or into the spinal theca.

The *intravenous* route has the advantage of rapid action, complete bioavailability and it can be used for drugs too irritant to be given intramuscularly. However, it is technically more difficult and an inadvertent intra-arterial injection can cause arterial spasm with resulting tissue damage. Today, some drugs, particularly if a prolonged and continuous effect is required, are given via an intravenous syringe-driver pump (see p. 119). These can be used by the patient at home as well as in hospital.

Intramuscular injection is easier. Absorption from the injection site is variable, being greatest from the deltoid muscle and least from the buttock. It depends on muscle blood flow and is increased by exercise and rubbing the injection site and reduced in shock. Slow-release formulations are available for a prolonged effect. Injection can be painful and 3 ml is the maximum acceptable volume. Rarely, it may result in abscess formation.

Subcutaneous injection is widely used. Absorption is slower than after intramuscular injection and is again influenced by local blood flow, being increased with exercise and decreased in shock. When a marked local effect is required (e.g. in local anaesthetics) a vasoconstrictor is added to the injection to prevent the drug being absorbed away from the injection site.

Intrathecal injection is used when it is necessary for the drug to reach the nervous system and bypass the blood/brain barrier. *It is all too easy to cause severe damage by using the wrong dose or the wrong drug. Special care, with repeated checks, is required if this route is used.*

Rectally

Certain drugs are absorbed from the rectum and may be given as suppositories or enemata.

By inhalation

Drugs may be inhaled either to produce a local action on the respiratory tract or because they are absorbed via the lungs and produce a general effect.

By local application

Drugs are applied locally as *lotions, liniments, ointments* or *creams* (see p. 329) to the skin, mucous membranes and wound surfaces and produce their action at the site of application.

Transdermal application

A number of drugs can be absorbed effectively via the skin. This is useful not only in the treatment of skin diseases, but, in some cases, where absorption is sufficient, in producing systemic actions.

The drug is applied to the skin as a plastic patch holding a container which releases it at a constant rate. There are regional variations in skin permeability—for example, the very thick skin of the palms or soles would not allow efficient absorption even if these were con-venient locations. Patches are usually applied to clean, unbroken skin on the trunk or the post-auricular area (behind the ear) where good vascularity enhances uptake. Examples of drugs which can be administered in this way include:

- Glyceryl trinitrate for angina
- Hyoscine for motion sickness
- Oestrogens for hormone replacement therapy
- Fentanyl for analgesia.

1. *Advantages.* One patch may be effective for a relatively long period so replacement can be made infrequently.

2. *Disadvantages.* Absorption can be variable. Occasionally there may be skin or adverse systemic reactions. If these occur, simply removing the patch will not halt the reaction immediately, as the drug that has been absorbed will continue to act for some time, depending on its nature and dose.

HOW ARE DRUGS PRODUCED?

Most drugs are made chemically in the laboratory or factory. Some are extracted from natural sources such as plants or fungi: for example, benzylpenicillin was obtained originally from a mould. After extraction, the chemical structure of the compounds may be modified to make them more effective.

With increasing understanding of both the nature of diseases and of drug action, it is now possible to design and synthesize drugs which have a specific action on the abnormality which causes the disease.

Certain substances which occur naturally (such as hormones) are proteins with a very complex structure. They are difficult to synthesize chemically and extraction from animals may be unsatisfactory and expensive and, in addition, if obtained from animal sources may not be identical to those found in humans. This problem is now being solved by *genetic pharmacy*.

The gene responsible for the production of a complex protein is isolated from human cells and inserted into other vector (carrier) cells (such as the bacterium *Escherichia coli* or a yeast) which divide rapidly and are manipulated to produce the required protein in large quantities. This method is responsible for the production of several protein hormones such as human insulin and erythropoietin. Similar techniques offer great possibilities for the future.

HOW DO DRUGS WORK? (PHARMACODYNAMICS)

In spite of a great deal of research it is still not known how some drugs produce their effect but it is possible to describe the way in which most of them act.

1. *The receptor theory.* It is believed that the cells in certain tissues contain structures called receptors. These combine with substances which are produced naturally in the body and the cells are stimulated or inhibited, the contraction of muscle fibres produced by acetylcholine being an example. The drug is thought to fit onto a receptor rather as a key fits a lock. It may then either stimulate the receptor and produce an effect similar to that of the naturally occurring substances and is called an *agonist*, or it may occupy the receptor without producing any effect by preventing any naturally occurring stimulation and is then called an *antagonist*. The blocking of acetylcholine by atropine is a good example (Fig. 1.10).

With some drugs the action on a receptor is immediate and direct, but with others the action on the receptor may initiate a chain of events before the final action of the drug is apparent. For example, corticosteroids may take an hour or more to become effective. The examples of the types of drug action given below are variable, but many of them depend ultimately on some type of receptor mechanism.

2. *Antimetabolites.* These drugs closely resemble substances which are used by cells for nutrition and, when absorbed, the cells cannot use them and so fail to multiply.

Several drugs used in the treatment of cancer act in this way. Thus methotrexate, which is similar to folic acid, a normal cell constituent, competes with folic acid for a vital step in the build-up of nuclear material within the cell and blocks the process so that the cancer cell dies.

3. *Enzyme inhibitors.* Enzymes are substances which speed up many chemical processes within

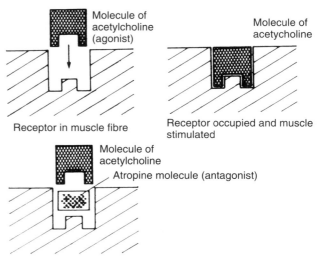

Figure 1.10 Stimulation of muscle by acetylcholine showing occupation of the receptor by the drug. After atropine the receptor site is blocked and no stimulation occurs.

the body. Some of these enzyme-activated processes are concerned with the transport of chemicals in and out of the cells. Certain drugs have the property of inhibiting their action and thus interfere with some of these processes. Diuretics are a good example as normally salt and water are transported out of the renal tubule back into the body, but this action requires enzymes and if they are inhibited by a diuretic, salt and water are not reabsorbed and pass out of the kidney with a resulting diuresis.

4. *Action on cell membranes.* The function of nerves and muscles depends on ions passing across the membranes surrounding these cells. Certain drugs interfere with the movement of these ions and thus prevent nerve or muscle function, as demonstrated by local anaesthetics which block impulses passing up a sensory nerve.

5. *Replacement of deficiencies.* In some diseases there is a deficiency of a substance which is necessary for the body to function normally. This may be a hormone (see p. 175) or some essential dietary factor such as a vitamin (see p. 263). By replacing the deficiency the disease can be controlled, but the replacement

drug will usually need to be taken for the rest of the patient's life.

6. *Cytotoxic effect.* Drugs may be used to kill bacteria or malignant cells without undue change to the patient's cells. The means by which this is brought about varies between drugs.

These are just a few of the ways in which drugs may work. It is probable that all drug action depends on their interference with cell activity, and when more is known about the processes within the cell, then more will be discovered about how they work.

FURTHER READING

Brodie M J 1988 Pharmacokinetics for the prescriber. Medicine International 59: 2408

Feeley J, Brodie M 1988 Practical clinical pharmacology. British Medical Journal 296: 1046

George C F 1984 Food, drugs and bioavailability. British Medical Journal 289: 1093

McPherson G 1993 Absorbing effects. Nursing Times 89: 30

Mucklow J C 1989 Accumulation. Prescribers Journal 29: 36

Rawlings M D 1988 Pharmacogenetics. Prescribers Journal 28: 64

Rees J, Ritter J M, Spector R 1994 Aids to clinical pharmacology and therapeutics, 3rd edn. Churchill Livingstone, Edinburgh

Ritter J M, Lewis L D, Mant T G K 1999 Clinical pharmacology, 4th edn. Edward Arnold, London

2

The role of nurses in drug administration

THE NURSE'S RESPONSIBILITIES

Drug therapy plays a major part in the treatment of patients. Traditionally, medicines have been prescribed by doctors and the nurse's responsibility has been to ensure safe and reliable administration and to monitor side-effects. For nurses in hospitals and those employed by general practitioners (practice nurses) this is still the case. However, in 1994 the law was changed to allow district nurses and health visitors employed in eight pilot sites throughout England to prescribe from a limited formulary. Most of the preparations they are able to prescribe are for over-the-counter preparations but it is likely that this will be extended in future. In 1998 the government announced plans to permit all appropriately qualified community nurses to prescribe. Irrespective of whether or not they are permitted to prescribe and the setting in which they are employed, however, all nurses need to help patients understand the purpose of their treatment and to promote compliance with taking medication.

The nurse must be aware that his or her responsibilities in giving drugs are governed by the Misuse of Drugs Act 1971, for controlled drugs, and the Medicines Act 1968, for prescription only medicines, together with additional regulations formulated by individual health authorities. All Hospital and Community Trusts have their own procedures and policies. The United Kingdom Central Council (UKCC) code of conduct, in laying down the general responsibilities of the nurse, stipulates that his or her actions should put the patient's safety and well-being first at all times.

In hospital, the custody and administration of drugs is the responsibility of the ward sister/charge nurse, who may delegate this responsibility as instructed by the employing authority's policy. Although it is usual for a qualified nurse to give drugs, with a second nurse checking to prevent error, the UKCC takes the view that registered nurses should be seen as competent to administer drugs on their own and be responsible for their actions. Student nurses will take part in drug administration and senior student nurses who have shown competence may be allowed to act as the senior person giving drugs. Intravenous drugs must also be given by two nurses, the senior of whom must be qualified and certified to do so. Requirements will vary between employing authorities and if a qualified nurse moves she must obtain a certificate for the new district. The status of the person checking the drug will also be designated by the employing authority. Nurses' actions in relation to drug administration will be legally covered by the employing authority when the rules are followed.

DRUG HISTORY

A reliable drug history should be obtained from the patient and, if necessary, from relatives or friends. This should include previous exposure to drugs, drugs being taken at the time and, in particular, any adverse effects resulting from their use. If the illness is of a recurrent nature, the efficacy of any drugs used in previous episodes should be noted.

It is important to remember that drugs include local applications, any over-the-counter or herbal remedies that may have been used and recreational drugs.

THE PRESCRIPTION

In hospital it is normal practice for all drugs to be prescribed. This enables the pharmacist to supply them and instruct the nurse in their administration. The prescription sheet, which is a primary document in the case records, must be headed with the patient's full name, age, number and ward. The prescription must be clearly and indelibly written and must contain the date, the approved name of the drug (preferably in block letters), the dose (using metric dosage), the route and frequency of administration with the validity period and signature of the medical practitioner. If any of these details are omitted the drug should not be given until the prescription has been amended. Frequency of dosage can be ordered by filling in allocated time spaces rather than using Latin abbreviations. Administration is recorded by initialling the relevant box on the prescription sheet. The exact format of this sheet will vary between districts, and nurses must familiarize themselves with documents in use when moving to a new district. On no account should a nurse write or alter a prescription in a hospital.

Controlled drugs

In hospital, controlled drugs (see p. 31) must always be given by two people and it is common practice for one to be a qualified nurse. Both nurses must sign the book following each administration *at the bedside* or *in the presence of the patient*. The prescription requires the number of doses in words and figures. An additional record is kept in a specially designed book so that every tablet or ampoule is accounted for when used, both nurses signing the book following each administration. The controlled drug record book is retained on the ward for 2 years after the date of the last entry. These are legal requirements for controlled drugs, but some hospitals apply similar rules to other drugs liable to misuse.

NURSING ASPECTS OF ADMINISTRATION

In the community most patients, or some member of the family, are responsible for drug administration, although the nurse or health visitor may have a role to play. Many people are now discharged within a few days or hours of surgery and the average length of stay for medical patients has also been reduced. People returning home are often still taking drugs which until recently would have been given only within the confines of a hospital, so monitoring for adverse effects is an increasingly important aspect of the community nurse's role. The nurse must also be aware that some drugs, even if stopped before discharge, may still exert an action or cause side-effects.

The nurse is responsible for interpreting the prescription accurately, recording that the drug has been given and observing the patient's response. Prior to administration the nurse must know the reason for, action and usual dosage of the drug; this should enable him or her to recognize and question mistakes in prescribing. When in doubt about a prescription, advice should be sought and, if necessary, the doctor should be consulted. Observations should be made for therapeutic and adverse effects. The nurse should realize that the patient's condition may alter the effect of a drug and that there may be interactions with concurrent treatment. The nurse is greatly assisted in these circumstances by the pharmacist, with whom a good working relationship will enhance the safety of patient care.

The Committee on Safety of Medicines requests that adverse reactions are reported (yellow cards) and, in addition, may require that a special watch is kept on certain preparations (see p. 302).

Ward administration of drugs

Drugs may be given to the whole ward by the same nurses or to a smaller group of patients by those directly involved in their care. The second method is preferable as timing is more accurate and the nurse will know the patients well and can cater for individual needs such as difficulty in swallowing medication. Time can be spent teaching patients about their drugs and student nurses can take part to gain experience in relating drugs to the patient's condition. In some hospitals experimental schemes have involved

patients being responsible for their own drugs, particularly if they need to take the same drugs when they go home. On the whole these have been successful and provided valuable opportunities for patient education. Where members of the family will be giving drugs they can be invited to the ward at the appropriate time to practise a technique (such as giving an injection) or to ask about any anticipated problems. An innovative approach on some wards has been in the timing of drug rounds so that medicines can be given nearer the time patients would take them at home. Many people have taken their drugs at home for years and may be upset by altered timing in hospital. Many schemes have abolished the early morning drug round to give patients longer to sleep.

For a few drugs flexibility is not possible; antibiotics are more effective if doses are spread evenly throughout the day, and insulin must be given before meals. Others such as nonsteroidal anti-inflammatory drugs (NSAIDs) are best given with or after food.

Whichever approach is taken, specific rules of drug administration must be followed to obviate errors. The underlying principles, to give the correct dose of the prescribed drug to the right patient, by the right route, at the right time, require the nurse's undivided attention. When two nurses are involved, instructions should be read aloud.

1. Read the patient's full name from the prescription sheet.
2. Read the prescription, checking the validity and time of last administration.
3. Read the name of the drug from the label when removing the container from the shelf.
4. Check the label of the container for the name, strength and dose of the drug, the route of administration where relevant and the expiry date against the prescription.
5. Measure or count the correct dose. Avoid contact with the drug as allergies can develop, particularly if the hands are damp.

When measuring liquids, shake the bottle, hold the measure at eye level placing the thumbnail on the meniscus and pour from the back of the bottle to keep the label clean. A calibrated measure should be used. When a fractional dose is required, calculations should be made independently before checking the dose.

6. Re-check the label before returning the container to the shelf.

7. Both nurses must verify the patient's identity by checking the details on the prescription sheet with the patient's identity bracelet. If this is absent, ask the patient to state his or her full name. If this is not possible identification must be confirmed by a member of the family or permanent staff.

8. Ensure the patient is in a fit state to receive the drug.

9. Give the dose and see that it has been swallowed.

10. Record the administration. Also record when a drug is not given and the reason.

Additional points. Patients who refuse to take a drug or show doubt or anxiety may have a good reason which will become apparent if the nurse takes time to listen to them.

Safety factors

- Do not leave the drug trolley unattended.
- Do not give drugs from memory, a prescription sheet must always be used.
- Do not give a drug from a container that is not correctly labelled.
- Do not give a drug prepared by anyone else.
- Do not return an unused dose to a stock bottle.
- Unused drugs may be returned to the pharmacy where they will be checked and used for another patient. Drugs returned by outpatients should be destroyed.

Aids to taking oral drugs

1. Ensure the patient is sitting up whenever possible to facilitate swallowing.

2. Prepare a drink before giving the drug, and see that an adequate amount of fluid is taken with the drug to prevent oesophageal irritation/ulceration.

3. Liquid preparations are given via a British Standard oral syringe. Soluble tablets should be dissolved completely before presenting them. If a patient has difficulty holding a tablet it should be introduced on a spoon.

4. If a patient has difficulty swallowing a tablet, remove it, give a drink and try again. Many drugs can be prepared and given in liquid form if necessary.

5. If a drug tastes unpleasant it may be followed by a flavoured drink or mouthwash.

Although many drugs will be given orally, the nurse will also administer them by the rectal and vaginal routes and by injection. In all cases the above rules must be followed.

Rectal drugs

These are given in suppository form using protective gloves and a small amount of lubricant to ease insertion. It is important that the method is explained to the patient beforehand and that correct positioning is used with the patient lying on their left side with hips and knees flexed. It has been shown that insertion of the blunt end of the suppository aids comfort and retention.

Long-term treatment may be given by this route in which case patients can be taught self-administration most effectively.

Vaginal drugs

Vaginal pessaries and creams are inserted with the patient lying on her side or back. Clean (rather than sterile) gloves are satisfactory except after delivery. A lubricant is used and the drug inserted into the posterior fornix of the vagina. In some circumstances a pad may be worn after insertion as leakage can occur. Again, patients can be instructed on self-medication by this method. Pessaries are best inserted last thing at night as they tend to become dislodged.

Injections

The nurse will be responsible for giving drugs by intradermal, subcutaneous and intramuscular routes. Qualified nurses may give drugs intravenously through an established route. Fractional dosage may be required in these circumstances and careful calculation is vital as errors in dose measurement can occur, the danger of this being compounded by the more rapid action of drugs by injection. When giving injections, sterile equipment must be used and strict aseptic techniques observed. Cleansing of the skin with an alcohol swab is still commonly used, but the benefits of this are questionable. However, where the skin is contaminated or the balance of flora changed as in debilitated patients it may be necessary. If used, the alcohol should be allowed to dry before inserting the needle. In most circumstances the site is massaged after removing the needle to aid absorption of the drug.

Intradermal injection. The two most common reasons for giving intradermal injections are testing for sensitivity to allergens and immunization. In the former situation there is a risk of an anaphylactic reaction, so adrenaline should be readily available. A very small amount of fluid (0.1 ml or less) is given using a 1 ml syringe, graduated in 0.1 ml divisions, through a short fine needle (26 gauge $\times \frac{3}{8}$ in; see Fig. 2.1). This is introduced just under the skin at an angle of 10–15°, which will raise a small weal. The area should not be massaged after removing the needle. The usual site of injection is the lightly pigmented area of the forearm where the reaction can be easily observed.

Subcutaneous injection. A subcutaneous injection is given into the fatty layer just under the skin (see Fig. 2.1). Small amounts of fluid are injected (0.5–2 ml) using a 25 gauge $\times \frac{15}{16}$ inch needle. A fold of skin is raised between the thumb and forefinger and the needle is inserted at an angle of 45° (see Fig. 2.1). After insertion the plunger is withdrawn slightly to ensure a blood vessel has not been entered. If this occurs the needle should be removed, pressure applied to the area and a new injection prepared. For injections of heparin and insulin shorter needles are used. These may be the very short fine needles integral with insulin syringes or 25 gauge $\times \frac{5}{8}$ needles. In these instances the needle enters the skin at 90°. The area is not massaged after withdrawing the needle but firm pressure is used to prevent haematoma formation when heparin is given and to ensure uniform absorption rates in patients with diabetes. Other modifications which may be made when giving insulin are discussed on page 193.

The usual sites for subcutaneous injections are the outer aspect of the upper arm, the outer aspect of the upper thigh and the skin of the abdominal wall (Fig. 2.2).

Intramuscular injection. This is given into muscle so larger amounts can be injected: 1–5 ml (Fig. 2.3). The best site is the outer aspect of the thigh, locating the area in the middle third of the space between the knee and greater trochanter of the femur. The upper outer quadrant of the buttock is also used (Fig. 2.3). It is vital to determine the sites carefully to avoid damage to the sciatic nerve and major blood vessels. Alternatively, the upper outer aspect of the arm may be used if the muscle is big enough. To aid relaxation the patient should be positioned comfortably; for buttock injections either lying on the abdomen with the toes turned in or lying on the side with the lower leg extended and the upper leg flexed. For thigh injections the limb should be slightly flexed and supported.

When preparing injections care should be taken to prevent skin contamination as contact dermatitis can occur. Gloves may be worn in some circumstances and the hands washed thoroughly after completion of the procedure. Drugs which may cause this reaction are penicillin, the aminoglycosides and chlorpromazine. Special precautions are taken when using cytotoxic drugs (see p. 283). When giving an intramuscular injec-

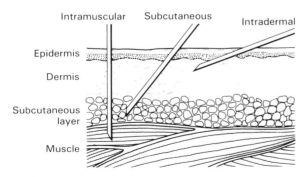

Figure 2.1 The position of the needle for intramuscular, subcutaneous and intradermal injections.

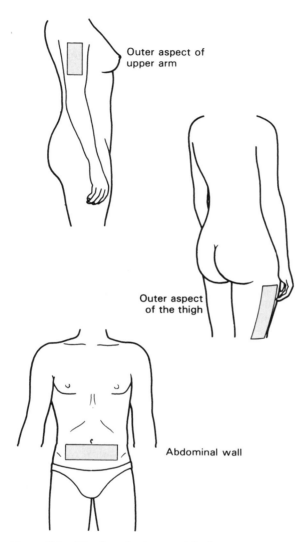

Figure 2.2 Sites for subcutaneous injections.

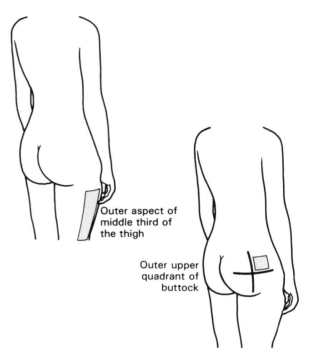

Figure 2.3 Sites for intramuscular injections.

tion the skin is held taut and a 21 gauge × 1½ inch needle introduced at 90° (Fig. 2.1). As in the subcutaneous technique the plunger is withdrawn to check for inadvertent puncturing of a blood vessel. The fluid is then injected slowly, the needle withdrawn quickly, pressure applied initially and then the area massaged gently.

When injecting substances such as iron, which cause skin discoloration, the Z track method can be used. In this technique the skin is pulled to one side before inserting the needle, a few seconds are allowed to elapse before it is with-

drawn, at which point the skin is released, thus achieving the Z track.

Intravenous injections and additives. It has been estimated that 12% of patients have an intravenous infusion at some time during their stay in hospital, usually for one or more of the following reasons: fluid replacement treatment, drug treatment, monitoring central venous pressure, hyperalimentation or to provide emergency access to a vein. Responsibility for drug administration by the intravenous route is now becoming part of the nurse's extended role, although in most health districts it is necessary to have attended a special training course and received a certificate of competence, which may not be valid in another institution. The intravenous route is most often used for heparin, cytotoxic drugs and antibiotics. Individual drugs may be given as a bolus or added to the infusion fluid, in which case careful mixing and labelling are vital and it is important to check that drugs do not interact with each other in the infusion bottle. Intravenous drugs need very careful monitoring and the nurse requires an adequate knowledge of potential side-effects. It is therefore essential that student nurses involved in checking and observing the effects of drugs given by this route are closely supervised. When the flow rate is mechanically controlled it is still necessary to check independently that the correct dose is being delivered. Any adjustment to dosage must only be undertaken by trained nurses.

Infection is a known hazard of intravenous cannulation and is increased when drugs or additives are given because the apparatus will be handled more often. Patients must therefore be observed for signs of local infection at the site of the cannula and their temperature monitored carefully. Continuous infusion of drugs by an infusion apparatus is not very accurate, although the use of a paediatric volume control administration device will render the flow rate more easily controllable.

60 microdrops (Soluset) = 1 ml
20 macrodrops (standard giving set) = 1 ml

For more satisfactory and accurate dosage an infusion pump should be used.

Nursing point

Needle stick injuries pose an occupational hazard to nurses and may result in the transmission of blood-borne infection—hepatitis B, hepatitis C or, more rarely, HIV. Risks can be reduced by disposing of the needle and syringe immediately after use, without attempting to recap the needle, as research studies indicate that recapping is particularly likely to result in injury. All sharps should be placed in a designated container which should be disposed of when no more than two-thirds full. Sharps should never be transported in the hands or in pockets and hands should never, under any circumstances, be inserted into the sharps container. Injuries, when they occur, should be recorded in accordance with local policy and medical opinion should be sought (see also p. 237).

Giving drugs to children

Obtaining cooperation from children is very important and a simple, honest explanation helps to achieve this. Children are more likely to take drugs from a familiar person and, where appropriate, parents and relatives can actually give drugs observed by the nurses who have prepared the medication. As paediatric doses are so different from those of adults it is important for nurses familiar with children's care to be involved in checking drugs, adhering to local policies. Fractional dosage is used and needs careful calculation to avoid error. Most drugs are given in liquid form. For very young children a medicine dispenser is useful. This is a special 1 ml syringe into which the required dosage is drawn via a special bottle adaptor. With the child sitting up, the dispenser is inserted into his or her mouth with the tip pointing to the inside of the cheek and the plunger is depressed slowly, allowing the drug to be swallowed naturally. For older children a special graduated syringe is used. Medicines should not be given in milk or food and it is important to praise the child for taking them.

Giving drugs to elderly patients

Many elderly patients dislike taking oral drugs and, to overcome this, adequate time should be taken for simple explanation. If swallowing tablets proves difficult it may be possible to prescribe the drug in liquid form or to use semi-solids such as ice cream as a vehicle for introducing medication. If there is doubt as to whether it has been swallowed, inspection of the mouth may be needed.

COMPLIANCE AND EDUCATION

In the past, giving drugs usually involved only passive participation by the patient with little information being offered unless it was requested. There is increasing evidence that adequate explanation to the patient increases the likelihood of adherence to a prescribed course of treatment. Indeed, according to the Patients' Charter issued by the Department of Health in 1991, every citizen has the right to a clear explanation of any proposed treatment—clearly this includes any drugs prescribed. In order to comply, an understanding and acceptance of the treatment is vital; failure to do so may be unintentional due to lapse of memory, or deliberate, when timing and dosage may be altered by the patient. Studies show that non-compliance is a major problem, resulting in omission or repetition of drug treatment which may require readmission to hospital. Unused drugs may be a potential danger to patients and relatives, increasing the risk of deliberate or accidental self-poisoning.

Education of the patient with regard to drug treatment is the responsibility of the doctor, pharmacist and nurse. However, this also applies to educating other health care professionals such as social workers, occupational therapists, physio-therapists, non-professional carers and the general public to improve overall understanding of the significance of the proper use of drugs as a part of treatment.

In hospital the nurse is in an expedient position to fulfil this role by being the person primarily involved in drug administration and having continued contact with the patient. The aim of teaching is to help the patient to gain insight into the way drugs can be used to treat his or her disorder. Implicit in this is the nurse's knowledge of the disease process and drug action. Answering patients' questions will impart a certain amount of information, but this must be accompanied by a more structured approach.

Teaching begins on the patient's admission when an understanding of his or her present treatment should be established. Poor literacy or language difficulties impede comprehension and any problems elicited will need sensitive dis-cussion. Anxiety about the harmful effects of chemicals and addiction to drugs may concern some patients and will hinder learning if not overcome. It is also important to ascertain whether any regular self-medication is occurring as this may influence the action of prescribed drugs, e.g. the use of antacids concurrently with tetra-cycline reduces absorption rates.

At this time drugs brought in by the patient are seen by the doctor and permission gained, if possible, to dispose of them, explaining the dangers of error if a different regimen is pre-scribed on discharge. Teaching should continue

during the hospital stay. It is common practice for the patient to be given brief, rather hurried instructions on drug treatment when being handed the bottles of drugs immediately before leaving the ward. At this time motivation and concentration may be low as the patient is more concerned with going home.

Teaching in preparation for discharge

Patients vary as to the amount of information they need so this must be tailored to individual requirements, but should include the following:

1. The name and purpose of the drug, stressing its positive effects.
2. Frequency and timing of administration according to home routine, including advice about 'as required' medications.
3. Method of administration with explanation where special equipment will be required for routes other than oral.
4. Proposed length of treatment—short or long term.
5. The importance of not stopping or starting drugs without advice and where to obtain that advice.
6. How to obtain further supplies and safely dispose of unwanted drugs.
7. Adverse effects to be reported and how to carry out special tests and observations to show if they are developing. The aim is to give adequate information without causing unnecessary alarm. Most drugs produce side-effects, some of which are minor, but others are potentially serious. In some cases it may be possible to advise on the relief of side-effects. If sufficient information is not given patients may just stop taking the drugs rather than report the adverse effects, or they may stop treatment when symptoms subside, as perhaps in the case of antibiotic treatment. A well-informed patient able to participate in his or her own care will feel more in control and thus more responsible, contributing to compliance.

Teaching should continue during the stay in hospital and should *include members of the patient's family as appropriate.*

Some wards have experimented with schemes

in which patients, under supervision, are responsible for their own drug administration. There is also evidence that a simple explanatory booklet given to patients on discharge reinforces teaching. Patients taking drugs such as steroids or anticoagulants should be given a card with information about dosage, etc.

Missed doses

The preceding discussion should have emphasized the importance of taking drugs in the correct dose, via the correct route and following particular instructions. It will also have highlighted the problem of non-compliance, which continues to be a major stumbling block in therapeutics. In hospital the nurse is in a strong position to influence patient compliance and to provide explanations and allay anxieties as they occur. Time spent listening to patients' points of view and exploring their concerns is helpful to both nurses and patients.

In the community patients are more likely to be left alone to cope with their drugs and, often, non-compliance occurs through forgetfulness or misunderstanding.

As nurse prescribing becomes a reality, those in a position to influence which drugs and doses patients should take must remember:

1. It is sensible to choose drugs whose efficacy is unlikely to be affected by the occasional missed dose.
2. Drugs should not be used at the limits of their duration of action—a drug with an intermediate duration of action is more efficacious if taken twice daily rather than stretched to once daily by taking a higher dose.
3. Drugs that are eliminated slowly and accumulate in the body are least impaired by poor compliance.

Additional useful points

1. Drugs prescribed for others should not be taken even if the problems appear similar.
2. Drugs may deteriorate from moisture if kept in bathroom cabinets.

3. Different drugs should not be put in the same container as errors may occur. The drugs may interact chemically.
4. All drugs should be kept out of the reach of children, preferably in a locked cupboard. They should never be referred to as 'sweets'.

Special problems of compliance may be found in patients with memory impairment, defects of sight or hearing and those with physical handicaps which interfere with mobility and dexterity. Elderly patients also form a group at particular risk as many of these problems may exist in one patient. Another group with special needs is those with diabetes or other endocrine disorders, psychiatric disorders, hypertension and tuberculosis, for whom long-term treatment is necessary. Some of the drugs may be unpleasant to take, may affect the whole way of life of the patient or give rise to particularly unpleasant side-effects. In these situations ongoing educational support is essential.

In all situations it is useful to have verbal information reinforced by written instructions as it is well known that anxiety limits retention of information. It is especially important that this is done where there is memory impairment. Instruction should be kept simple; memory aids such as tear-off calendars and recording cards can be of value. Special dose boxes, e.g. the Dosett pill dispenser, which hold up to 1 week's supply of drugs can be used, but may be too complicated for some patients and still require another person to fill them.

Containers need to be labelled with adequate sized lettering and/or colour coding. Information on the label as to the purpose of the drug, e.g. 'heart tablets' or 'water tablets', may be helpful for elderly patients. Braille labels can be used for blind patients.

Drug manufacturers could also contribute to compliance by appropriate packaging and presentation of drugs. The container should be easy to open; child-resistant containers are used increasingly, but are very difficult for elderly patients and those with arthritis to handle. Many people are unaware that ordinary screwtop bottles are available. Caps with wings can be supplied where necessary; the occupational therapist will be able to assess the patient's need and offer other helpful suggestions.

Despite these aids there will still be some patients who are unable to cope with drug administration independently. In these situations education of other family members, friends, neighbours or 'home-helps' will be necessary. A number of trials of self-administration of drugs in elderly patients have been carried out in some parts of the country in preparation for discharge from hospital and to improve compliance. These programmes aim to identify individual patient problems well before discharge, but require the total commitment of all staff involved and continued counselling and follow-up in the community. It appears that these programmes have proved useful in training elderly patients and it may be that special self-administration programmes could have a wider application.

Medication errors

Occasionally medication errors are made by nursing staff. Such episodes not only have the potential to endanger patients, but they also have a serious effect on the self-esteem and confidence of the nurse and need to be investigated fully and objectively so that any lessons learnt can be used to reduce the risk of future errors.

Reasons for medication errors include:

1. *The patient.* Failure to understand self-administration systems or to recognize adverse effects if they occur. Poor compliance. Interactions with self-administered alternative treatment.

2. *The nurse.* Failure to take an adequate drug history with particular reference to previous adverse effects. Failure to identify the patient correctly. Failure to educate the patient adequately. Lack of knowledge of the properties and actions of the drug involved. Confusion over the names of drugs. Errors in calculation or measurement of the dose or in the mode and site of administration.

3. *Organizational.* Inadequate control of ordering and storing of drugs. Errors in labelling, inaccurate prescriptions. Failure to guard constantly against errors and to investigate the cause if they occur and to take steps to prevent recurrence.

NURSE PRESCRIBING

Nurse prescribing has been under professional consideration for over a decade. The idea was mooted in 1986 that community nurses should be able to prescribe prescription-only medications (POMs) from a limited list. In 1989 an advisory group set up by the Department of Health recommended that 'suitably qualified nurses working in the community should be able—in clearly defined circumstances—to prescribe from a limited range of items and to adjust the timing and dosage of medication within a set protocol'.

Nurse prescribing in law and as a professional task applies only to district nurses, midwives and health visitors in the community. These people may do so only from the limited list of items included within the Nurse Prescribers' Formulary (Table 2.1) having undertaken special training. In legal terms 'prescribing' is taken to mean the ability to make a personal, professional and independent assessment of the patient. Based on this, a free choice is made from the Nurse Prescribers' Formulary of the most appropriate drug or treatment. A doctor's opinion is unnecessary. The nurse signs the prescription form and remains professionally and legally accountable for his or her actions.

Research studies have indicated that despite initial lack of confidence, nurses have responded well to the challenge of prescribing and numerous benefits have been reported, including an improvement in patient care, more efficient use of nurses' time, and clarification of professional responsibilities, which have resulted in better communication between members of the primary health care team.

Currently, there are plans for the government to extend nurse prescribing from the pilot sites and to increase the number of items within the Nurse Prescribers' Formulary. A decision to extend nurse prescribing to all appropriately qualified community nurses was taken by the government in spring 1998.

Table 2.1 Some items included in the Nurse Prescribers' Formulary

Gastrointestinal system
Laxatives
  Senna tablets and granules
Ispaghula granules
  Docusate sodium
Sterculia
  Co-danthramer
Bisacodyl suppositories
Glycerol suppositories
Lactulose
Phosphate enema
Sodium citrate enema

Stoma care products
  Adhesives and adhesive removers
  Deodorants
  Skin protectives and cleaners

Analgesia
  Aspirin
  Paracetamol

Anthelmintics
  Piperazine
  Mebendazole

Antifungal agents
  Nystatin oral suspension and pastilles
  Clotrimoxazole cream

Urinary tract
  Preparations for maintaining indwelling urinary catheters

Mouthwashes and gargles
  Thymol

Skin care
  Emollient and barrier creams
  Emollient bath additives
  Magnesium sulphate paste (for boils)
  Skin disinfectants
    aqueous solution of 10% povidone-iodine
    sodium chloride
  Desloughing agents
    iodosorb
    varidase topical (streptokinase, streptodornase)

Anaesthesia
  Lidocaine hydrochloride for topical use

Parasitical preparations
  All *British National Formulary* items except Benzyl benzoate

The full list is also given in the *British National Formulary*. It will no doubt be modified with increasing experience.

Protocols versus nurse prescribing

'Protocols', often known as clinical guidelines or standards, have long been used in hospital and community settings to provide written documentation for an agreed method of performing a particular procedure, to achieve continuity and to standardize care. Today it is common practice for drugs to be administered according to protocols in hospital and the community; for example, nurses may administer immunizations or oral contraception under protocol. The use of a protocol is distinct from nurse prescribing as the nurse is unable to make an independent choice of medication or treatment—this will already have been specified within the protocol. The protocol is operating as a substitute prescription authorized and signed by a doctor who remains legally and professionally accountable for the treatment of the patient. Nevertheless, the nurse remains professionally and legally accountable for his or her decisions within the use of the protocol.

Breakdown of communication is possible after the patient is discharged from hospital and when drugs may be prescribed by more than one person. The new prescribing–dispensing process will mean greater contact between the nurse and pharmacist, especially when problems arise. It has been recommended that prescribing records are stored in the patient's home as district nursing records are already kept. The prescribing record contains details of previous and current drugs, including any additional over-the-counter products and drug allergies. When prescribing, the nurse will need to consider psychosocial as well as physical factors and the need for patient education must be recognized. The record should monitor the response to drugs and reasons for discontinuing their use.

NON-PRESCRIPTION DRUGS

For years social scientists have been interested in the 'sick role' phenomenon and the factors which cause people to decide they are ill and behave accordingly by taking drugs or going to bed. It has also become apparent that some people visit their doctors more frequently than others, whereas some diagnose themselves as not ill enough to 'trouble' a doctor or nurse but, nevertheless, take some form of drug. Indeed, few households are without some mild form of analgesic or antiseptic. Most people who travel abroad wisely purchase antidiarrhoeal drugs and every year large numbers of people dose themselves for coughs, motion sickness and constipation. Health care professionals need to know what the patient is taking and this extends to over-the-counter as well as prescribed drugs. Aspirin is widely available, but many people do not realize the full range and potency of its therapeutic effects. Paracetamol, another mild analgesic, can cause severe and fatal liver damage in overdose. Both these drugs are incorporated into numerous proprietary medicines, for example, several forms of Anadin are marketed containing different amounts of aspirin and in some cases paracetamol, with its implications in overdose or if prescribed drugs are needed. *When the nurse assesses the patient on hospital admission or the initial community visit he or she should not only enquire about prescribed drugs but any medication and, if possible, see it.* The commercial preparation Lomotil for diarrhoea contains atropine, which in overdose may cause atropine toxicity or interact with other drugs. Some expectorants induce drowsiness and a few contain appreciable amounts of alcohol. Patients need to be aware of the likely side-effects and actions of these drugs as much as of those which are prescribed.

With nurse prescribing now a reality, a sound knowledge of non-prescription drugs is essential for all who provide care in hospital or the community.

FURTHER READING

Bird C 1990 Drug administration; a prescription for self-help. Nursing Times 24(43): 54–57

Britten N 1994 Patients' ideas about medicines—a qualitative study in a general practice population. British Journal of General Practice 44:387: 465–468

Carlisle D 1996 Errors but no trials. Nursing Times 92(42): 50–51

Collingsworth S, Gould D J, Wainwright S P 1997 Patient self-administration of medication: a review of the literature. International Journal of Nursing Studies 34: 256–269

Department of Health 1989 Report of the Advisory Group on Nurse Prescribing. DoH, London

Department of Health 1991 The Patient's Charter. HMSO, London

Drug Administration 1988 A nursing responsibility, 2nd edn. Royal College of Nursing, London

Editorial 1991 Helping patients to make the best use of medicines. Drug and Therapeutics Bulletin 29(1): 1–2

Elliott-Pennells C J 1997 Nurse prescribing. Professional Nurse 13(2): 114–115

George C 1994 What do patients need to know about prescribed drugs? Pharmaceutical Journal 252: 7–8

Gould D 1988 Called to account. Nursing Times 84(12): 28–31

Howell M 1996 Prescription for disaster. Nursing Times 92(34): 30–31

Lapham R, Agar M 1995 Drug calculations for nurses. Headline, London

Lipley N 2000 Nurse prescribing. Nursing Standard 14(16): 12

Nixon P 1996 Homing in on drug rounds (medicine administration in nursing homes). Nursing Times 92(16): 59–60

Parker S 1999 Nurse Prescribers. Journal of the MDU 15: 21

United Kingdom Central Council for Nursing, Midwifery and Health Visiting 1992 Standards for the administration of medicines. UKCC, London

Walker R 1982 Suppository insertion. World Medicine 18: 58

Williams A 1996 How to avoid mistakes in medicine administration. Nursing Times 92(13): 40–43

Woodrow P 1998 Numeracy skills. Nursing Standard 12(30): 48–55

3

Nurses and the pharmaceutical service

In hospital the overall responsibility for the care and supply of drugs lies with the pharmacist, who will advise on their handling and use. The nurses' responsibilities for the handling of drugs fall into seven areas: they will *obtain drugs, possibly prescribe them, store them, prepare and administer them to patients, record the administration, and observe their effects*, in accordance with the requirements of the law and with hospital protocols and procedures. In all of these activities they are able to call upon the pharmacist for help and advice.

A close working relationship can be built up between nurses and pharmacists where there is an active clinical pharmacy service attached to the ward. The usual practice is for the pharmacist to visit the ward once or twice a day, to see the prescription sheets, initiate the dispensing of any drugs required, raise any queries on dosage, availability or incompatibility with the doctor, and offer any drug information required by the doctor or nurse. By doing this, the pharmacist very quickly becomes familiar with the requirements of the ward both in terms of supply and information, and can play a considerable part in ensuring the safe handling and use of drugs. Many pharmacists in hospital attend ward rounds as part of the clinical team to ensure that pharmaceutical care is provided appropriately to patients from admission to discharge.

DRUG SELECTION AND DOSAGE

The selection of a drug is the responsibility of the doctor, advised as appropriate by senior colleagues or the pharmacist. Many hospitals now have their own drug formularies, which combine treatment guidelines and recommend a 'best-buy' drug from the often bewildering range available, and give information on dosage, routes of administration, costs, contraindications and side-effects. Hospital pharmacies usually stock only those drugs listed in the formulary.

Nurses are now permitted to prescribe some preparations as further development of their extended role (see p. 24).

DRUG SUPPLY

Drugs in frequent use in a ward, or likely to be required in an emergency, are usually supplied as ward stock. Traditionally, the nurse has been responsible for ordering stock drugs, either by writing out a list of items required or by using a pre-printed order form, in each case basing requirements on the empty containers in the cupboard or trolley. In most hospitals the pharmacy now operates a top-up system with a pharmacy technician checking and supplying drugs to an agreed stock level on a weekly basis, thus removing the responsibility of ordering from the nurse. Whichever system is used, the aim must be to avoid both wasteful overstocking and running out at times when the pharmacy is closed.

Individual patient dispensing is used for less frequently required drugs and in cases where the preparation is tailored to the patient's particular requirements. Although most drugs are manufactured by industry, hospital pharmacies are always able to prepare different doseforms or strengths; for example, a mixture for a patient unable to take solids, a paediatric mixture where the child needs a lower dose, or a suppository if the oral route is contraindicated. Some hospitals are able to prepare injections of novel or little used chemicals, or formulate a chemical substance into preparations suitable for administration by a variety of routes. These more expert services, although concentrated in a few hospitals, are available to all through service contracts. The ward pharmacist can always advise on a suitable preparation and arrange for it to be made available.

The law requires that drugs of addiction, known as controlled drugs, must be supplied only against the signature of the sister or nurse in charge of the ward, and that the requisitions for these drugs must state precisely the name, form, strength and quantity of the drug required. Controlled drugs most likely to be met by the nurse include *morphine, diamorphine (heroin), papavertum (Omnopon), cocaine, pethidine, methadone, dextromoramide, buprenorphine* and *fentanyl*. In addition, some hospitals place similar controls on other drugs liable to misuse, such as *night sedatives, tranquillizers* and *antidepressants*, and on spirits such as *whisky* and *brandy*.

DRUG STORAGE

All drugs are potentially dangerous and all must be stored in locked cupboards reserved specifically for drugs. Ward sisters are legally authorized to possess controlled drugs for use on their wards (but not for any other purpose) and these and all other drugs issued to the ward are in their custody. Keys to the drug cupboards must be held by a sister, staff nurse or nurse in charge of the ward at the time. Drugs in current use may be stored in drug trolleys provided that these are locked and immobilized between drug rounds. Topical preparations such as ointments, lotions and disinfectants are also dangerous if misused, and these too must be locked in cupboards. This has been mandatory for many years in children's wards. More specific policies may be developed to suit local situations.

Storage conditions are important for most drugs and it is the pharmacist's responsibility to ensure that the label on the container bears adequate instructions such as 'store in a refrigerator'. Drugs which need cool or cold storage will begin to deteriorate if left at room temperature for more than a few hours, and if this happens the pharmacist's advice must be sought—it is not sufficient to put the drug in the fridge after 2 days and hope for the best.

All injections and many tablets have expiry dates assigned by the manufacturer, and if a drug is nearing this date the nurse should mention the fact to the ward pharmacist, who may be able to arrange for it to be used elsewhere. Drugs contained in emergency kits should be checked regularly and procedures in place to ensure timely replacement of preparations before reaching their expiry date. A nurse should not administer a drug which has passed its expiry date unless advice has been sought of the pharmacist who, with knowledge of the drug, may authorize its use. Similar constraints apply if the nurse feels that the condition or appearance of the drug is unusual or unsuitable.

DRUG PREPARATION

Nurses are required to do little in the way of preparation of drugs except for reconstituting injection solutions and making additions to intravenous infusion fluids. The practice of crushing tablets and mixing them with jam or sugar to get a child to take them, or of crushing tablets to put down a nasogastric tube, should be used only on specific pharmaceutical advice as many tablets are carefully formulated to give a sustained release of the drug, while others have the drug protected by a film, sugar or enteric coating to disguise a bitter taste or prevent gastric irritation; these characteristics will be destroyed if the tablet is crushed. The pharmacist can always prepare a suitable formulation for a particular patient.

Reconstitution of injection solutions from vials of sterile powder is taught as a nursing procedure. Reconstitution of certain drugs, such as the cytotoxic agents, can be hazardous to the nurse, and local precautions, including the use of protective clothing, must be obeyed. Only specially trained nurses undertake this activity, and most cytotoxic injections are being reconstituted centrally by pharmacy staff in cabinets designed to protect the product from microbial contamination and the operator from the drug. Such centralized services can save money by avoiding wastage of residues from reconstituted vials. Repeated contact with antibiotics can cause skin sensitization, and care must be taken to avoid skin or mucous membrane contact when these are being handled (see p. 243). Reconstitution of any drug should be carried out immediately before use, using the diluent recommended in the package leaflet or advised by the pharmacist, and in general any reconstituted solution remaining should be discarded. In the case of very expensive preparations it may be possible to store and re-use the residue, but great care must be paid to storage conditions and expiry, both of which will differ from those of the dry powder. Local policies and procedures must be followed. Limitation on re-use are that the reconstituted solution must never be stored in a syringe, must not be used for intravenous or intrathecal injection and must be used within 6 hours. In cases of doubt, the pharmacist will advise.

The majority of drugs for single parenteral use are for intramuscular or subcutaneous injection, but where a very rapid effect is required, or the drug is too irritant for intramuscular injection, or if it is desired to give the drug at a constant rate over several hours, the intravenous route may be used, either by direct intravenous injection, by injection as a bolus into the intravenous giving set, by addition to an intravenous infusion fluid or the use of a syringe pump.

The addition of drugs to intravenous infusion fluids has become an acceptable procedure for nurses who have been specially trained and authorized. Authorization is restricted to first level nurses with practical experience, but requirements will differ between hospitals. Problems which may arise in this procedure are microbial contamination of the infusion fluid, incomplete mixing of the drug and the fluid, and chemical incompatibilities (not always visible) between the drug and the fluid or between two drugs added to the same fluid. The first two are a result of faulty technique, while the third may be prevented by reference to incompatibility data which will be available through a pharmacist. Most hospitals provide a 24-hour advisory service from the pharmacy, and many have a resident phamacist.

DRUG LABELS

The style and content of labels will vary from hospital to hospital, but some typical labels for drugs dispensed for inpatients and outpatients are shown in Figure 3.1. In each case the name

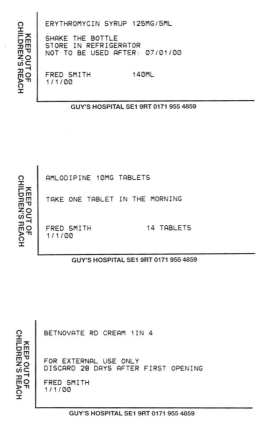

Figure 3.1 Typical labels for drugs dispensed for patients.

and strength of the drug appears at the top with directions on the frequency and method of administration for the patient on the outpatient label. Inpatient labels do not normally include directions for use, as the dosage frequency and administration often changes in hospitalized patients. Warnings on storage conditions and precautions are shown on all labels. The patient's name, quantity dispensed and date of dispensing also appear on each label. Patient information leaflets are also dispensed with the medication for patients to take home and read.

DRUG ADMINISTRATION

Drugs are administered under the supervision of the ward sister or staff nurse, and great responsibility rests on the nursing staff to ensure that there is no error. The principles behind the

rules are that the right patient must receive the right dose of the right drug in the right form by the right route at the right time, and that the fact is duly recorded. Local policies and procedures must be followed. A full discussion of the nurse's role may be found on page 16.

It is important that the precise directions for dose, time and frequency are followed. With some potent drugs, variations in times of dosing may lead to a loss of efficacy. Taking medication before, during or after food can also significantly alter its clinical effect.

Many hospitals are rewriting their drug policies to permit administration of drugs by a nurse without this being checked. Hospitals are developing computer systems on which the doctor will prescribe and the nurse record the administration of drugs, avoiding the traditional medicine sheets. This will provide an excellent tool for audit and costing purposes.

Schemes for self-administration of drugs by patients prior to discharge are being implemented in many hospital wards and involve training and assessment by pharmacists and nurses together.

If a nurse thinks a prescribed dose is unusually high (or low), the nurse in charge should be informed, the dosage checked in the *British National Formulary* and hospital formulary and the doctor contacted if necessary. When in doubt, the nurse must seek advice before giving the dose: it may be too late afterwards.

It is often assumed that once a patient leaves the ward he or she will continue to take the drugs provided in accordance with the directions, but this is frequently not the case. There should be an ongoing preparation of the patient for discharge, including an explanation of how drugs should be taken or used, the importance of following the dosage instructions, and details of any precautions which should be observed. This can result in a significant improvement in patient adherence to a medication regime. Written instructions and background information reinforce verbal explanations, particularly for patients and their carers.

Patients receiving steroid, insulin or anticoagulant treatment or being treated for depression with monamine oxidase inhibitors must be issued with cards describing precautions to be taken, and instructed to show the card to their doctor, dentist or pharmacist when receiving treatment or purchasing proprietary medicines. Such cards are usually available on the wards or from the pharmacy.

Some hospitals now issue patients with cards detailing their drugs, which are shown to the patient's GP and amended by him or her if the treatment changes. In this way, any practitioner treating the patient will be presented with an up-to-date drug profile.

OBSERVING THE EFFECTS OF DRUGS

Having given the drug, nurses are required to observe its effect by taking measurements, such as recording temperature, monitoring pulse rate or blood pressure, measuring urine output or testing urine for glucose, proteins, etc. Such observations are part of the ward routine and contribute to building up a picture of the patient's condition and progress. Nurses are in an ideal position to observe their patient's progress throughout the day so they should know the desired effect of the drug, its side-effects, its possible interaction with other drugs and how its effect might be modified by the patient's condition; it is in this area that the pharmacist can play an important part advising nurses.

INFORMATION NEEDS OF NURSES

During training nurses will acquire a basic knowledge of therapeutics and pharmacology which will probably have been extended by reading textbooks. It is possible, however, that they will be very familiar with only a limited number of drugs, usually those in widespread use in the hospital wards where they are allocated during clinical placements. It is certain that during their professional career they will meet new drugs—either those which have been recently introduced, or those which are only occasionally used for common disease, or those which are used to treat rare disorders. The ward

pharmacist is an ideal source of information about the handling and administration of new and rarely used drugs.

Most large hospital pharmacies have *drug information units*, which provide information on request to doctors, nurses and other health workers.

The ward pharmacist should provide a link between nurses and the drug information unit, supplying appropriate information. Some hospitals are also providing information cards or files which are kept on the wards and contain concise nurse-oriented information on drugs likely to be encountered, although the range of drugs covered in this way will not be complete. Computer databases are sometimes available on the wards, although care must be taken to select concise and appropriate information for inclusion. In addition, ward pharmacists will willingly talk to groups of nurses about any aspects of drugs and their use. Students who are given projects involving drugs are also encouraged to seek the help of the drug information unit.

LEGAL RESPONSIBILITY OF NURSES AS REGARDS DRUGS

The laws affecting drug supply and use are the Misuse of Drugs Act 1971 and the Medicines Act 1968, together with Regulations made under these Acts. The Misuse of Drugs Act governs the drugs of addiction, termed 'controlled drugs', whereas the Medicines Act governs the manufacture, marketing and supply of all drugs. The Secretary of State for Health is empowered under the National Health Services Act to make regulations concerning aspects of practice, including the prescribing and administration of drugs.

Under the Misuse of Drugs Act and Regulations, the *sister* or *acting sister* in charge of a ward, theatre, or other department in a hospital or nursing home may possess controlled drugs supplied to him or her by the pharmacist, and may administer them in accordance with the directions of a doctor or dentist. Midwives have additional authority under the Act to obtain, possess and administer *pethidine* in the practice of their profession. A doctor may not prescribe diamorphine (heroin) or cocaine for the treatment or relief of addiction unless licensed to do so by the Home Office.

Drugs may not be marketed without a product licence, which is granted by the Secretary of State on the advice of the Committee on Safety of Medicines, an expert body which considers evidence on the safety and efficacy of each new product.

Since April 1985, doctors, whether in hospital or general practice, have not been able to prescribe certain blacklisted drugs and drug preparations on a National Health Prescription. This restriction was imposed by the Secretary of State for Health to reduce public expenditure on drugs which were considered by their advisers to be unnecessary, or for which a cheaper alternative was available. The drugs banned included some antacids, laxatives, vitamins and cough and cold remedies, and are listed in the *Drug Tariff* (HMSO, published monthly).

The Medicines Act and its Regulations permit a *hospital nurse* to obtain and possess 'prescription only' medicines, i.e. those which are only available to patients on the prescription of a practitioner, for use on their ward, and to administer them in accordance with the directions of a doctor or dentist. Hospital rules usually extend this control to all drugs whether they are legally 'prescription only' or not. *Midwives* are permitted under the Act to administer a specified range of drugs in the practice of their profession. *Nurses in hospitals* have no authority to administer drugs except on the directions of a doctor or dentist, whether these are in the form of a specific prescription for a patient or as part of a written procedure accepted by the hospital authority. Any nurse doing so may face disciplinary action and, if harm comes to the patient, may be liable to civil action. Hospital policies are based on *Guidelines for the safe and secure handling of medicines* (The Duthie Report, Department of Health, 1988) and the *UKCC Standards for the Administration of Medicines* (October 1992).

Certain procedures in the administration of drugs which were formerly performed by doctors only are now regarded as part of the extended role of the nurse. Policy varies from hospital to hospital, but two examples are the addition of drugs to intravenous infusion fluids and the intravenous injection of drugs as a bolus via an intravenous line, which are sometimes undertaken by nurses who have been specially trained and authorized. This applies particularly to trained nurses working in Accident and Emergency Departments, Theatres, Intensive Care and Cardiac Units where an extended role may be practised.

IN THE COMMUNITY

Nurses now have considerable experience in the community before they qualify. The new roles of the district nurses and health visitors are discussed on page 24. In the community, the local pharmacist has the same role as in a hospital, supplying prescribed drugs and ensuring their safety and appropriateness. Pharmacists become well acquainted with their regular clients and are required to maintain their medication records on a computer. This means that the pharmacist can check new prescriptions against current drugs and other details such as known adverse effects. Nurses who prescribe should develop good relationships with pharmacists, who often provide advice about over-the-counter drugs, and their knowledge and records may also be of value to the prescriber nurse in preventing possible interactions.

Nurses working in the community, and private nurses, have authority to possess controlled drugs only to administer them in accordance with the directions of a doctor or dentist. Unlike nurses in hospitals, they may not hold a 'stock' of controlled drugs, but may obtain them only on prescription for a specific patient.

Similarly *nurses in community or private practice* have no authority to obtain or possess 'prescription only' medicines except on prescription, or to administer them to patients except in accordance with the directions of a doctor or dentist.

DOSAGE CALCULATIONS

Patients may be prescribed doses of a drug which

are not precisely equivalent to a single tablet, ampoule or 5 ml spoonful. In this case, it is necessary to calculate the quantity of drug preparation which will contain the dose prescribed, and this is a common source of error in drug administration. *The ward pharmacist should always be asked to annotate the prescription with the precise quantity of drug preparation which will contain the prescribed dose.* If the dose must be given before the ward pharmacist has seen the prescription, then any calculation made must be checked by a second person, and if there remains any doubt, advice must be sought before the drug is administered. Remember that the most common error when calculating drug dosage is a misplaced decimal point, i.e. the patient receives 10 times too much or only one-tenth of the dose.

Dosage calculation is a worry to nurses (and others!) and they may find it helpful to read *Drug calculations for nurses* (1995) by R Lapham and H Agaz, published by Arnold, London.

SUMMARY OF PHARMACEUTICAL SERVICES AVAILABLE TO NURSES

1. Supply of drugs for use on the ward.

2. Preparation of unusual formulations or doses of drugs.

3. Advice on storage conditions and expiry dates.

4. Advice on legal responsibilities.

5. Ward pharmacy services providing a ready point of contact and enquiry.

6. 24 hour service or on-call service.

7. Advice on preparation and reconstitution of drugs.

8. Advice on addition of drugs to intravenous infusion fluids.

9. Information on physical, chemical and pharmacological properties of drugs.

10. Information on dose, method of administration, effects, side-effects, precautions and contraindications associated with drugs.

11. Information on drug costs and drug usage in a particular hospital.

12. Seminars and discussions on drugs and their uses.

13. Information to assist with drug projects.

14. Advice about prescribing in the community.

15. Education and training for dosage calculation and administration.

4

The autonomic nervous system. Asthma. 5-Hydroxytryptamine. Migraine

The autonomic nervous system is that part of the nervous system which supplies the viscera as distinct from the voluntary muscles. The viscera include the gastrointestinal tract, the respiratory and urogenital systems, the heart and blood vessels, the intrinsic muscles of the eyes and various secretory glands.

The autonomic nervous system consists of two divisions and most viscera are supplied by nerves from both these divisions. They are called the *sympathetic* and *parasympathetic* systems and in general it may be said that they have opposite effects on the various viscera which they supply and that they also differ both in their anatomical arrangement and mechanism of function.

ANATOMY

The *sympathetic* system consists of the chain of ganglia lying on either side of the vertebral column and extending from the cervical to the lumbar vertebrae. Sympathetic nerve fibres, after passing out from the spinal cord, leave the anterior nerve root and pass to one of these ganglia. Here they form a synapse or junction with further nerve cells whose fibres are distributed to the viscera. Some sympathetic fibres, after leaving the spinal cord, pass through the ganglia and form their synapses in ganglia situated peripherally—the group of ganglia surrounding the coeliac artery is a good example of this arrangement.

The *parasympathetic* fibres leave the central nervous system and are distributed with certain

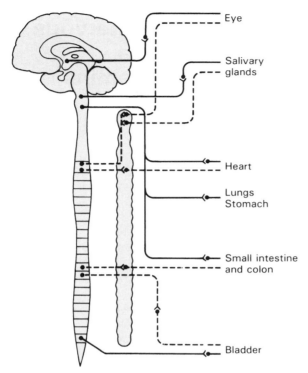

Figure 4.1 The anatomy of the autonomic nervous system. Sympathetic as broken line, parasympathetic as solid line.

PHYSIOLOGY

Stimulation of a nerve liberates a substance at the nerve ending which activates a receptor in the organ supplied or in another nerve cell. This is known as the *chemical transmission of nerve impulses* and is an important concept because many drugs act by interfering with this process. In the autonomic nervous system transmission occurs in this way in both the sympathetic and parasympathetic divisions, but the substances involved differ.

The parasympathetic system
(see Fig. 4.2)

Following stimulation of a parasympathetic nerve, a substance called *acetylcholine* is liberated at the nerve ending which acts on a receptor in the organ supplied. To prevent the effect of acetylcholine being too prolonged and powerful there is also present at the nerve ending a substance called *cholinesterase*, which rapidly breaks down the acetylcholine and terminates its effect.

cranial nerves (III, VII, IX and X) and with the sacral nerves. The relay ganglia of the parasympathetic system are situated peripherally near the organs supplied (Fig. 4.1).

The autonomic system also carries a large number of sensory nerves which supply the various organs. These nerves enter the spinal cord where they may form a spinal reflex arc with the autonomic nerves leaving the cord or they may ascend to the brain where more complex reflexes are built up which may be influenced by impulses arising from the higher levels of the brain. It is a matter of common experience that some visceral sensation may enter consciousness and that events in consciousness may themselves stimulate various visceral effects. The rapid beating of the heart after a fright is a typical example.

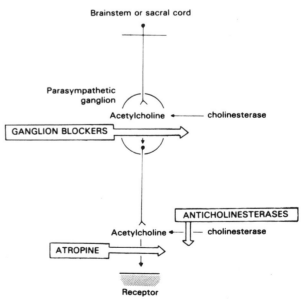

Figure 4.2 Physiology of the parasympathetic nervous system and its modification by drugs.

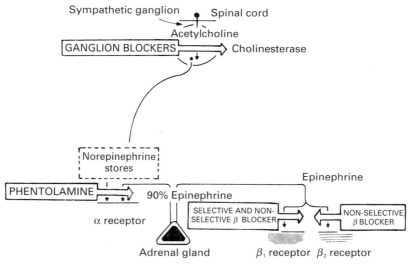

Figure 4.3 The sympathetic nervous system, showing naturally occurring stimulating agents and drugs which block their action.

The sympathetic system (see Fig. 4.3)

The sympathetic system is rather more complicated because two substances may be liberated and there is more than one type of receptor. The sympathetic nerves release *norepinephrine* from stores at the nerve endings in the peripheral tissues. In addition, the sympathetic system releases *norepinephrine* and *epinephrine* from the medulla of the adrenal glands; these substances enter the bloodstream and produce widespread effects. There are several types of sympathetic receptors.

α *receptors* are stimulated by norepinephrine released at sympathetic nerve endings and by epinephrine.

Stimulation produces:

1. Constriction of blood vessels particularly at the skin, causing a rise in blood pressure and reflex slowing of the heart.
2. Dilatation of the pupil.

Stimulation of α receptors is blocked by several drugs (see p. 47).

β_1 *and* β_2 *receptors* (see Figs 4.4 and 4.5) are both stimulated by isoprenaline and epinephrine. In addition, norepinephrine acts as a β_1 stimulator

on the heart, and the drug salbutamol produces a β_2 response largely on the bronchi. The effects are:

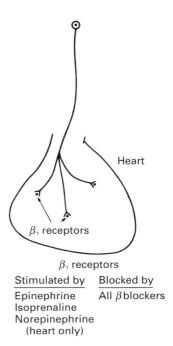

β_1 receptors	
Stimulated by	Blocked by
Epinephrine	All β blockers
Isoprenaline	
Norepinephrine	
(heart only)	

Figure 4.4 Important β_1 receptors, showing agonists (stimulators) and blocking agents.

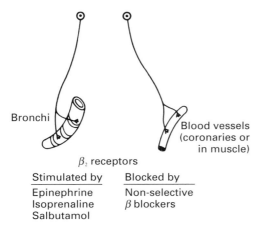

β₂ receptors

Stimulated by	Blocked by
Epinephrine	Non-selective
Isoprenaline	β blockers
Salbutamol	

Figure 4.5 Important β₂ receptors, showing agonists (stimulators) and blocking agents.

1. β_1 responses. Increase in rate and excitability of the heart with increased output of blood.

2. β_2 responses. Dilatation of bronchi and blood vessels.

Stimulation of β receptors can be blocked by drugs known as β *blockers*. Some of these are termed *selective* as they block the stimulation of β_1 receptors only, whereas others are *non-selective* and block the stimulation of both β_1 and β_2 receptors (see p. 47).

Overactivity of the sympathetic nervous system produced by fright or anger causes a mixed picture due to stimulation by norepinephrine and epinephrine of α, β_1 and β_2 receptors (see Table 4.1).

Transmision at autonomic ganglia

Acetylcholine is also liberated at the synapses of both sympathetic and parasympathetic ganglia and is responsible for the transmission of nerve impulses between nerve endings and ganglion cells.

SYMPATHOMIMETIC DRUGS

Sympathomimetic drugs have effects similar to those produced by activity of the sympathetic nervous system.

Table 4.1 The chief effects of sympathetic and parasympathetic activity

	Sympathetic activity	Parasympathetic activity
Heart rate	Increased	Slowed
Blood vessels	Constricted	Dilated
Stomach and intestine	Decreased activity and secretion	Increased activity and secretion
Salivary and bronchial glands	Decreased secretion	Increased secretion
Urinary bladder	Body relaxed, sphincter contracted	Body contracted, sphincter relaxed
Bronchial muscle	Relaxed	Contracted
Blood sugar	Raised	
Eye	Pupils dilated	Pupils constricted Accommodates for near vision

Epinephrine (adrenaline). Epinephrine is one of the substances produced by sympathetic activity; for medical use it is, however, prepared synthetically. It acts on the sympathetic receptors of the visceral organs. Epinephrine is destroyed by stomach acid and is therefore not effective if taken orally. It is usually given by subcutaneous or intramuscular injection, its effects being produced more rapidly from the latter site. Following injection, its various actions become apparent within a minute. They are:

1. An increase in the force and rate of contraction of the heart (β_1 effect), so that the patient may report palpitation.

2. A rise in systolic blood pressure due to the increased output of blood by the heart (β_1 effect). The diastolic pressure shows little change as epinephrine produces vasoconstriction only in the skin and in the splanchnic area (mixed α and β_2 effects) and vasodilatation in arteries in muscle (β_2 effect).

3. Epinephrine relaxes smooth muscle, including that of the bronchial tree.

4. Epinephrine raises blood sugar by mobilizing glucose from tissues.

Following injection, epinephrine is rapidly broken down in the body by *amine oxidase* and *methyl-O-transferase*, and its effects only last a few minutes.

Therapeutics. Epinephrine is used less now than in former times. It is still the best immediate treatment for serious anaphylactic reactions (see p. 297). By causing constriction of blood vessels it relieves oedema and swelling. The usual dose is 0.5 ml of a 1 : 1000 solution, intramuscularly, and it is important not to inject this dose of the drug into a vein by mistake as a sudden intravenous injection can precipitate a fatal cardiac arrhythmia.

It can, however, be given as an intravenous bolus in a dose of 1 mg (10 ml of a 1 : 10 000 solution) as a stimulant to the heart in cardiac arrest.

Note: Do not inject into the same intravenous line as sodium bicarbonate.

Norepinephrine (noradrenaline). Norepinephrine is closely related to epinephrine and is produced in the body by sympathetic activity. It can also be prepared synthetically. Its most important action is to produce widespread vasoconstriction and thus a rise in both systolic and diastolic blood pressure (α effect). Norepinephrine is rapidly inactivated by the body and, therefore, to produce a continuous effect on the blood pressure it is given by intravenous infusion.

Therapeutics. Norepinephrine has been used in the treatment of various forms of shock associated with a very low blood pressure. There are two solutions available:

1. *Injection of norepinephrine acid tartrate* contains 4 mg of norepinephrine base in 4 ml and is diluted before infusion.

2. *Special injection of norepinephrine acid tartrate* contains 400 micrograms of norepinephrine base in 4 ml.

Note: 4 mg of norepinephrine base = 8 mg of norepinephrine acid tartrate.

For preparation of solutions for infusion, the reader is referred to the *British National Formulary*. A patient receiving norepinephrine requires careful nursing and observation with frequent estimations of blood pressure, which may fluctuate widely with small changes in the rate of infusion. Care should be taken to avoid extravasation which can cause necrosis.

Opinion has moved against using norepinephrine to raise blood pressure except in extreme circumstances, for although a satisfying rise in blood pressure can be obtained due to vasoconstriction, this also reduces the blood flow in essential organs, particularly the kidney, with troublesome results.

Isoprenaline is related to epinephrine but it stimulates only β_1 and β_2 receptors. It is well absorbed from the buccal mucosa and following inhalation. It relaxes smooth muscle, including that of the bronchial tree, and also stimulates the heart, but has little or no effect on the blood pressure. It is important to avoid over-dosage as it can cause dangerous cardiac arrhythmias. It is rapidly inactivated after absorption and its effects are short-lived.

Therapeutics. Isoprenaline was formerly used in the treatment of asthma, both by inhalation and orally. Because its action of cardiac stimulation can precipitate fatal arrhythmias, it has now been replaced for this purpose by the safer β_2 agonists. It can also be given by infusion in severe bradycardia.

Adverse effects include palpitation, nausea, headaches and tremors.

Selective β_2 agonists

These stimulate predominantly β_2 receptors so that although they are effective bronchodilators they have minimal effect on the heart. This is an important improvement over drugs such as isoprenaline as the risk of cardiac arrhythmias is removed.

Salbutamol is the most widely used β_2 agonist and a powerful bronchodilator. It can be given by various routes, but if given orally a considerable proportion is broken down in the liver (first pass effect). Its action lasts about 4 hours. In large doses it may cause tremor and tachycardia and occasionally night cramps.

Therapeutics. Salbutamol is used to treat bronchospasm due to asthma or bronchitis. It may be taken to relieve an attack or, on a regular basis, to control the spasm. It can be given:

1. Orally in doses of 2–4 mg three or four times daily. Note that a relatively large dose is required because of the large first pass effect and side-effects are frequent.

2. Slowly, intravenously in doses of 4 micrograms/kg body weight to treat a severe asthmatic attack. *This is rarely necessary as a nebulizer is very effective. It also requires careful monitoring for cardiac arrhythmias.*

3. Inhalation is the most commonly used route of administration and given in this way in the treatment of bronchospasm it is possible to get the maximum effect on the bronchi with minimal effect elsewhere. Even so, only 10% of the dose reaches the bronchial tree, the rest being swallowed (Fig. 4.6).

There are various delivery systems for inhalation (see Fig. 4.7). The dose by aerosol inhaler is 100 micrograms per puff (usually one or two puffs are given); by rotahaler it is 200 or 400 micrograms per capsule; or by nebulizer—nebules containing 2.5–5.0 mg of salbutamol, which can be diluted with sterile 0.9% saline, are used. If inhalations are given on a regular basis they are required 4–6 hourly.

In addition to its use in asthma, salbutamol is used to *inhibit premature labour* (see p. 208).

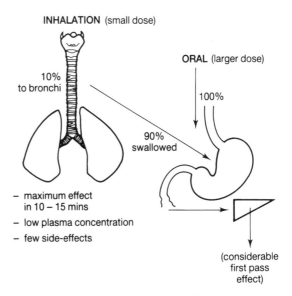

Figure 4.6   Comparison of inhalation and oral dosage of salbutamol.

There are other selective β_2 agonists which are very similar to salbutamol (Table 4.2).

Salmeterol and **eformoterol** are long-acting β_2 agonists. They are effective after about 30 minutes and their action lasts for about 12 hours;

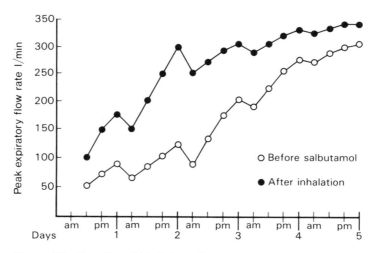

Figure 4.7   The effect of inhalations of salbutamol on a patient with severe asthma. Note the progressive improvement in respiratory function and the morning dips which are characteristic of asthma.

Table 4.2 Other β_2 agonist bronchodilators

Drug	Dose by aerosol	Special features
Terbutaline	250–500 micrograms (250 micrograms/puff) 3–4 times daily	Small first pass effect useful orally. Slightly longer action than salbutamol (6 h)
Fenoterol	100–200 micrograms (100 micrograms/puff) 1–3 times daily	Less β_2 selective
Reproterol	0.5–1.0 mg (1–2 puffs) up to 3 times daily	
Bambuterol	10–20 mg once daily orally	Prodrug of terbutaline

therefore they should not be used for rapid effect in treating an acute attack, but given twice daily, by inhalation, as a preventative. Although it has been claimed they have some anti-inflammatory action as well as relieving bronchospasm, this is controversial and they may be combined with an inhaled steroid.

Inhalation delivery systems

Inhalation is a useful and effective way of giving some of the drugs used to treat asthma and other forms of bronchospasm.

1. *Pressurized aerosol inhalers* are the most convenient systems for home use. The drug is dissolved or suspended in a propellant and on pressing the plunger a standard amount is released in the form of fine particles measuring 2–5 μm. It is essential that the patient is taught the technique of using the inhaler if the treatment is to be effective (Fig. 4.8).

Nursing point

Many patients require repeated instruction in the use of aerosols particularly the young and the elderly. Inhalers containing a placebo are available for teaching.

---

a. Remove the cap from the mouthpiece and shake the inhaler.

b. Breathe out slowly but not fully.

c. Place the mouthpiece in the mouth and close the lips around it.

d. Breathe in slowly and at the same time depress the plunger thus releasing the drug.

e. Hold the breath for at least 10 seconds and longer if possible.

f. If a second inhalation is required, wait for 1 minute.

g. If steroids and β_2 agonists are both prescribed give the β_2 agonist first and wait for 5 minutes.

Spacers. Some patients lack the coordination required to use a pressurized aerosol. A spacer is a reservoir between the aerosol and the mouthpiece. Pressing the plunger releases the drug into the reservoir from whence it may be inhaled.

2. *Rotahalers* are used for those who find the pressurized aerosols difficult to operate. Capsules containing the drug in powder form are placed in the rotahaler which opens the capsule and delivers the drug to be inhaled. The capsules may become soft and fail to function and some patients find the powder an irritant. The *Diskhaler* is a similar arrangement where the powdered drug is carried in blisters on a disc. The apparatus releases the drug, which is inhaled.

3. *Nebulizers* are used in severe asthma and chronic bronchitis and enable a larger dose to reach the bronchi. Air, or oxygen, is driven through a solution of the drug and the resulting mist is inhaled via a mask. It is important to have the correct particle size and it is best obtained by using an air flow rate of 6–8 litres/minute. Piped air or oxygen may be used or various mechanical compressors are available which some patients use at home. *It is important that these are cleaned regularly to prevent bacterial contamination.*

Alternative drugs used in asthma and other types of bronchospasm can be given by inhalation including β_2 agonists, corticosteroids (see later), sodium cromoglicate and ipratropium bromide.

4. *Delivery systems for children.* Asthma is a common disease in childhood, affecting about 10% of children. It usually disappears in adolescence.

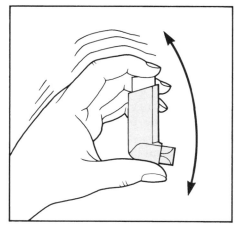

1 Remove the cover from the mouthpiece, and shake the inhaler vigorously.

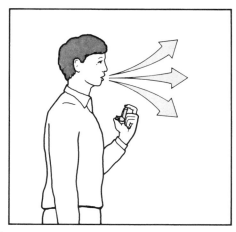

2 Holding the inhaler as shown above, breathe out gently (but not fully) and then immediately...

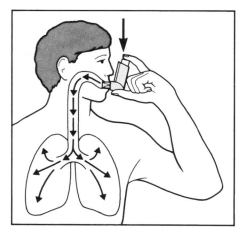

3 Place the mouthpiece in the mouth and close your lips around it. After starting to breathe in slowly and deeply through your mouth, press the inhaler firmly as shown above to release the medication and continue to breathe in.

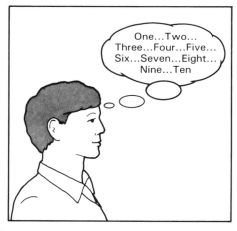

4 Hold your breath for 10 seconds, or as long as is comfortable, before breathing out slowly.

5 If you are to take a second inhalation you should wait at least one minute before repeating steps 2, 3 and 4.

6 After use replace the cover on the mouthpiece.

Figure 4.8 How to use an inhaler properly.

Drug treatment with inhalers may be required but may be difficult to administer.

Less than 18 months — Nebulizers cannot be used.
18 months–2 years — Nebulizer can be used.
2–5 years — Nebulizer and spacers can be used.
5–10 years — As above with the addition of rotahalers.
Over 10 years — As for adults.

The drug treatment of asthma

Asthma is a common disorder causing considerable morbidity and some mortality so the correct use of drugs either given *regularly to prevent* an attack or *intermittently to relieve* one plays an important part in its management (Fig. 4.9).

The attack of asthma, with its characteristic wheeze, is due to narrowing of the bronchi by:

1. Spasm of the circular muscle in the bronchial wall
2. Inflammation with oedema of the bronchial mucosa.

Patients with asthma have an *inherent* sensitivity of the bronchi that is probably partially inherited. The attacks are precipitated by *trigger* *factors* such as infection, exercise, various allergies and psychological factors which release substances in the bronchial wall causing spasm and inflammation.

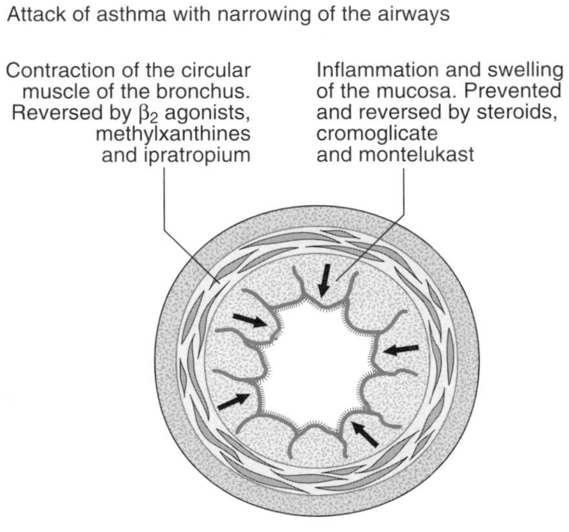

Drugs can prevent or relieve attacks by:

a. Relaxing or —β_2 agonists
   preventing the   methylxanthines
   bronchospasm   ipratropium
b. Reducing   —corticosteroids
   inflammation   sodium cromoglicate
   and oedema   nedocromil
                     leukotriene modifiers

1. **Bronchodilator** drugs play an important part in the treatment of asthma.

a. *Inhaled β_2 agonists* are widely prescribed. They are given by inhalation to treat a developing attack or to prevent an attack when it seems likely (e.g. exercise-induced asthma). Their *regular use* alone as a preventive is more controversial. They do not control the inflammatory component of asthma and there is some evidence that their regular use can lead ultimately to more severe and sometimes fatal attacks. If regular use of a β_2 agonist is required to control asthma most authorities advise that a corticosteroid should be added to the regimen.

Oral salbutamol tablets are not very efficient, but salbutamol controlled-release tablets, one at night, have a prolonged action and are useful in preventing nocturnal attacks of asthma.

b. **Methylxanthines** are a group of drugs which inhibit the enzyme phosphodiesterase in the bronchial muscle, causing it to relax and thus relieve the bronchospasm.

Aminophylline and *theophylline* belong to this group and, although they are effective, they require careful use as there is only a small difference between the therapeutic and toxic dose. In addition, their rate of elimination depends on a number of factors including weight, sex, age, concurrent disease and other medication and may vary considerably (Fig. 4.10).

Aminophylline can be given slowly intravenously as a single dose of 250 mg to terminate an acute attack. It can also be given as a loading dose followed by an infusion by pump or micropipette. If the infusion is prolonged plasma

Attack of asthma with narrowing of the airways

Contraction of the circular muscle of the bronchus. Reversed by β_2 agonists, methylxanthines and ipratropium

Inflammation and swelling of the mucosa. Prevented and reversed by steroids, cromoglicate and montelukast

Figure 4.9 The asthma attack and its control by drugs.

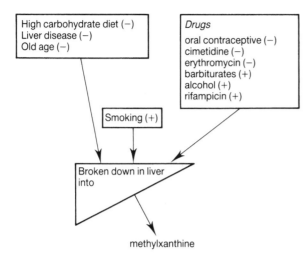

+ = (low blood levels) increased clearance,
− = (high blood levels) decreased clearance

Figure 4.10 Factors altering the blood level and activity of methylxanthines.

levels should be measured at intervals as a guide to dosage. High plasma levels may result if oral and intravenous administration are combined and this can be dangerous. *Therefore, before giving intravenous aminophylline, always ask if the patient is already taking a methylxanthine orally.*

Taken orally, aminophylline and theophylline may be nauseating but this can be overcome by using slow-release preparations which only require 12-hourly administration and avoid peaks in the plasma levels and are thus less likely to cause side-effects. *Slow-release preparations must be swallowed whole to avoid interfering with the slow delivery system.*

Because of interindividual variation, fixed dose regimens are not ideal and it is better to control dosage by measuring blood levels to obtain optimal results.

Available preparations include:

Phyllocontin Continus — contains aminophylline
Theo Dur — contains theophylline
Slo-phylline — contains granules which can be sprinkled on food for easier administration.

Adverse effects are dose related and include nausea, anxiety, tachycardia and arrhythmias and convulsions. Interactions are common and effects are increased by cimetidine, erythromycin and oral contraceptives.

c. **Ipratropium bromide** is related to atropine and acts as a bronchodilator by virtue of its anticholinergic action. It is given via an inhaler or a nebulizer and any of the drug which is swallowed is not absorbed from the intestine. It thus has a powerful local action on the bronchi but avoids the unwanted side-effects of atropine (see p. 50). It should be used for those patients who have not responded to β_2 agonists. Its bronchodilator effect begins after about 45 minutes and lasts for 3–4 hours; therefore, it is best if taken regularly to *prevent* an asthmatic attack. It may be combined with a β_2 agonist or corticosteroids.

Adverse effects are an unpleasant taste and a dry mouth.

2. **Corticosteroids (steroids)** reduce the inflammatory and allergic aspects of asthma and decrease bronchospasm in severe and persistent asthma. *Beclomethasone* (a steroid well absorbed from mucous surfaces) can be given by inhalation. Three strengths are available (50, 100 or 200 micrograms per puff). The usual dose is 100–400 micrograms twice daily. In resistant asthma this may be increased to 800–2000 micrograms daily. This enables the maximum concentration to be obtained in the bronchi with minimal systemic side-effects. *Budesonide* in doses of 200 micrograms twice daily is similar. *Fluticasone* has less systemic effect for the same benefit. Occasional candida infection of the mouth may occur, presumably due to the lowering of local resistance by the steroid, and occasionally a hoarse voice develops due to weakening of the vocal cords. This effect usually disappears if the drug is stopped or the dose reduced.

Corticosteroids given by inhalation in doses up to 400 micrograms a day for children and 800 micrograms a day for adults do not produce the systemic side-effects associated with oral steroids, and even with higher doses the systemic effects are usually minimal. However, children on high doses may show a reduced growth rate.

In a few resistant cases of asthma oral prednisolone will be required, at the minimal effective dose.

3. **Sodium cromoglicate** prevents asthmatic attacks by stopping the release of substances from mast cells in the bronchi which are responsible for bronchospasm. It is given regularly by pressurized aerosol or rotahaler. The usual dose is four inhalations daily. It is most effective in young patients with asthma with an allergic history but is of some use in non-allergic asthma.

Nedocromil is also a mast cell stabilizer and anti-inflammatory drug and is very similar to sodium cromoglicate. It is given as a pressurized aerosol, the starting dose being 4.0 mg twice daily, and is used to prevent rather than treat attacks.

4. **Leukotriene modifiers.** Leukotrienes are substances, produced by inflammatory white cells, which cause spasm of the bronchial muscle. Asthmatic subjects appear to be very sensitive to this action which plays an important part in the asthmatic attack. Drugs are becoming available which prevent spasm either by blocking the action of leukotrienes or by preventing inflammation. They also diminish hyperactivity of the bronchial mucosa and reduce inflammation.

Montelukast can be given orally to adults and children over six. At present it is used as a continuous treatment for mild-to-moderate asthma and may reduce the need for other drugs. It is also useful in preventing exercise-induced asthma and that due to aspirin.

Adverse effects appear mild.

Management of chronic asthma

The management of asthmatic patients is not easy in spite of the number of remedies available and the various guidelines drawn up to advise on which therapy should be used. It is important that the management involves a partnership between the patient (or for children, including the parents) and the health professional, whether nurse or doctor.

Drug therapy will depend on the age of the patient and the severity and pattern of attacks. The use of drugs in chronic asthma may be looked on in stages, with the patient starting at the appropriate level and moving up or down according to the response to treatment. For adults and older children, the following programme is widely used:

Stage 1. The patient has occasional episodes of wheezing—these can be treated with an inhaled bronchodilator (usually a β_2 agonist). Bronchodilators can also be used as a preventative before some known precipitating trigger, e.g. exercise. If several inhalations are required daily a move is made to the next stage.

Stage 2. Regular inhaled low-dose steroid or sodium cromoglicate is given and a β_2 agonist used as required. If this fails to prevent attacks treatment should proceed to stage 3.

Stage 3. There is some difference of opinion as to the best drug combination at this stage:
either high-dose inhaled steroid + a β_2 agonist as required
or low-dose inhaled steroid + a long-acting β_2 agonist (e.g. salmeterol).

Stage 4. High-dose inhaled steroid + *regular* bronchodilator (e.g. β_2 agonist, methylxanthine or ipratropium used as is most appropriate).

Stage 5. Oral steroids are added to the regime.

In young children both the diagnosis of asthma and its management present special problems which are beyond the scope of this book.

Management of status asthmaticus

A prolonged and severe attack of asthma can be very distressing to the patient and may be dangerous. The immediate treatment is:

1. Ensure adequate hydration of the patient if necessary by infusion as this will prevent the sputum becoming sticky.

2. Use bronchodilators:

a. Salbutamol, 5.0 mg diluted with sterile 0.9% saline, given by nebulizer every 4 hours.

b. In very severe attacks salbutamol 250 micrograms or aminophylline 250 mg can be given i.v. over 10 minutes. Aminophylline can also be given by continuous infusion.

3. Hydrocortisone 200 mg i.v. every 6 hours or prednisolone 30–60 mg orally reduces inflammation. Corticosteroids, even if given intravenously, take several hours to be effective.

4. No sedation owing to risk of respiratory depression.

5. Amoxycillin 250 mg three times daily as chest infection frequently complicates the attack.

6. Oxygen as required.

7. Occasionally, patients who respond poorly will require artificial ventilation.

Special points for patient education

It is very important that the patients learn to manage their own disease as far as possible and for children the parents should be fully involved. This means that they should be taught to:

1. Modify their lifestyle as far as possible to avoid attacks, yet lead a normal life.
2. Understand the use of their drugs, whether they are for an acute attack or used prophylactically.
3. Understand the care and maintenance of their home nebulizer if they use one.
4. Learn to monitor their disease by means of a peak flow meter and adjust their treatment accordingly. A peak flow of <70% of normal requires step-up treatment. With a peak flow of <50% of normal, the patient's doctor should be called and corticosteroids started.
5. Recognize (both nurses and patients) the signs of dangerous deterioration in asthma. A rapid pulse (> 110 per minute), rapid respiration (> 25 per minute), exhaustion and inability to complete a sentence require that the doctor should be called urgently and indicate that the patient will probably require hospital admission.

Nursing points

Do not forget that β blockers can make asthma worse and should be avoided in patients with asthma, and that NSAIDs may precipitate an attack.

Chronic obstructive airways disease

This common disease differs from asthma in that it is progressive rather than intermittent, affects older people and is clearly related to smoking and air pollution. The small bronchi are obstructed by inflammation and excess mucus production (chronic bronchitis) and in addition, there is destruction of the walls of the alveoli (emphysema).

Treatment is not very satisfactory and is aimed at minimizing progressive lung destruction and treating acute exacerbations as they arise. It is essential that the patient gives up smoking and avoids air pollution as far as possible.

Bronchodilators are used as for asthma but their efficacy is variable and ipratropium may be better than β_2 agonists. Inhaled or systemic steroids are worthy of a trial but if there is little or no improvement over a short course they should be tailed off.

Exacerbation occurs, particularly in winter, due to infection of the bronchi and will require antibiotic treatment. Ultimately, a proportion of patients will progress to respiratory failure.

OTHER SYMPATHOMIMETIC DRUGS

Amfetamine and dexamfetamine are similar drugs whose main effect is on the central nervous system. They produce some euphoria, abolish fatigue, increase activity and reduce appetite. They are taken orally. They carry a considerable risk of dependence and their use is now confined to:

1. Narcolepsy, starting dose 5.0 mg twice daily.
2. Some hyperactive children on whom, paradoxically, they have a sedative effect.

They should not be used for appetite control.

ADRENERGIC BLOCKING AGENTS

It is possible to block α and β adrenergic receptors.

α adrenergic blockers

α adrenergic blocking drugs are used in the treatment of *hypertension*. By removing the vaso-constrictor action of norepinephrine these drugs dilate arterioles and thus lower blood pressure. They are considered on p. 67. They are also used in the diagnosis of *phaeochromocytoma* (a rare tumour of the adrenal gland) when *phentolamine* is used.

α adrenergic receptors control the smooth muscle round the neck of the bladder. By block-ing these receptors it is possible to relax this muscle and partially relieve *bladder neck obstruction* due to an enlarged prostate. Several α blockers including *doxazosin* and *terazosin* can be used when surgical treatment is contraindicated.

β adrenergic blockers

This group of drugs which block the effects of epinephrine and norepinephrine on β adrenergic receptors is widely used. In general, their thera-peutic effects and uses are very similar, but individual members of the group show minor differences:

1. Some block predominantly β_1 receptors (i.e. cardiac receptors) and are called *selective* β blockers, others block both β_1 and β_2 receptors (i.e. cardiac + bronchial + peripheral blood vessel receptors) and are called *non-selective* β blockers.

2. Members of the group differ in their speed and site of elimination and in their duration of action.

General actions of β blockers (Table 4.3)

1. By blocking β_1 receptors in the heart the rate is slowed, the output of blood from the heart is reduced and the work done by the heart is thus decreased. This is particularly marked when there is increased activity of the sympathetic nervous system such as occurs with excitement or exercise. In addition, the excitability of heart muscle is reduced.

2. By blocking β_2 receptors β blockers cause bronchospasm, particularly in patients with asthma. This is particularly marked with non-selective β blockers as selective β blockers have less effect on β_2 receptors. This is usually of little consequence in normal subjects, but in patients with asthma may make bronchospasm worse and increase dyspnoea.

3. β blockers lower blood pressure.

4. Some β blockers have metabolic effects and they prevent the rise in blood glucose which normally follows increased sympathetic activity.

5. It is believed that at least some β adrenergic blockers penetrate the central nervous system. Some sedation is fairly common in patients receiving β blockers and occasionally this may be severe. In addition, vivid dreams and more rarely hallucinations occur.

6. Many of the symptoms of anxiety such as palpitations, sweating and tremor are mediated

Table 4.3 Features of some β blockers in common use

Drug	Selectivity	Elimination hepatic	Renal	Half-life (hours)
Propranolol	$\beta_1 + \beta_2$	+	−	3
Oxprenolol	$\beta_1 + \beta_2$	+	−	2
Sotalol	$\beta_1 + \beta_2$	(+)	+	12
Timolol	$\beta_1 + \beta_2$	(+)	(+)	5
Nadolol	$\beta_1 + \beta_2$	−	+	16
Metoprolol	$\beta_1 > \beta_2$	+	−	4
Pindolol	$\beta_1 > \beta_2$	(+)	+	4
Acebutolol	$\beta_1 > \beta_2$	(+)	(+)	6
Atenolol	$\beta_1 > \beta_2$	−	+	12
Bisoprolol	$\beta_1 > \beta_2$	(+)	(+)	10
Betaxolol	$\beta_1 > \beta_2$	?	(+)	16
Esmolol	$\beta_1 > \beta_2$	?	?	Very short

via the sympathetic nervous system. These symptoms can often be relieved by β blockers. Whether this is only a peripheral action or whether in addition there is some other effect on the brain is not known.

Therapeutics. β blockers are used to treat:

1. Angina of effort (see p. 83) because they reduce the work of the heart especially on effort or excitement.

2. Cardiac arrhythmias because they reduce the excitability of the heart.

3. Hypertension as they lower blood pressure, perhaps by setting the regulation of blood pressure at a lower level.

4. Thyrotoxicosis and anxiety because they reduce the increased sympathetic activity which occurs in these disorders.

5. Essential tremor, a rare familial condition characterized by severe intention tremor.

6. Prevention of migraine attacks.

Adverse effects other than exacerbation of heart failure and of bronchospasm can be troublesome, but are not usually serious. Occasionally they cause vivid dreams and hallucinations, and by decreasing cardiac output they reduce the blood flow to the extremities, which may feel unduly cold, and are best avoided in peripheral vascular disease. They mask the usual warning symptoms of hypoglycaemia and can be dangerous in patients with diabetes who are taking insulin (see p. 192). Active people may feel less energetic whilst taking these drugs.

Labetalol and *carvedilol* are combined α and β blockers which are used in treating hypertension (see p. 71).

PARASYMPATHOMIMETIC DRUGS

Parasympathomimetic drugs have effects similar to those produced by activity of the parasympathetic nervous system.

Acetylcholine. *Acetylcholine* is released from the *parasympathetic nerve endings* throughout the body and also from motor nerve endings in *voluntary muscle*. Its effects as a result of parasympathetic release are shown in Table 4.1 and, in addition, it activates voluntary muscle when a motor nerve is stimulated and is essential for all voluntary movements. Its action is very short-lived as it is quickly broken down by *cholinesterase* so it is not used therapeutically. However, a prolonged effect can be produced either by giving an acetylcholine-like drug which is not broken down or by using a drug which inhibits the action of cholinesterase, thus prolonging and intensifying the actions of naturally occurring acetylcholine. This type of drug is called an *anticholinesterase*.

Carbachol is a synthetic substance chemically related to acetylcholine. Its actions resemble those of parasympathetic stimulation. It is not broken down by the body cholinesterases and its actions are therefore much more prolonged than those of acetylcholine.

After subcutaneous injection, flushing and sweating appear in about 20 minutes, followed by increased intestinal peristalsis sometimes with colic and contraction of the bladder muscle. These actions last up to an hour. Carbachol may be given by subcutaneous injection or by mouth.

Therapeutics. The most important therapeutic use of carbachol is in the treatment of urinary retention following surgical operation or childbirth when there is no obstruction. It causes contraction of the bladder muscle resulting in the passage of urine.

Adverse effects include colic, diarrhoea and a marked fall in blood pressure. They are controlled by atropine.

Bethanechol is similar.

Pilocarpine is used only as eyedrops, where it causes constriction of the pupil.

The anticholinesterases

These drugs prevent the breakdown by cholinesterase of acetylcholine produced at nerve endings throughout the body. The actions of acetylcholine are thus intensified at their two sites of action.

1. The parasympathetic nerve endings.
2. The nerve endings in voluntary muscle.

It can thus be seen that the final picture produced by these groups of actions is mixed. The action at the parasympathetic nerve endings usually predominates and the action on nerve endings in voluntary muscle is only seen under special circumstances.

The most important effects of anticholinesterases are:

1. *The eye.* Some anticholinesterases are absorbed through the conjunctiva and following application to the eye cause constriction of the pupil and spasm of accommodation.

2. *Intestinal tract.* Anticholinesterases cause increased tone and motility.

3. *Urinary tract.* They cause contraction of the bladder.

Several anticholinesterases are used to treat a variety of disorders depending on where their actions are most pronounced.

Neostigmine is a synthetic anticholinesterase with actions very similar to those of physostigmine, but with an effect on the neuromuscular junction of voluntary muscle and less on the eye and cardiovascular system. It is rapidly effective following subcutaneous or intramuscular injection and is also absorbed after oral administration, although larger doses are required by this route.

Therapeutics. Neostigmine is used widely in the treatment of disorders in the neuromuscular junction of voluntary muscle (e.g. myasthenia gravis) (see p. 145), and has been used in cases of paralytic ileus and atony of the bladder.

Pyridostigmine and edrophonium are anticholinesterases used in the treatment of myasthenia gravis.

Distigmine has widespread actions and may be used for urinary retention and myasthenia gravis. It can be given orally or by injection.

There are a number of other anticholinesterase preparations which are not used therapeutically but which are extensively employed as *insecticides* and are also *potential lethal weapons* for use in war. As some are absorbed through the intact skin and produce powerful anticholinesterase effects, they have been termed 'nerve gases'.

The *adverse effects* of the various anticholin-esterases are similar. The symptoms include intestinal colic and diarrhoea, sweating and salivation, the pupils are constricted, the pulse slow and the blood pressure low. The immediate treatment is atropine 1 mg intravenously.

There are now a number of drugs available which will reactivate cholinesterase by separating it from anticholinesterase. *Pralidoxime* is the best known.

DRUGS INHIBITING THE ACTION OF ACETYLCHOLINE

The drugs which inhibit the action of parasympathetic nerve endings belong to the belladonna group or are synthetic substitutes.

All these drugs produce their effect by blocking the action of acetylcholine on the cholinergic receptors in the organ concerned.

Atropine. Atropine is well absorbed from the intestine after oral administration; it can also be given subcutaneously, intramuscularly or intravenously. Atropine is largely broken down by the liver. Its effects last 2 hours or longer.

As a result of blockade of the parasympathetic system the following are observed.

Gastrointestinal tract. Diminished motility of the stomach and both small and large intestines with relief of spasm. Decrease in salivary secretion and reduction of gastric acid secretion.

Heart. Diminished cardiac vagal tone leading to an increase in pulse rate.

Lungs. Blockade of vagal (parasympathetic) action leading to some relaxation of the bronchial muscle. Diminished secretion from the bronchial glands.

Involuntary muscle. Relaxation of other involuntary muscles, notably those of the biliary and renal tracts.

The eye. Blockade of the parasympathetic nerve supply to the eye, leading to dilatation of the pupil and paralysis of accommodation with an inability to see near objects clearly.

Warning. It is important that atropine or similar drugs should not be given to those with a tendency to glaucoma. In this disorder the drainage of fluid from the eye is reduced and the pressure rises within the eyeball. Atropine further reduces the flow of fluid from the eye and may precipitate an acute attack of glaucoma (see p. 323).

Therapeutics. Atropine has several therapeutic uses, the more important of which are:

1. *Relief of involuntary muscle spasm.* Most forms of smooth muscle spasm are relieved by atropine, 600 micrograms subcutaneously or intravenously being useful in the relief of intestinal, biliary or renal colic.

2. *Eye conditions.* Atropine may be applied locally to the eye as an eye drop to dilate the pupil in a variety of conditions. *Homatropine* is often used in 2% solution for this purpose as its effects are not so prolonged as those of atropine.

3. *Preoperative medication.* Atropine is given preoperatively in doses of 600 micrograms subcutaneously to dry up the salivary and bronchial secretions and to protect the heart from undue vagal depression.

4. *Bronchial spasm.* An atropine derivative (*ipratropium*) is given by inhalation to relieve bronchospasm in asthma (see p. 44).

Adverse effects are dose related. Dry mouth, constipation, difficulty with micturition (in the elderly) and paralysis of ocular accommodation are common. With higher doses restlessness, hallucination and delirium can occur.

Hyoscine (scopolamine). The peripheral actions of hyoscine are the same as those of atropine. Its action on the central nervous system differs, however, in that hyoscine, even in small doses, is a central nervous system depressant leading to drowsiness and sleep.

Therapeutics. Hyoscine is particularly used for its central as well as peripheral effects. It is used preoperatively in doses of 400 micrograms by injection and can be taken orally as an antiemetic.

THE SYNTHETIC SUBSTITUTES

These drugs are now rarely used to treat peptic ulcers but are still given to patients with the irritable bowel syndrome and related disorders and occasionally for nocturnal enuresis.

Among those available are:

Dicycloverine
Mebeverine
Propantheline

Adverse effects are similar to those of atropine.

Oxybutynin 5 mg twice daily and **flavoxate** relax the muscle of the bladder and are used in patients with frequency and other urinary problems.

Tolteridine is used for similar problems.

5-HYDROXYTRYPTAMINE (5-HT, SEROTONIN)

5-Hydroxytryptamine is an important chemical transmitter and stimulant with actions in the nervous system and elsewhere but it is not part of the autonomic nervous system. 5-Hydroxytryptamine is released by nerves and other structures and reacts with several types of receptor. Its action depends on the class of receptor which is stimulated and the organ involved.

Drugs are available which can activate or block 5-HT receptors and abnormalities in the actions of 5-HT are involved in several disorders:

Brain	— depression
Brain and gut	— vomiting caused by certain cytotoxic drugs
Cranial blood vessels and nerves	— migraine

Carcinoid tumours produce large amounts of 5-HT which cause a variety of symptoms.

MIGRAINE

Migraine is characterized by recurrent attacks of moderate-to-severe headache, often unilateral and pulsating, which may be associated with vomiting and preceded by visual disturbances (the aura). Its often familial attacks may be precipitated by 'trigger' factors such as certain foods, alcohol, stress and hormonal influences (the Pill). The aura is caused by a wave of depressed activity passing over the cerebral cortex associated with changes in the cerebral circulation. The headache is due to activation of the trigeminal nerve with release of substances which cause dilation of local blood vessels, leading to pain. Stimulation of 5-HT receptors in this area reverses the vasodilation and thus relieves the headache.

Treatment of the acute attack

Non-specific drugs. The headache often responds to simple analgesics such as aspirin 600–900 mg for an adult or paracetamol 0.5–1.0 g. NSAIDs can also be used. They should be started early in the attack. Metoclopramide (see p. 107) may be given 30 minutes before the analgesic to prevent vomiting and increase the rate of gastric emptying and thus hasten absorption and relief of pain.

Tolfenamic acid is a NSAID which, given orally, may be particularly effective but, at present, it is expensive.

It often helps to lie down in a quiet, darkened room and some patients find a small dose of diazepam useful in promoting sleep.

If these measures fail, as they do in about 20% of subjects, a specific remedy should be used.

Sumatriptan stimulates 5-HT receptors in the wall of the dilated blood vessels surrounding the brain and on the trigeminal nerve, resulting in vasoconstriction and, thus, relieving the headache.

Therapeutics. It is given by *subcutaneous* injection as soon as possible after the onset of symptoms and relieves the headache, in most patients, within 1 hour. Its action lasts about 2 hours after which the headache may return. It can be repeated once, after 1 hour, if necessary. It is also available for oral use, the dose being 50–100 mg and as a nasal spray. It is effective in about 85% of patients by injection and 60% if given orally.

Adverse effects are rare but a few patients report tightness in the chest. Although clinical evidence of myocardial ischaemia is very rare, it should not be given to patients with coronary artery disease in view of the risk of arterial spasm and it should not be combined with ergotamine. It may also cause dizziness and nausea.

Sumatriptan is undoubtedly effective for treating a migraine attack but it is rather expensive.

Naratriptan and **Zolmitriptan** are similar and are given orally.

Ergot is a fungus which grows on rye and contains two substances which are pharmacologically active—ergometrine (see p. 206) and ergotamine.

Ergotamine is an α sympathetic stimulant that causes constriction, particularly, of small arteries. It may also react with 5-HT receptors. It is not an analgesic but relieves the migraine headache by its vasoconstrictive action.

Therapeutics. Ergotamine has been widely used to treat migraine headaches but due to its adverse effects and the introduction of newer remedies its popularity has declined. It is frequently combined with caffeine as Cafergot (1.0 mg/tablet), the initial dose being 1–2 tablets which can be repeated to a maximum of 4 tablets in 24 hours (not to be repeated for 4 days) and 8 tablets in a week. It is also available combined with cyclizine as Migril 2 mg/tablet). Ergotamine is also absorbed rectally and via the respiratory passages and an aerosol inhaler is available.

Adverse effects include vomiting, diarrhoea and peripheral vasoconstriction which can be severe enough to cause gangrene if an overdose is given. Tingling and numbness are an indication to stop treatment immediately. Withdrawal of the drug, particularly after heavy dosage, may itself cause headaches. It is contraindicated in coronary disease and pregnancy and vasoconstriction is increased in patients taking β_2 blockers.

Prevention of migraine attacks

Frequent attacks of migraine can be very debilitating and seriously interfere with living a

---

Special points for patient education in migraine

1. Patients must be taught which drugs are used to relieve an acute attack and which are used for prevention.

2. It must be stressed that ergotamine should only be taken to relieve attacks and for a limited number of doses, not taken regularly for prevention as this will lead to serious side-effects and may actually cause headaches.

3. Migraine attacks may be precipitated by a variety of external factors, such as certain foods and the 'Pill'. The patient should learn to recognize these and avoid them if possible.

---

normal life. If, after excluding trigger factors, the attacks occur more than once a week it may be necessary to use continuous drug treatment as a preventative measure.

At present there is no clear-cut best drug so the choice is a matter of weighing efficacy against side-effects for a particular patient.

β blockers prevent or reduce attacks in about half the patients. They probably act by reducing vasodilation and there is no preferred β blocker for this purpose. When they are prescribed, their contraindications must be remembered and they should not be combined with ergotamine.

Pizotifen is concerned with the action of 5-HT and prevents migraine attacks by reducing the constriction and dilatation of blood vessels. It can cause drowsiness and the initial dose should be given at night. Its main adverse effect is weight gain and it may take up to a month to be effective.

Sodium valproate (see also p. 169) is an antiepileptic agent which can also be used to prevent migraine attacks. It should not be used in pregnancy, owing to the risk of fetal malformation, and, rarely, it can cause liver damage and a reduction of platelets in the blood.

Antidepressants. Dothiepin and amitriptyline are effective, even if the patient is not suffering from depression.

Methysergide blocks the action of 5-HT on receptors in smooth muscle. It is effective but has serious adverse effects and should only be used when safer treatment has failed.

Nursing point

The overuse of simple analgesic drugs, particularly when combined with caffeine or opioids, can itself cause headaches and nurses should enquire about analgesic consumption in those with frequent headaches.

FURTHER READING

Barnes P J 1995 Inhaled glucocorticosteroids for asthma. New England Journal of Medicine 332: 868

Chapman K R, Keston S, Szaiai J P 1994 Regular versus as-needed inhaled salbutamol in asthma control. Lancet 343: 1379

Cross S 1997 Revised guidelines for asthma management. Professional Nurse 12: 408

Editorial 1987 Nebulisers in the treatment of asthma. Drug and Therapeutics Bulletin 25: 101

Editorial 1997 Using β$_2$ stimulants in asthma. Drug and Therapeutics Bulletin 35: 1

Editorial 1998 Leukotriene modifiers in the treatment of asthma. British Medical Journal 316: 1257

Editorial 1994 Treating mild asthma—when are inhaled steroids indicated? New England Journal of Medicine 331: 737

Ferrari M D 1998 Migraine. Lancet 351: 1043

Goadsby P J, Olesen J 1996 Diagnosis and management of migraine. British Medical Journal 312: 1279

Leach A 1994 Making sense of peak-flow recordings of lung function. Nursing Times 90: 34

Lipworth B J 1997 Treatment of acute asthma. Lancet supplement 350: 18

Pearce L 1998 A guide to asthma inhalers. Nursing Times supplement March 1998

Rees J, Price J 1995 Treatment of chronic asthma. British Medical Journal 310: 1459

5

Drugs affecting the cardiovascular system

DRUGS ACTING ON THE HEART

There are three major disorders of the heart itself which can be treated by drugs. They are:

1. Cardiac failure
2. Cardiac arrhythmias
3. Cardiac ischaemia.

CARDIAC FAILURE

The heart is a muscular pump receiving blood from the systemic and pulmonary veins and driving it, under pressure, into the pulmonary arteries and the aorta. The volume of blood passing through the heart each minute is known as the *cardiac output*. This is largely determined by four factors:

1. The pressure in the venous system filling the heart and stretching the heart muscle, which is known as the *preload*. In health, a rise in venous pressure causes a rise in cardiac output.

2. The arterial pressure that is the resistance against which the heart must pump, known as the *afterload*.

3. The heart rate—an increase in rate leads to an increased output, except in heart failure when an increased rate decreases cardiac efficiency.

4. The contractile efficiency of the heart muscle.

In good health the cardiac output varies considerably depending on the needs of the body, being low at rest and rising with exercise. The healthy heart has a great functional reserve and can cope with demands for increased output which occur from time to time.

In cardiac failure the contractility of the heart muscle is reduced so the ventricles fail to empty properly. The muscle becomes thicker and stiffer and, in diastole, fails to relax completely; thus, filling of the ventricles is diminished. The heart and neck veins become distended with blood and cannot respond to the increased filling pressure (preload) by raising output. At first this is only apparent on exercise but, later, occurs at rest. The pump becomes insufficient for the needs of the body and various organs receive an inadequate blood and oxygen supply. This is particularly important in the kidney, where it activates the angiotensin/renin system (see p. 67), causing the kidney to retain salt and water. Oedema of dependent parts and lungs develops, the latter being responsible for marked dyspnoea (shortness of breath), which is a common feature of cardiac failure. Angiotensin is also responsible for arterial constriction, which increases the work (afterload) of an already labouring heart. This is further aggravated by an increase in sympathetic activity causing additional vasoconstriction and tachycardia.

The low cardiac output carries less oxygen to the tissues. The oxygen supply to the heart and brain is kept up at the expense of other organs which are starved of oxygen and this accounts for the fatigue which may be a prominent symptom (Fig. 5.1).

There are many causes of cardiac failure. The heart muscle may be damaged by previous coronary thrombosis or by cardiomyopathy, or an increased workload over a long period due to high blood pressure or valve disease ultimately causes it to fail.

Drugs in congestive cardiac failure

Five main groups of drugs are used:

1. Diuretics, which cause the kidney to excrete excess salt and water (see p. 213).

2. ACE inhibitors, which act by suppressing the angiotensin/renin mechanism (see p. 69) which is overactive in cardiac failure.

3. Drugs which improve the function of the myocardium so the heart contracts more powerfully and empties more completely, thereby raising the cardiac output. This is called a *positive inotropic effect*. The only drug of this type which is used successfully in chronic cardiac failure is digitalis; other drugs of this type are used in cardiac shock (see p. 59).

4. Vasolidators, which lower peripheral resistance and thus reduce cardiac work.

5. β blockers, which reduce inappropriate sympathetic activity.

Diuretics

These are considered in detail on page 213. Both thiazide and loop diuretics are used in cardiac failure. By increasing the excretion of salt and water they help to get rid of oedema and pulmonary congestion and by reducing blood volume they relieve distension of the heart. However, the reduced blood volume tends to activate renin release by the kidney and this may partially reverse their beneficial effects by stimulating the kidney to retain fluid and, by vasoconstriction, to increase the work of the heart. Nevertheless, the benefits usually outweigh the disadvantages and they are widely used for the relief of chronic cardiac failure. For mild heart failure thiazide diuretics may be adequate but more severe heart failure will require a loop diuretic such as frusemide.

Both thiazide and loop diuretics increase potassium loss via the kidney. If small doses are used this is unlikely to require correction but:

1. If large doses of diuretic are used
2. If dietary potassium is deficient (e.g. in the poor or elderly)
3. If concurrent digitalis is given

potassium deficiency increases digitalis toxicity. Supplementary potassium or a potassium sparing diuretic should be added to the regimen (see p. 217). In all cases the plasma potassium concentration should be monitored and kept above 3.2 mmol/litre.

Interactions. NSAIDs will reduce the efficacy of diuretics.

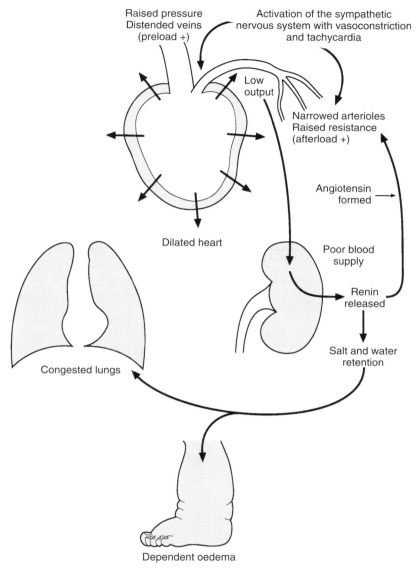

Figure 5.1 Processes in cardiac failure.

Angiotensin converting enzyme (ACE) inhibitors (see p. 69)

This group of drugs, which is also used to treat hypertension, has emerged as an important addition to the management of chronic heart failure. By blocking the overactive renin/ angiotensin mechanism (see p. 69) they reduce the retention of salt and water by the kidneys and, in addition, by dilating arterioles they lower the resistance to blood flow from the heart (afterload), reduce cardiac work and raise cardiac output.

Therapeutics. ACE inhibitors have considerably improved the treatment of cardiac failure and have prolonged survival. However, the initiation of treatment requires much care and should be started in hospital. The main danger is a profound fall in blood pressure after the first dose, especially liable to occur in patients already taking diuretics, and is due to vasodilation and a low blood volume resulting from the diuretic treatment.

The initial dose of ACE inhibitor should be low and the blood pressure should be closely monitored (4 hourly) for 24 hours. ACE inhibitors should not be given to patients with renal failure or in pregnancy. Renal function should be measured at regular intervals for those on long-term treatment.

Adverse effects. See p. 69.

Nursing point

When monitoring the blood pressure following the first dose of an ACE inhibitor, it should be remembered that the fall after captopril only lasts a few hours but that after enalapril may be delayed for up to 8 hours and last up to 30 hours.

Interactions. ACE inhibitors cause a decrease in potassium excretion by the kidney. Great care is therefore necessary if they are combined with potassium-sparing diuretics or supplementary potassium as dangerous hyperkalaemia can develop. They are less effective when combined with NSAIDs.

Vasodilators

Several vasodilators have been used with some success in cardiac failure and include sodium nitroprusside (see p. 70) and nitrites (see p. 82). They reduce the work of the heart by lowering peripheral resistance and, by dilating the veins, lower the venous pressure and allow the heart to beat more effectively. However, they are less effective than ACE inhibitors and are usually only used for short-term emergencies.

Digitalis

This drug has been used by doctors for hundreds of years. In 1785 William Withering of Birmingham described its use in dropsy and noted that it appeared to act on the heart.

There are two types of digitalis in common use—*digoxin* which is obtained from the white foxglove and *digitoxin* from the purple foxglove. Both drugs are usually given orally, but they can be injected intravenously. They are well absorbed and become attached to the heart muscle where they improve its function. Digoxin is excreted by the kidneys; this is important as accumulation occurs in patients with poor renal function unless a lower dose is used. Digitoxin is broken down by the liver.

	Maximal effect after oral dose	*Duration of action*
Digoxin	6 hours	2 days
Digitoxin	12 hours	7 days

It will be noted that the action of these drugs lasts for several days. This is not due only to slow elimination, but because, once bound to heart muscle, their action is prolonged.

The effects seen in the failing heart are:

1. Depression of conduction in the AV node and the bundle of His (see Fig. 5.2). This action does not affect the heart in sinus rhythm, but in atrial fibrillation it decreases the number of impulses reaching the ventricles from the fibrillating atria, and thus decreases the rate of ventricular contraction.

2. Slowing of the heart rate, partially due to increased activity of the vagus nerve and partly to a direct action on the sinu-atrial node.

3. Increased force of contraction of the ventricular muscle. This action is due to an increase in calcium ions in the heart muscle cells. In large doses this may be associated with increased excitability of the ventricle.

The most important of these three actions is slowing of the ventricular rate, particularly in atrial fibrillation where the slower and more regular contractions allow the heart to function more efficiently and raise cardiac output. The *positive inotropic effect* is less important and if the heart is in sinus rhythm the benefits are minimal.

Therapeutics. Treatment is started with a full dose of the drug until a satisfactory response is obtained as judged by the general condition of the patient, a ventricular rate of 60–80 per minute and a diuresis followed by reduction of oedema.

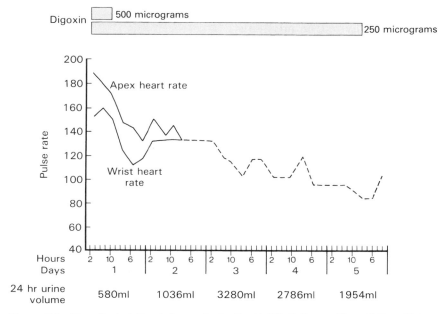

Figure 5.2   The effect of digoxin in a patient with atrial fibrillation and heart failure. Note the difference between the heart rate at the apex and the rate at the wrist due to weak contractions failing to produce a pulse at the wrist. This difference disappears on treatment with digitalis.

This usually starts about 6 hours after dosing (see Fig. 5.2).

If the patient has atrial fibrillation the apex rate is the best guide because the pulse rate at the wrist may appear to be slower as weak beats may not be felt.

The initial dose for an adult should be 500 micrograms of digoxin orally, followed by 250 micrograms three times daily for a day or two until a full therapeutic response is achieved. Thereafter the maintenance dose to replace the day-to-day loss will usually lie between 125 and 250 micrograms daily. Elderly patients and those with impaired renal function require smaller doses to avoid accumulation of the drug and in these patients 62.5 micrograms daily or less may be sufficient.

The introduction of powerful and fast-acting diuretics has reduced the need for rapid digitalization but 250–500 micrograms of digoxin can be given *slowly* intravenously. It is important to ensure that the patient is not already receiving digitalis or overdose may occur.

Plasma levels of digoxin can now be measured, the correct therapeutic range being between 0.9 and 2 micrograms/litre (the sample is taken at least 6 hours after dosing). There is, however, considerable interperson variation and the estimation of plasma levels is more useful to confirm non-compliance or overdose than in the control of treatment where clinical observation is usually adequate.

Digitalis may also be used in certain *cardiac arrhythmias*, even if they are unassociated with heart failure.

Atrial fibrillation. By suppressing conduction between the atria and ventricles digitalis controls the ventricular rate in atrial fibrillation whether there is associated cardiac failure or not. It does not, however, abolish the fibrillation.

Atrial flutter. Digitalis may change the arrhythmia into atrial fibrillation. If the drug is then stopped, normal sinus rhythm may be restored.

Adverse effects. There is only a small difference between the therapeutic dose of digitalis and the toxic dose so dosage should be carefully regulated. Elderly patients, those with renal impairment and with hypothyroidism are more liable to suffer adverse effects. *The nurse should keep a watch for toxicity* and should know the common manifestations of overdose. They are:

1. Undue slowing of the heart due to excessive effect on the conducting system or the sinu-atrial node. A pulse rate below 60 indicates that the drug should be omitted for a day or two.

2. Coupled beats. These are due to ventricular extrasystoles following normal beats. They are felt at the wrist as a double pulsation followed by a pause. The extrasystoles result from increased excitability of the ventricles and are an indication to omit the drug. Continued overdosage may lead to ventricular paroxysmal tachycardia or even ventricular fibrillation, which is rapidly fatal.

3. Sometimes a combination of complete heart block with a ventricular rate of about 100 is seen. This disorder is difficult to diagnose without an electrocardiogram.

4. Nausea and later vomiting. This is due to stimulation of the vomiting centre in the medulla by digitalis. However, as heart failure itself may produce vomiting, it is not a very reliable symptom of overdosage.

5. Rarely, coloured vision may be found in overdosage.

6. In elderly patients digitalis may cause confusion.

It is also important to remember that *lowering the level of potassium in the blood increases the toxicity of digitalis*. This may occur with certain diuretics (p. 215) and their administration may result in the appearance of signs of digitalis overdosage in a patient who has been satisfactorily treated for a long time.

Interactions:

1. The action of digoxin is increased by verapamil, diltiazem and amiodarone and the dose should be halved if these drugs are introduced.

2. Any drug which lowers plasma potassium (i.e. diuretics) potentiates the toxicity of digoxin.

β blockers

The use of β blockers to treat cardiac failure is more controversial. In this condition there is increased activity of the sympathetic nervous system which may be inappropriate and, by reducing the effect of this activity, β blockers have a therapeutic action. However, because of their depressing action on cardiac function, they can exacerbate cardiac failure. At present, there is probably a place for small and carefully controlled doses of β blockers in certain patients provided their heart failure is not too severe or of recent onset.

The treatment of cardiac failure

The three main objectives in treating cardiac failure are to increase the efficiency and output of the heart so that there is sufficient blood and oxygen supply to the various organs, to reduce congestion and oedema and to try where possible to remove or diminish the factor or factors which caused the heart to fail.

Patients with cardiac failure are nursed in a sitting position so that the accumulated oedema fluid drains away from the lungs and abdominal viscera to the legs and does not therefore embarrass respiration. Although the legs may be slightly elevated on a stool when the patient is sitting out of bed, they should not be raised above the horizontal as this may shift fluid to the abdomen and lungs. Constipation may be a problem requiring modification of diet and, sometimes, a purgative or suppository.

These patients usually require easily digested and light foods. Retention of salt is as important as retention of water by the kidneys in producing oedema. Modern diuretics will usually

---

Nursing point

Mistakes with digitalis dosage are not uncommon. Three strengths of digoxin tablet are currently available—62.5, 125 and 250 micrograms. The paediatric elixir contains 50 micrograms/ml. To avoid confusion, the dose should be written in micrograms.

enable the kidneys to excrete salt and a low-salt diet is rarely required. Opinions vary as to the correct fluid intake but it is not usually necessary to restrict it. However, in severe heart failure or when sodium deficiency has developed as a result of prolonged and intensive diuretic treatment, intake should be cut to 1500 ml daily and the regime arranged to minimize the patient's discomfort.

In mild or moderate heart failure treatment is usually started with *diuretics*, either thiazides for minimal failure or loop diuretics for more severe failure. They are given once daily by mouth. Patients should be weighed regularly at the same time of day and in the same clothes to assess the efficacy of treatment. This may be sufficient treatment and can be carried out at home under the patient's GP.

There is a tendency to introduce *ACE inhibitors* into the therapeutic regime early in treatment. They should certainly be used if the response to diuretics is not satisfactory or if cardiac failure is severe, but many doctors think there is a place for their use even in moderate failure, and there is evidence that they not only control symptoms but also prolong life.

Digitalis was formerly used extensively in heart failure both to stimulate contraction of the heart and to slow the pulse rate, thus raising the cardiac output. It is now realized that the effect on the contraction is short-lived and less important than it was once considered to be, so its main use in heart failure is to slow the pulse rate, particularly in atrial fibrillation.

Various ancillary drugs may be used in the treatment of cardiac failure. A hypnotic drug may be required if the patient cannot sleep. In the very restless and ill patient, morphine is extremely useful, particularly in acute failure of the left ventricle, but it must be used with care in patients who are cyanosed as depression of respiration may occur. If cyanosis is a marked feature, *oxygen* is given at full concentration unless the patient has concurrent chronic respiratory disease, in which case the concentration should be controlled.

Patients in bed with cardiac failure are liable to develop venous thrombosis and it is common

practice to give prophylactic treatment with *heparin* 5000 units subcutaneously twice daily.

It is not so easy to remove the cause of the cardiac failure, but some of the precipitating factors can now be treated. High blood pressure can be reduced by drugs, and advances in cardiac surgery have enabled many defects of the valves of the heart to be relieved.

Acute failure of the left ventricle, which commonly occurs in patients with high blood pressure or following a cardiac infarct, leads to rapidly developing oedema of the lungs with distress and shortness of breath. It is best treated with a rapidly acting *diuretic* (frusemide 10–40 mg i.v. either as a bolus or by infusion pump), *morphine* 5–10 mg i.v. or diamorphine 2.5–5.0 mg i.v. which sedates the patient and also, by dilating veins, reduces congestion of the lungs. If necessary, they may be combined with *prochlorperazine* 12.5 mg deep i.m. to control vomiting.

Vasodilators may also be used. Glyceryl trinitrate dilates the veins and reduces the filling pressure and distension of the heart. Sodium nitroprusside, in addition, relaxes the arterioles thus reducing cardiac work. Both drugs are usually given by intravenous infusion and dosage requires careful monitoring.

Drugs in shock

In a state of shock the output of blood from the heart is acutely reduced, the blood pressure is low and circulation to the organs of the body is inadequate. Clinically, the patient is pale, sweating and confused, the pulse is rapid, the blood pressure low and the limbs cold; kidney failure may supervene. This state may occur for three main reasons:

1. *Sudden reduction of blood volume*, usually due to bleeding, which is treated by replacing the lost fluid by infusion.

2. *Reduced pumping action of the heart* (pump failure) following damage (e.g. after a myocardial infarct).

3. *Septic shock*, usually due to infection with Gram-negative bacteria (see p. 220), which is commonly found in patients receiving steroids

---

Nursing point

Calcium antagonists may make cardiac failure worse and should be avoided if possible in this disorder; NSAIDs reduce the effect of diuretics and can cause fluid retention with oedema.

Special points in patient education

Unless the underlying cause can be removed, most patients with chronic heart failure will require some medication for the rest of their lives. It should be explained to them that the main objectives of treatment are to give them a reasonable exercise tolerance and to keep them free of oedema. The importance of taking their drugs regularly should be stressed. They should be told of the main adverse effects, particularly those producing symptoms (e.g. nausea in digitalis overdose). All patients with chronic heart failure should be seen regularly, either as outpatients or by their family doctor.

---

or cytotoxic drugs. Bacterial toxins cause vasodilation and leaking of fluid from the circulation, which reduces the blood volume, combined with a falling cardiac output. In addition to the usual measures to combat shock, rapid and vigorous treatment with the appropriate antibiotic is necessary as the condition may prove fatal.

Various drugs are being tried to neutralize the bacterial toxin involved but, at present, there is no preferred regime.

If the main fault is pump failure, drugs can be given to increase the force of contraction of the heart muscle (**positive inotropic effect**) and thus improve cardiac output and circulation and raise the blood pressure.

Digitalis is not effective in these circumstances and may precipitate a dangerous cardiac arrhythmia. The most commonly used drugs are dopamine and dobutamine. This type of treatment requires careful monitoring, usually in an intensive care ward.

Dopamine is a naturally occurring substance which is changed to norepinephrine in the body. However, it has actions of its own and is used to treat shock which may follow cardiac infarction or major cardiac surgery.

It is a β_1 stimulant and also increases the release of norepinephrine in the heart, thus causing the heart muscle to contract more powerfully. In addition, dopamine stimulates receptors in the renal blood vessels, causing them to dilate and increase both renal blood flow and urinary output. This action is used as shock often causes a decline in renal function.

Dopamine is given by continuous intravenous infusion (via a central line). In doses of 2–5 micrograms/kg/minute it affects mainly the kidneys and is used to improve their function, often combined with a diuretic.

Higher doses should not be used as the intense vasoconstriction which develops may cause gangrene of the extremities.

Interactions. Patients receiving monoamine-oxidase inhibitors should be given one-tenth of the usual dose of dopamine.

Dobutamine is similar to dopamine but has no effect on the kidneys. It is, however, less likely to cause cardiac arrhythmias.

Dopamine and dobutamine may be combined: a low dose of dopamine being used for its effects on the kidneys and dobutamine for its cardiac action.

Both dopamine and dobutamine should be infused via a central vein to minimize peripheral vasoconstriction.

Other cardiac stimulants

Efforts are continually being made to find a drug which will stimulate heart muscle to raise the cardiac output. Several have been introduced but as yet there is no really effective newcomer.

CARDIAC ARRHYTHMIAS

In the normal heart the initial stimulus of contraction starts in the sinu-atrial node (the pacemaker of the heart) situated at the junction of the superior vena cava and the right atrium. The rate of discharge from the node is under control of the vagus and sympathetic nerves. Vagal activity slows the heart rate and

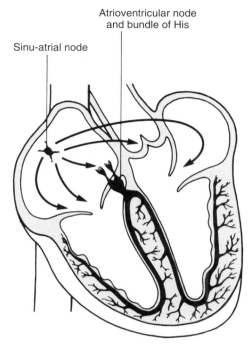

Figure 5.3   The heart, showing the sinu-atrial node and conducting system (atrioventricular node and bundle of His).

sympathetic activity increases it. The wave of contraction spreads over both atria forcing blood into the ventricles. The stimulus then pauses for a fraction of a second at the *atrioventricular (AV) node* before passing down the *bundle of His* and spreading through the muscles of both ventricles, which contract and drive blood into the pulmonary artery and the aorta (Fig. 5.3). The heart then relaxes, refills with venous blood and awaits the next stimulus for contraction. Under certain circumstances this cycle may be disturbed.

Disorders of cardiac rhythm can be divided into those due to overexcitability of the heart, which are by far the most common, and those due to conduction defects in the bundle of His.

Arrhythmias due to overexcitability

Extrasystoles (ectopic beats). These are caused by an excitable focus either in the atria or ventricles which stimulates the heart to contract while relaxed and awaiting the next normal stimulus. This normal stimulus then falls on a heart in the unresponsive or refractory phase which immediately follows a contraction and there is a pause before normal rhythm is resumed. Extrasystoles are very common in healthy people and although they may be associated with heart disease they are usually of little significance. They may be related to excessive smoking or to the consumption of tea, coffee or alcohol. They rarely require treatment other than reassurance.

Paroxysmal tachycardia may arise from the ventricle (*ventricular*) or from the atria or atrio-ventricular node (*supraventricular*). In ventricular tachycardia an excitable focus in the ventricle stimulates the ventricle to contract regularly at about 160–180 times a minute. It frequently occurs in diseased hearts, for instance after a cardiac infarct (Fig. 5.4).

Supraventricular tachycardias are believed to have a rather different mechanism. They are usually due to a rapid circus movement within the AV node which fires off ventricular contractions via the bundle of His at about 160/minute. This is known as a *re-entrant phenomenon*. If the circus movement is suppressed, the heart returns to normal rhythm. Less commonly, there is an accessory pathway between the atria and the ventricles which is involved in the re-entrant phenomenon (see Wolfe–Parkinson–White syndrome, p. 66).

Attacks of paroxysmal tachycardia may last for anything from a few seconds to hours or even days. They may occur in quite healthy people or they may complicate heart disease.

Atrial flutter. Sometimes the atria may contract at an even higher speed, usually about 240–300/minute. This is called atrial flutter. Under these circumstances the ventricles are unable to 'keep up' with the atria and therefore respond to every other or perhaps every third atrial contraction, a condition known as 2 : 1 or 3 : 1 heart block.

Atrial (auricular) fibrillation. In atrial fibrillation each individual bundle of muscle fibres in the atria contracts individually at a rate of about 450 contractions/minute. This results in complete disorganization of atrial contraction, and furthermore the ventricles are bombarded, via

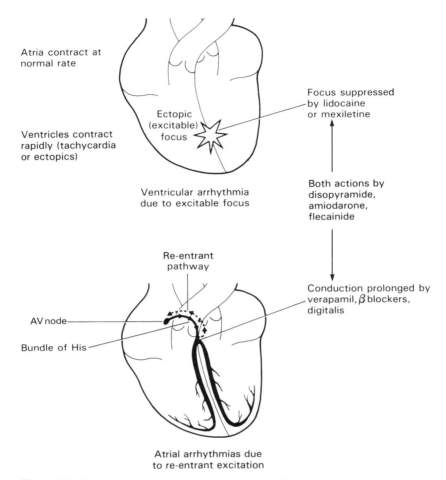

Figure 5.4 The mechanisms of paroxysmal tachycardias.

the bundle of His, with rapid and irregular stimuli and are unable either to fill properly with blood or to contract satisfactorily. Atrial fibrillation, which may be persistent or paroxysmal, is usually associated with heart disease (coronary disease, hypertension, cardiomyopathy and valvular disease). It can complicate thyrotoxicosis, various acute illnesses and alcoholism. Sometimes, there is no apparent cause.

Arrhythmias due to conduction defects

Heart block. Sometimes the bundle of His may fail to transmit the impulse from the atria to the ventricles. This condition is known as heart block.

If there is no association between atria and ventricles, the block is said to be *complete* and, if only a proportion of impulses get down the bundle, the block is said to be *partial*.

Cardiac arrhythmias are not necessarily associated with cardiac failure, but certain arrhythmias, commonly atrial fibrillation, may, by throwing an extra strain on the heart, either precipitate or augment cardiac failure.

Drugs used to treat arrhythmias

Cardiac arrhythmias can be terminated and normal rhythm restored by drugs. If, however, the heart is functioning poorly it is safer to stop the arrhythmia by DC cardioversion or, if it is a conduction defect, to use electrical pacing.

Arrhythmias due to overexcitability

When the arrhythmia is due to an excitable focus in the heart muscle (usually in the ventricle), drugs which reduce excitability are appropriate and include:

- Lidocaine
- Mexiletine.

When the arrhythmia is due to a circus movement, as in supraventricular tachycardias, drugs which slow conduction in the AV node are used. They include:

- Adenosine
- Verapamil
- β blockers
- Digitalis.

See also Wolfe–Parkinson–White syndrome (p. 66).

In addition, three drugs which have both actions and can therefore be used in both types of arrhythmia are:

- Disopyramide
- Amiodarone
- Flecainide.

Lidocaine (lignocaine) suppresses the excitability of the ventricular muscle with only moderate depression of the heart's action. It is not likely therefore to cause cardiac arrest or a fall in blood pressure except in overdose.

Therapeutics. Lidocaine is used to treat arrhythmias due to ventricular excitability which are liable to occur in the first few days after a cardiac infarct. It must be given intravenously because if it is given by mouth it is very rapidly broken down by the liver after absorption from the intestine (*first pass effect*). Unfortunately its action only lasts about 20 minutes. The initial dose is 50–100 mg injected over 2 minutes, and this may be followed by an intravenous infusion of a solution containing 1.0 mg of lidocaine in 1.0 ml of 5% dextrose solution (0.1%) at the rate of 1–4 mg of lidocaine/minute. In patients with cardiac failure or shock the breakdown of lidocaine by the liver is much slower, and dangerous

accumulation can occur with continuous infusion. In these circumstances the infusion rate should not exceed 1 mg/minute.

Contraindications and adverse effects. Lidocaine should be avoided in shocked patients when it may further depress cardiac function. It should not be given if the conducting system of the heart is damaged as may happen after cardiac infarction.

The most common adverse effects are caused by stimulation of the central nervous system with restlessness, tremor and possibly fits. It can also cause a fall in blood pressure and bradycardia, particularly if heart function is already compromised.

Interactions. A low plasma potassium level reduces the effectiveness of lidocaine and the plasma potassium concentration should be kept above 4 mmol/litre.

Mexiletine is similar in its action to lidocaine. It suppresses cardiac arrhythmias and it is particularly valuable because it is effective when given orally.

Adverse effects include nausea and dizziness and are frequent.

Verapamil (see p. 69). Verapamil blocks the flow of calcium ions into the muscle cells of the heart. This reduces the force of contraction of the heart muscle and slows conduction in the AV node, and is thus useful in supraventricular tachycardia as it breaks the circus wave of stimulation. Because of its depressing effect on cardiac muscle contraction *verapamil should not be used if a β blocker has been given in the preceding 24 hours* as the combination can seriously reduce cardiac efficiency and may cause cardiac arrest. For the same reason verapamil should not be used in cardiac failure. It may also be combined with digoxin to improve the control of atrial fibrillation.

The intravenous dose to terminate an attack of supraventricular tachycardia is 10 mg given over 3 minutes. It is then given orally to prevent further attacks in doses of 40–120 mg three times daily or as a slow-release preparation.

Interactions. Verapamil reduces the excretion of digoxin, so if the two are combined the dose of digoxin should be reduced.

β blockers. The general pharmacology of this group of drugs is considered on page 47. By preventing the stimulation of adrenergic receptors by epinephrine, these β blockers decrease the excitability of the heart and thus stop arrhythmias due to an excitable focus or to a supraventricular circus movement as in tachycardia.

It must be remembered that in reducing adrenergic drive to the heart and depressing the heart muscle, these drugs may exacerbate or precipitate heart failure in those whose hearts are under stress from some disease. β blockers should not be used in cardiac failure, except under special circumstances (see p. 58).

Therapeutics. β blockers can be used to prevent ectopic beats or supraventricular tachycardia and to improve the control of atrial fibrillation by digoxin. They are frequently prescribed after myocardial infarction where they improve the prognosis.

Dosage:

- Propranolol 20–40 mg three times daily, orally
- Atenolol 50–100 mg once daily.

Sotalol is believed to have an additional action which is useful in ventricular arrhythmias.

Interactions. β blockers may also exacerbate the depressing effect on heart muscle of such drugs as verapamil.

Adenosine suppresses conduction through the AV node and is used to terminate supraventricular arrhythmias. It is given intravenously, the usual dose being 3–6 mg. Its action begins very rapidly and only lasts a very short time, but this is usually sufficient to restore sinus rhythm.

Adverse effects are flushing, chest pain and dyspnoea coming on immediately after injection and lasting up to 30 seconds.

Digitalis. In addition to its use in heart failure, digitalis is sometimes useful in supraventricular arrhythmias, where by slowing conduction it may abolish the arrhythmia or control the ventricular rate.

Disopyramide. This drug decreases excitability and slows conduction so it can be used for both supraventricular and ventricular tachycardias. It can be given either orally or intravenously.

Disopyramide is excreted via the kidneys and reduced dosage is necessary if renal function is impaired.

Adverse effects include dry mouth, worsening of glaucoma and difficulty with micturition, all due to an anticholinergic action. Disopyramide may also cause nausea, vomiting and diarrhoea.

Amiodarone. This most interesting drug is effective in both ventricular and supraventricular arrhythmias. It acts by prolonging the refractory period of heart muscle: this is the short period after each contraction of the heart when the muscle will not respond to any stimulus. Its other important property is that, unlike most anti-arrhythmic drugs, it has little depressing effect on cardiac function. The initial oral dose is 200 mg three times daily and this is reduced after 1 week to a satisfactory maintenance dose, usually 200 mg daily. This unusual dosage scheme is required because it is very readily bound by the tissues and only when these binding sites have been saturated does it produce its effect on the heart. This also means that it is slowly eliminated and its actions continue for some time after dosage has stopped. Amiodarone can be used intravenously but it must be given over at *least 20 minutes* and preferably longer via a *central venous line*; otherwise, it may cause a considerable fall in blood pressure.

Adverse effects are common and to some extent limit its use. They include:

1. Photosensitivity rash and bluish grey pigmentation of exposed areas.

2. Amiodarone contains a high concentration of iodine and may cause both hypothyroidism or thyrotoxicosis. Thyroid function tests (TSH, T3 and T4) should be performed every 6 months in those on long-term treatment.

3. Pulmonary fibrosis requires chest X-rays every 6 months.

4. Deposits in the cornea of the eye occasionally cause visual haloes.

5. Rarely, liver damage and neuropathy.

6. Rapid i.v. injection causes marked hypotension.

Interactions. Amiodarone potentiates the actions of warfarin and digitalis.

Flecainide reduces excitability and slows conduction in the AV node and bundle of His, so it can be used for both ventricular and supraventricular arrhythmias including those complicating the Wolfe–Parkinson–White syndrome.

Therapeutics. Flecainide can be given by slow intravenous injection (over 10 minutes) to terminate arrhythmias. Given orally, it is useful in preventing ventricular arrhythmias.

Although flecainide is an effective drug it can induce dangerous arrhythmias in patients who have poorly functioning or damaged ventricular muscle, particularly following myocardial infarction, and should be avoided in this group.

Adverse effects. Dizziness is not uncommon. Flecainide has some depressant effect on heart muscle and should be used with care, if at all, in patients with conduction defects on a pacemaker. Rarely, it actually provokes, rather than diminishes, ventricular arrhythmias.

Propafenone is effective in suppressing both ventricular and supraventricular arrhythmias and those complicating the Wolfe–Parkinson–White syndrome. It can be given orally in divided doses and has also been used intravenously. Its efficacy appears similar to that of lidocaine and flecainide. The dose may need to be individualized as there is considerable interindividual difference in the blood levels for a given dose due to variations in drug metabolism. It has a weak β-blocking action and should be avoided in patients who are subject to bronchospasm.

Direct current cardioversion

A direct current (DC) shock is applied to the heart via electrodes placed on the chest. This shock obliterates the ectopic focus or circus movement which causes the arrhythmia and allows normal rhythm to be resumed. This form of treatment has been widely and successfully used in treating atrial fibrillation and about 70% of these patients can be converted to sinus rhythm. Unfortunately, in spite of maintenance treatment with anti-arrhythmic drugs many patients relapse within a few months. It is also useful in other arrhythmias.

Electrolytes and arrhythmias

A low plasma potassium concentration (hypokalaemia) increases the risk of developing an arrhythmia and makes the arrhythmia more difficult to terminate. This is particularly liable to occur after an infarct or in patients taking diuretics. Following an infarct the plasma potassium level should be kept above 4.0 mmol/litre.

Magnesium deficiency also predisposes to arrhythmias and in some units magnesium sulphate is infused immediately after a myocardial infarct to reduce cardiac excitability.

Treatment of individual arrhythmias

In *persistent atrial fibrillation* an attempt is usually made to restore sinus rhythm, the most effective method being DC cardioversion. The patient should be anticoagulated for 4 weeks before and after conversion to reduce the risk of thrombi forming in the atria and becoming emboli. Unfortunately, relapse will occur within a year in about half these patients but maintenance treatment with amiodarone or quinidine reduces the risk. If attempts at DC cardioversion fail or relapse cannot be prevented, the ventricular rate can be controlled with digitalis at about 70–90 per minute. Better control may be obtained if digitalis is combined with verapamil or a β blocker. In persistent fibrillation, the ever present risk of emboli arising in the atria requires that, if possible, patients be anticoagulated with warfarin. Regular aspirin can also be used but is less effective.

In *paroxysmal atrial fibrillation* amiodarone or sotalol, taken regularly, may prevent attacks.

Atrial flutter. Digitalis may restore normal rhythm. It may, however, produce atrial fibrillation which can then be treated as above.

Ventricular tachycardia or extrasystoles. Intravenous lidocaine damps down the excitable focus and usually stops this type of tachycardia. DC shock is also very effective and may be preferred if the facilities are available, particularly if the heart is showing signs of strain. Disopyramide or amiodarone or sotalol given orally are used to prevent extrasystoles, although often no treatment is necessary.

Supraventricular tachycardia. Acute attacks are terminated by depressing conduction through the AV node and thus breaking the circuit. This may be achieved by the patient performing the Valsalva manoeuvre (expiring against the closed glottis), which causes reflex vagal stimulation and slows AV conduction. A similar effect can be produced by pressure over *one* carotid sinus.

Adenosine 3 mg given as a rapid intravenous injection under ECG monitoring is the treatment of choice.

The alternative drug is verapamil 5–10 mg i.v. given over 5 minutes but there is some doubt as to its safety.

Amiodarone, given slowly i.v., can be tried if other drugs have failed.

β blockers are used by some but due to their negative inotropic effect (depression of the heart muscle) *they must not be combined with verapamil.*

If drug treatment fails DC shock may be used.

Attacks may be prevented by oral β blockers or verapamil.

Nursing point

The Valsalva manoeuvre or carotid massage should be carried out with the patient lying flat when it is more effective and he or she is less liable to faint.

The Wolfe–Parkinson–White (WPW) syndrome

The WPW syndrome is an interesting congenital abnormality occurring in about 0.2% of the population. It is due to an extra (accessory) conducting system between the atria and the ventricles. In itself it causes no trouble but is associated with supraventricular arrhythmias due to re-entry (i.e. down one bundle and up the other) and atrial fibrillation, which are occasionally dangerous.

In treating these arrhythmias it must be remembered that the accessory bundle may not respond to drugs in the same way as the normal conducting system. In particular, digoxin and verapamil enhance rather than depress conduction through the accessory bundle and are therefore contraindicated. Depending on cir-

cumstances amiodarone, disopyramide or flecainide are used.

Arrhythmias due to conduction defects

Conduction defects can sometimes be relieved by sympathomimetic drugs (p. 39). Isoprenaline is most commonly used; however, in most patients with conduction defects, rhythm will have to be maintained by a *pacemaker.*

Bradycardia, particularly when it occurs following a coronary thrombosis, may be due to failure of the cardiac pacemaker (SA node). Atropine 0.6 mg i.v. is useful to restore normal function of the pacemaker.

Nursing points

Much of the treatment of cardiac arrhythmias takes place in hospital with continuous monitoring, often in an intensive care unit. Careful observation is required and changes in rhythm must be noted as they may indicate the need to stop a drug or change treatment.

Remember that no mechanical system is perfect and the nurse should check all mechanical aids, particularly infusion pumps administering drugs, at regular intervals.

DRUGS USED TO LOWER BLOOD PRESSURE

The blood pressure depends on:

1. The peripheral vascular resistance
2. The output of blood from the heart
3. The volume of blood within the circulation.

By decreasing one or more of these factors it is possible to lower the blood pressure.

The *peripheral vascular resistance* depends on the cross-section of the smaller arteries (arterioles). The walls of these arteries contain circular muscle fibres which are controlled by the sympathetic nervous system (p. 37). Stimulation of this system releases *norepinephrine* which causes these muscles to contract and leads to narrowing of the arterioles and a rise in blood pressure. In addition, the cells lining blood vessels are continually producing *nitric oxide* which acts as a vasodilator and thus tends to lower blood pressure.

Angiotensin (see below) also causes constriction of blood vessels and a rise in blood pressure.

The *cardiac output* depends on several factors, but one important control is again the sympathetic nervous system which, by releasing *epinephrine*, causes a rise in pulse rate and output of blood.

The *volume of blood within the circulation* is ultimately controlled by the kidneys. There are receptors which 'sense' changes in the blood volume and if it falls the kidney secretes a substance called *renin* which, via a complex series of changes, leads to retention of salt and water by the kidneys (Fig. 5.5) and the formation of angiotensin II, which causes vasoconstriction, both of which raise the blood pressure.

HYPERTENSION

In certain people the blood pressure is consistently raised above normal limits. This is chiefly due to a raised peripheral resistance secondary to vasoconstriction, although the kidneys also play a part. The condition is known as *hyper-*

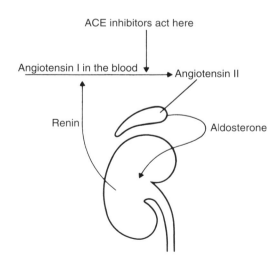

Figure 5.5 Renin released from the kidney acts on angiotensin I in the blood to form angiotensin II. Angiotensin II constricts blood vessels and raises the blood pressure. Angiotensin II also releases aldosterone from the adrenal cortex causing salt and water retention by the kidney. The net result is a rise in blood pressure.

tension. In the majority of patients the cause is not known although there are probably inherited and environmental factors and the condition is then called *essential hypertension*. Much more rarely it is secondary to kidney or endocrine disorders. The actual elevation of blood pressure, unless severe, rarely produces symptoms but over a period of time it damages the heart, blood vessels and kidneys, which leads to coronary thrombosis, heart failure, strokes and less often to renal failure.

It is therefore logical to prevent these complications by lowering the blood pressure and this can be achieved by drugs which:

- Lower peripheral resistance
- Lower cardiac output
- Decrease blood volume
- Act centrally.

DRUGS WHICH LOWER PERIPHERAL RESISTANCE BY DECREASING SYMPATHETIC ACTIVITY

As stated above the peripheral vascular resistance is maintained by the sympathetic nervous system. It therefore follows that a drug which blocks the action of the sympathetic system will decrease peripheral resistance and lower blood pressure.

α sympathetic blocking drugs
(see Fig. 5.6)

Prazosin, doxazosin and terazosin block the vasoconstrictor sympathetic nerve supply to the small arteries (α_1 receptors) and the resulting vasodilatation causes a fall in blood pressure. With these drugs there is little compensatory rise in pulse rate or cardiac output. The fall in blood pressure is inclined to be postural (greater on standing than lying). Prazosin is short-acting and dosage is required two or three times daily, which makes even control of blood pressure difficult. Doxazosin and terazosin have a longer action so once a day dosage is adequate.

Therapeutics. The initial dose can sometimes cause a profound fall in blood pressure, with fainting, so it is advisable that this dose is given before retiring and that it should be low. Subsequent doses rarely provoke this problem, but the blood pressure should be taken standing and lying down to assess any postural fall. The dose is increased at weekly intervals until satisfactory control is achieved. These drugs may be combined with other hypotensive agents. α blockers also improve the flow of urine in patients with bladder neck obstruction and are used in mild cases of prostatic enlargement.

Prazosin	500 micrograms initially then 1.0 mg three times daily up to 20 mg daily.
Doxazosin	1.0 mg daily increased to 4.0 mg daily.
Terazosin	1.0 mg daily increased up to 10 mg daily.

Adverse effects are unusual except for postural hypotension. Occasionally, these drugs cause urinary incontinence, particularly in women.

DRUGS WHICH ACT DIRECTLY OR INDIRECTLY ON THE ARTERIOLE
(see Fig. 5.6)

Hydralazine. Hydralazine lowers the blood pressure by relaxing the blood vessels. It acts directly on the muscle and not via the sympathetic nervous system. Unfortunately it also causes a rise in pulse rate and cardiac output, which to some degree cancels its hypotensive action. This problem can be overcome by combining hydralazine with a β blocker which will prevent the rise in pulse rate and cardiac output and thus increase the fall in blood pressure. The

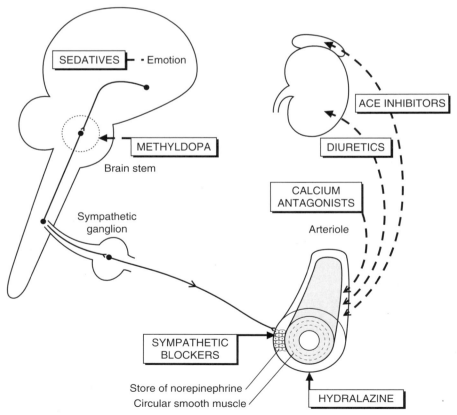

Figure 5.6 Site of action of some hypotensive drugs.

initial dose is 25 mg twice daily. Hydralazine has now been largely replaced by new hypotensive drugs, but is still used in serious hypertension in pregnancy.

Adverse effects include headache and rashes, and arthritis similar to systemic lupus erythematosus can be troublesome with high dosage.

Calcium antagonists. This group of drugs blocks the entry of calcium ions into the muscle cells in the arterial walls, resulting in relaxation of the muscle and dilatation of the arteries. Calcium antagonists are used to lower blood pressure in hypertension and to dilate coronary arteries in angina (see p. 84). In addition, verapamil slows conduction in the AV node and is used in treating cardiac arrhythmias (see p. 63).

Therapeutics. Although their actions and uses are similar they differ in detail. They are all given orally and broken down by the liver.

Short-acting used for hypertension or angina:

Nifedipine Retard	10 mg twice daily. Slow-release preparations are available needing only one or two doses daily.
Nicardipine	Three times daily.
Diltiazem	Three times daily.

Long-acting used for hypertension or angina:

Amlodipine	5–10 mg once daily.
Felodipine	Once daily.

Hypertension only:

Isradipine	Twice daily.
Lacidipine	Once daily.

Used for hypertension, angina and cardiac arrhythmias:

Verapamil	240–480 mg daily orally. 5–10 mg slowly i.v. for arrhythmias

At present there is no clearly preferred drug for hypertension although the longer-acting preparations are more convenient.

Calcium channel blockers may be used alone or combined with other hypotensive drugs; for example, nifedipine + a β blocker is a popular combination.

Adverse effects. Headache, flushing and ankle oedema due to vasodilatation can occur with all these drugs, but are more common with nifedipine and nicardipine.

Constipation, only with verapamil.

Depression of heart muscle function. Marked with verapamil and to a lesser extent with others. Verapamil should not be given intravenously to patients receiving β blockers.

Great care is necessary if calcium channel blockers are given to patients with heart failure as this may be made worse.

There is some evidence of increased mortality in patients taking large doses of the short-acting preparation of nifedipine, particularly in patients with coronary artery disease. The longer-acting preparations appear safe but ACE inhibitors are to be preferred in hypertensive patients with diabetes.

Interactions. The action of nifedipine and nicardipine is increased by cimetidine.

The blood levels (and therefore the action) of carbamazepine, theophylline and digoxin are increased by these drugs.

Angiotensin converting enzyme (ACE) inhibitors. ACE inhibitors inhibit the conversion of angiotensin I to angiotensin II in the circulation. This reduces the vasoconstricting effect of angiotensin II and by inhibiting the release of aldosterone causes less sodium retention. The overall effect is a fall in blood pressure (see Fig. 5.6). They are used in treating hypertension and cardiac failure (see p. 55) and may actually improve the structure of thickened arteries and failing hearts. They also reduce proteinuria in diabetic patients with kidney disease and slow the decline in renal function.

Several of these drugs are now available, with similar actions and uses.

Therapeutic use. An ACE inhibitor may be used as a single drug to lower blood pressure or combined with other hypotensive drugs such as diuretics. ACE inhibitors are particularly useful if hypertension is complicated by heart failure (see p. 55). *Captopril* was the first to be introduced and is still widely used. It is rapidly absorbed when given orally; its action starts after half an hour and lasts up to 8 hours. The initial dose is 12.5 mg (6.25 mg for the elderly) twice daily before meals and this may be increased, if necessary, to 50 mg twice daily.

Enalapril is a prodrug and is itself inactive, but is converted into an active metabolite in the liver. It therefore takes longer to act (3 hours) but its effects are prolonged (24 hours). The initial dose is 5.0 mg once daily and is increased to 40 mg daily if necessary.

Other ACE inhibitors are:

Drug	Prodrug	Dosage frequency	Special points
Cilazapril	+	Daily	
Fosinopril	+	Daily	Hepatic and renal excretion
Lisinopril	−	Daily	
Perindopril	+	Daily	
Quinapril	+	Daily or b.d.	
Ramipril	+	Daily	

A marked fall in blood pressure occurs occasionally with the first dose of an ACE inhibitor especially if the patient is already taking a diuretic. For this reason the initial dose should be low and taken before retiring; patients should be warned of the possibility of a sharp fall in blood pressure if they get up in the night.

ACE inhibitors are contraindicated in pregnancy as they may damage the fetus and the dose should be kept as low as possible in renal impairment.

Before starting treatment, electrolytes and renal function should be measured.

Adverse effects and interactions:

1. A few patients develop renal failure with ACE inhibitors. This is particularly liable to happen in elderly patients and those with stenosis of the renal arteries. Plasma creatinine should therefore be measured in the first few weeks of treatment and thereafter at 6-monthly intervals.

2. Dry cough (10%). Bronchospasm (5%).

3. Fatigue, headaches, diarrhoea.

4. Rashes, change in taste (captopril).

5. Captopril may produce proteinuria and neutropenia, though rarely with the lower doses now used.

6. Hyperkalaemia in patients with renal disease or who are taking potassium-sparing diuretics or supplementary potassium.

7. Declining renal function if combined with NSAIDs.

Losartan and **valsartan** block the action of angiotensin II at the receptor site. Their hypotensive action is thus very similar to that of the ACE inhibitors and trials suggest that they have much the same efficacy.

Adverse effects are those of the ACE inhibitors though they are much less liable to cause a cough.

Sodium nitroprusside must be given intravenously and is therefore only suitable for treating a hypertensive crisis and some patients with acute heart failure. It is given by infusion and it is usual to start at the lower end of the dose range and increase it until the blood pressure is satisfactorily controlled. This will require close observation and is usually carried out in an intensive care unit.

There are five important practical points in its use:

1. The contents of the ampoule (50 mg) should be dissolved in 2 ml of 5% dextrose solution and then diluted in dextrose or saline.

2. The infusion must be protected from the light and discarded after 24 hours.

3. It should also be discarded if the colour changes from pale orange to dark brown or blue.

4. Infusion should not be continued for more than 72 hours.

5. With prolonged infusion, blood cyanide and thiocyanate levels should be measured to guard against the development of cyanide poisoning.

Adverse effects. Headaches, dizziness, palpitations and chest pain.

Minoxidil is a powerful vasodilator and thus causes a fall in blood pressure. Its use is confined to patients who are resistant to more usual treatment (see below).

Therapeutic use. When minoxidil is given it should be combined with:

1. A diuretic, otherwise it will cause salt and water retention.

2. A β blocker, or it will cause the heart rate to rise.

Adverse effects. Increasing hairiness is a strange but common and upsetting complication.

In addition to salt and water retention, pericardial effusions sometimes develop.

DRUGS WHICH LOWER CARDIAC OUTPUT

β blockers. β blockers will lower the blood pressure to a satisfactory level in about 40% of patients with hypertension, but the hypotensive effect may be delayed for several weeks after starting treatment. It is not known exactly how these drugs produce this effect. By interfering with the sympathetic nervous system they certainly prevent the rise in cardiac output and blood pressure which occur with excitement or effort. It may be that this damping down of the circulation ultimately causes a permanent fall in blood pressure. In certain circumstances β blockers decrease renin release by the kidney which would tend to lower the blood pressure (see p. 67) and some of them (particularly propanolol) have some central sedative action.

The effect of some β blockers is predominantly on the heart (β$_1$ receptors) and they are called 'selective' β blockers; others also affect the bronchi and possibly the peripheral circulation (β$_2$ receptors) and are known as 'non-selective' β blockers though this selectivity is not absolute.

Therapeutic use. There is no evidence that any particular β blocker is more effective in lowering blood pressure, but if the patient is prone to obstructive airways disease a selective β blocker is preferred. Among those used are:

Selective β blockers	Non-selective β blockers
Metoprolol 50–200 mg daily	Propranolol 80–320 mg daily
Atenolol 50–100 mg daily	Oxprenolol 80–320 mg daily
	Nadolol
	Timolol
	Pindolol

Atenolol, pindolol and nadolol can be given once daily. The others are usually given two or three times daily, although such frequent dosage may not be necessary to control blood pressure.

There are also slow-release preparations available of propranolol, oxprenolol and metoprolol.

Serious adverse effects are not common. Patients with bronchospasm from asthma or chronic bronchitis may get worse when receiving β blockers, which should be *avoided in patients with asthma* and used with care in patients with bronchitis, for which a selective β blocker is indicated (see above). They may also exacerbate heart failure and should be used with care in this disorder (see p. 58).

Patients with diabetes receiving insulin are at some risk as β blockers mask the symptoms of hypoglycaemia and this should be explained to them.

Apart from these three dangerous effects β blockers have other side-effects which, although not dangerous, may interfere with the quality of life—an important consideration if treatment is to be continued over long periods. Some patients report lacking energy and aggression and feel tired and depressed. Others may report vivid dreams and, occasionally, hallucinations.

Owing to the fall in cardiac output, the peripheral circulation decreases and this results in cold hands and feet and can be a serious problem in patients with *peripheral vascular disease*, in whom β blockers should be avoided.

Occasionally, the resting pulse rate is considerably reduced by β blockers. Provided it does not fall below 50/minute this is not usually a matter of concern. Lower rates require a change to oxprenolol or pindolol, which allow a rather higher pulse rate at rest.

Interactions:

1. Myocardial function is reduced if combined with intravenous verapamil.

2. β blockers increase the peripheral vasoconstricting action of ergotamine (see p. 51).

3. The action of some β blockers is increased by cimetidine.

Esmolol is a very short-acting selective β blocker used for cardiac arrhythmias and when a controlled reduction of blood pressure is required. It is given by intravenous infusion.

Labetalol combines β-blocking activity with some α-blocking effect. The result is that the cardiac output is decreased and at the same time there is some peripheral vasodilatation. This leads to a fall in blood pressure.

Therapeutic use. The initial dose is increased gradually until satisfactory control is achieved. Dosage requirements are variable and this makes treatment difficult. It can also be given i.v. to control a hypertensive crisis.

Adverse effects. Labetalol should be used with care in patients with heart failure as it may exacerbate the condition, and be avoided in patients with asthma. Other side-effects include stuffy nose, lethargy, vivid dreams and tingling of the scalp.

Celiprolol and **carvedilol** combine a selective β_1-blocking action on the heart with a stimulating β_2-action on the blood vessels causing vasodilatation. Theoretically this dual action should be advantageous in lowering blood pressure; however, clinical trials suggest that their efficacy is similar to that of other β blockers. They may also play a minor role in treating heart failure (see p. 58).

DRUGS WHICH DECREASE BLOOD VOLUME

Diuretics (see also p. 213) are still considered by many to be the drug of first choice to treat mild-to-moderate hypertension, provided they are not contraindicated by some concurrent disease or pregnancy. The fall in blood pressure is due to a reduction in blood volume and to a vasodilating effect on the walls of the arterioles. They are cheap, relatively easy to use and serious side-effects are rare.

Therapeutic use. Thiazide diuretics are the most suitable and there is no preferred preparation. The dose should be low (e.g. bendrofluazide 2.5 mg daily); raising the dose causes little further fall in blood pressure but increases the incidence of adverse effects.

Contraindications and adverse effects:

a. In gout, diuretics cause uric acid retention
b. In diabetes, diuretics decrease glucose tolerance and thus make control of the disease more difficult

c. In pregnancy, diuretics may damage the fetus.

They also cause impotence in about 20% of males. High dosage can lead to hypokalaemia, due to increased urinary loss of potassium. This is rare with low dosage but the blood potassium should be checked 1 month after starting treatment.

Interactions. NSAIDs reduce the efficacy of diuretics. Blood levels of lithium are raised by diuretics and the dose of lithium may require adjustment.

Indapamide is similar to the thiazides and offers no particular advantage.

DRUGS WHICH ACT CENTRALLY
(see Fig. 5.6)

Methyldopa. This drug lowers blood pressure by an action on the brain which results in decreased activity of the sympathetic system.

Therapeutics. Methyldopa was formerly used widely in the treatment of hypertension. It is effective and easy to use because the fall in blood pressure is not precipitous. However, it has a number of adverse effects which patients sometimes find unacceptable and its use has declined considerably. It is still, however, widely used in treating *pregnancy-related hypertension*.

The initial dose is 250 mg orally three times daily and this can be increased to 1.5 g daily. Further increases in dosage do not seem to enhance its effect.

Adverse effects are rather common. Drowsiness and depression often occur early in treatment but may pass off after a few weeks; more rarely, fluid retention producing oedema can be troublesome but is controlled by a diuretic. Haemolytic anaemia and drug fever have also been reported.

Moxonidine acts centrally to reduce activity of the sympathetic nervous system. At present, it is indicated if other hypotensive agents are not satisfactory and is given orally, once or twice daily.

Adverse effects include tiredness, headache and nausea.

THE TREATMENT OF HYPERTENSION

When raised blood pressure is detected, it is important to exclude underlying renal or endocrine causes, although essential hypertension is responsible in more than 90% of cases. Hypertension, by itself, rarely causes any symptoms and the object of treatment is to prevent the development of complications, e.g. stroke, coronary thrombosis, cardiac and renal failure. Many hypertensive patients live for years without these complications and this means that the drugs used in treatment should be safe and as free as possible from adverse effects. Unfortunately, no hypotensive drug entirely fulfils these criteria. It is generally accepted that severe hypertension carries a poor prognosis and adequate treatment considerably reduces morbidity and mortality. It is in patients with milder degrees of hypertension that a decision to embark on drug treatment is more difficult.

In healthy subjects with no evidence of cardiac, vascular or renal complications it is justifiable to observe the patient with regular measurement of blood pressure for 3–6 months because, in some people, it may return to normal levels, particularly when they become used to visiting the doctor. At this stage, non-drug measures may be considered (see under Special points for patient education, p. 74). If, however, the blood pressure remains persistently above 150/90 and particularly if there are special risk factors (hyperlipidaemia, diabetes, smoking or a family history of cardiovascular disease) it is usual to start treatment with a single drug and, if this fails, a combination should be given. The aim is to maintain the blood pressure around 140/85, though below 160/90 is acceptable.

Ideal blood pressure readings are not easy to achieve and a substantial proportion of treated subjects still have blood pressures well above 140/85.

There have been many trials of hypotensive drugs in this group of patients and the results can be roughly summarized as follows:

1. There was some reduction in overall mortality—probably about 20%.
2. The incidence of stroke was halved, but there was less reduction of coronary thrombosis.
3. In elderly patients the incidence of stroke was reduced by about 35% and there was some reduction in the occurrence of coronary thrombosis (20%).

It should be realized, however, that most trials to date have used diuretics or β blockers. Although it is logical to believe that other hypotensive drugs would confer similar benefits, the complete proof is only just emerging.

A variety of agents is now available and the best drug or combination of drugs for treatment is still being investigated. The usual approach is to start with β blockers in younger or middle-aged patients.

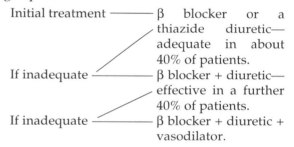

Initial treatment ———— β blocker or a thiazide diuretic—adequate in about 40% of patients.

If inadequate ———— β blocker + diuretic—effective in a further 40% of patients.

If inadequate ———— β blocker + diuretic + vasodilator.

Some authorities prefer to start treatment with a diuretic and this approach is to be preferred in elderly patients and in Afro-Caribbeans, who respond poorly to β blockers.

There is increasing concern about the quality of life of patients receiving treatment for hypertension as these regimes may be associated with various adverse effects which, although usually minor, can be troublesome. ACE inhibitors, though not entirely trouble-free, do not make life a burden and have a place in initial treatment, especially for diabetics in whom they help to preserve renal function. α blockers and calcium channel blockers may also be used and there are numerous possible combinations where the effects are at least additive. It is usually possible to plan a regime which is therapeutically effective without interfering with the patient's lifestyle.

Elderly patients are a little more prone to side-effects, but usually tolerate treatment well. Low-dose thiazides, ACE inhibitors and calcium channel blockers are all satisfactory.

ACE inhibitors are indicated if there is any evidence of *heart failure* or *diabetes* and α blockers may be helpful if there is prostatic obstruction.

A few patients require admission to hospital so that they can be fully investigated and when treatment is started, frequent observation of blood pressure can be made. In milder hypertension, with no complicating disease, treatment can be started and carried through on an outpatient basis. When adequate control is obtained, further supervision is required by the GP or hospital outpatients' department.

Occasionally, it may be necessary to reduce a *very high blood pressure rapidly*. Sodium nitroprusside (see p. 70) is the drug of choice for initial treatment. Great care must be taken when lowering a very high blood pressure as a precipitate fall may cause renal failure or cerebral damage due to a sudden reduction of the blood supply to the kidney and brain. The early stages of this treatment should be carried out in an intensive care unit if possible and the blood pressure monitored at frequent intervals. The aim of treatment should be to reduce the diastolic blood pressure slowly to around 100 mmHg. Thereafter treatment for hypertension should be carried out in the normal way (see above).

If facilities for intensive monitoring are not available and if the clinical situation is less acute, bed rest and a β blocker or slow-release nifedipine are satisfactory and should avoid a precipitous fall in blood pressure.

Hypertension in pregnancy presents a special problem as occasionally it may progress to preeclampsia and eclampsia, with serious risk to both mother and child. Mild transient elevation of blood pressure occurring towards the end of pregnancy rarely needs drug treatment. More severe hypertension, particularly if the patient was hypertensive before the start of her pregnancy, may require drugs to lower the blood pressure. Methyldopa has been found satisfactory for many years. β blockers are also used, but may retard fetal growth. In severe hypertension hydralazine orally or intravenously is effective. *Diuretics and ACE inhibitors should be avoided.*

Measuring blood pressure

Nurses frequently measure blood pressure. The technique is beyond the scope of this book, but there are some important points to remember when treating hypertension.

1. The blood pressure should usually be recorded with the patient both *lying* and *standing* as some hypotensive drugs cause a much greater fall in blood pressure when the patient is standing than when he or she is lying down. In certain cases it should also be recorded after exercise.

2. Some patients are nervous when visiting the doctor and this may cause their blood

---

Special points for patient education

1. Some patients do not realize that once drug treatment is started it will probably continue for the rest of their lives, although it may be altered or attenuated with advancing years.

2. There are several non-drug ways of lowering blood pressure. Adding no salt to food or cooking will reduce blood pressure and enhance the effect of drugs, but some patients find that this spoils the joy of eating. Various forms of relaxation, meditation and stress reduction produce a small but useful fall in blood pressure in many subjects.

3. It is very important that 'risk' factors which increase their liability to the complications of hypertension be avoided, so the following advice should be given:

   a. Stop smoking.
   b. Reduce weight if obese and correct blood lipids if abnormal (see p. 87).
   c. Reduce alcohol consumption if excessive (this actually lowers blood pressure).
   d. The place of diet and exercise in lowering blood pressure is more controversial, but a diet which is low in fat and contains plenty of fruit and vegetables, combined with an exercise programme within the competence of the patient, may help.

4. Patients should be warned of the main adverse effects of the drugs prescribed for them.

5. It is impossible for patients to know and understand all the possible interactions, but if given a new drug they should remind the prescriber that they are already receiving medication.

6. Some patients can be taught to take their own blood pressure and thus obtain a more accurate assessment of day-to-day levels.

Nursing point

Nurses are often involved in treating hypertension. They may work in special outpatient clinics or it may be part of their duties as general practice nurses and they will often be responsible for taking blood pressures and arranging attendances, etc. They should be familiar with the drugs being used, particularly their adverse effects so that they can advise the patient and, if necessary, together with the doctor, change the treatment. Remember that failure to respond to treatment or apparent relapse may be due to poor compliance or to an interaction with another drug, usually an NSAID.

---

pressure to rise, the so-called 'white coat' hypertension. Quiet reassurance and a rest period of 5 minutes is necessary before measuring the blood pressure. Sometimes it is helpful to teach intelligent patients to take their own blood pressure so a home record can be obtained which will give a better idea of day-to-day fluctuations. Because smoking may alter the blood pressure temporarily, patients should be asked to avoid it for 30 minutes before having their blood pressure measured.

3. A well-applied cuff and a good stethoscope are necessary for accurate readings.

4. Measurements of blood pressure tend to show 'observer bias'. This may happen in trials of new drugs and it is necessary in these circumstances to use a special sphygmomanometer in which the blood pressure is recorded 'blind' so that the recording is not known by the observer.

5. It is now possible to record patients' blood pressure as they go about their daily life, with an apparatus they can wear over a long period. This gives a much better assessment of their overall blood pressure and is useful in evaluating 'white coat' hypertension, stress response or the apparent failure of treatment. However, the apparatus is expensive, requires training to use and is not yet in general use.

DRUGS USED IN THE TREATMENT OF PERIPHERAL VASCULAR DISEASE

For many years various drugs, which in normal subjects dilate arteries, were used in vascular disease in the hope that they would increase the blood supply to the ischaemic limb. Unfortunately, vascular disease usually affects the large arteries and these diseased arteries were unresponsive to vasodilators, which are now recognized as being useless in this condition.

They are, however, useful in Raynaud's disease, which is due to spasm in the small arteries of the hands and feet brought on by cold.

Therapeutics. Nifedipine (see p. 69) used as for hypertension is the most useful drug. Other measures include keeping warm in cold weather. Do not forget that β blockers, ergotamine and smoking make peripheral vascular disease worse.

FURTHER READING

Bennett N E 1994 Hypertension in the elderly. Lancet 344: 447
Cobbe S M, Rankin A C 1988 Drug treatment of cardiac arrhythmias. Prescribers Journal 28: 48
Cohn J N 1996 The management of chronic heart failure. New England Journal of Medicine 335: 490
Dahlof B et al 1991 Morbidity and mortality in the Swedish trial in old patients with hypertension. Lancet 338: 1281
Editorial 1995 Who needs nine ACE Inhibitors? Drug and Therapeutics Bulletin 33: 1
Editorial 1989 Treating mild hypertension. British Medical Journal 298: 694
Editorial 1990 Do drugs help intermittent claudication? Drug and Therapeutics Bulletin 28: 1

Editorial 1991 Hypertensive emergencies. Lancet 338: 229
Editorial 1995 Losartan—a new antihypertensive. Drug and Therapeutics Bulletin 33: 73
Editorial 1998 Calcium channel blockers. British Medical Journal 316: 1471
Editorial 1998 Treatment of hypertensive patients with diabetes. Lancet 351: 689
Editorial 1999 β Blockers for mild to moderate heart failure. Lancet 353: 2
Editorial 1999 The evidence for β blockers in heart failure. British Medical Journal 318: 814
Ganz L L, Friedman P L 1995 Supraventricular tachycardias. New England Journal of Medicine 332: 162

Harrison L et al 1998 Hypertension optimal treatment (HOT) trial. Lancet 351: 1755

Jordan S, Torrance C 1998 Hypertension. Nursing Times 94: 50

Kitchen I 1984 Congestive cardiac failure and cardiogenic shock. Nursing 2nd series 25: 743

Magee L A et al 1999 Management of hypertension in pregnancy. British Medical Journal 318: 1332

Petrie J C et al 1997 British Hypertension Society Recommendations on Blood Pressure Measurement, 2nd edn, London

Prasad N, Isles C 1996 Ambulatory blood pressure monitoring. British Medical Journal 313: 1535

Roberts C, Banning M 1998 Managing risk factors for hypertension in primary care. Nursing Standard 12: 39

Simon J R 1996 Treating hypertension: the evidence from clinical trials. British Medical Journal 313: 437

Vallance P, Moncada S 1994 Nitric oxide—from mediator to medicines. Journal of the Royal College of Physicians 28: 209

6

Atheroma and thrombosis. Anticoagulants and thrombolytic agents

COAGULATION AND THROMBOSIS

When the wall of a blood vessel is damaged the blood coagulates and thus arrests bleeding. Clotting is a complex process which involves numerous enzymes and other chemicals called clotting factors. Most are present in the blood plasma, some are released by the platelets and thromboplastin is released from damaged cells. When blood clots, each clotting factor is activated in sequence as part of a cascade of reactions, as shown in Figure 6.1.

The key stages of this series of reactions are:

1. The formation of Factor Xa by the clotting cascade which, when activated, converts prothrombin to thrombin.

2. Thrombin forms fibrin strands from soluble fibrinogen, which then form a network over the damaged area.

At the same time, platelets become activated, assisting in the clotting process and aggregate to form clumps which become enmeshed in the fibrin network. The resulting clot plugs the defect in the blood vessel.

Coagulation or thrombosis may sometimes occur in blood vessels which have not been injured and in these circumstances blockage of the vessel concerned may have serious consequences. There are two types of thrombosis:

1. Venous thrombosis (phlebothrombosis)
2. Arterial thrombosis.

Although both may result in obstruction to a blood vessel they occur under different circum-

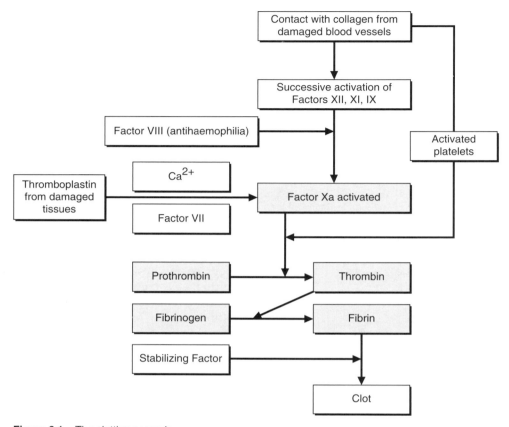

Figure 6.1 The clotting cascade.

stances, have different mechanisms and differ in their treatment.

VENOUS THROMBOSIS (PHLEBOTHROMBOSIS)

This usually occurs in the deep veins of the legs. It is due to stagnation of blood in the veins when a patient is lying still after an operation (particularly if the pelvis or hip is involved), associated with pregnancy or during a severe illness. The risk is increased in obese patients, in patients with malignancy or who have a history of previous thrombosis. *Oral contraceptives* containing estrogen are also a risk factor and should be stopped 6 weeks before a major operation or any surgery involving the pelvis or hip. It is also apparent that there are genetic factors which predispose to thrombosis. The danger of this

type of thrombosis is that part of the clot may break off, forming an *embolus* which is swept back via the heart to the lungs where it blocks a branch of the pulmonary artery, an event which can be fatal.

In atrial fibrillation a thrombus may develop in the left atrium because of impaired blood flow and fragments can become detached, resulting in emboli to the brain and elsewhere. Anticoagulants, which interfere with the clotting (coagulation) of blood, can be used either to prevent the formation of thrombi or to treat established venous thrombosis.

ANTICOAGULANTS

These drugs, by interfering with clotting, are used to prevent and treat venous thrombosis.

Heparin

Heparin is a complex substance. It is not absorbed by mouth and is usually given by intravenous or sometimes by subcutaneous injection. Heparin is an anticoagulant. Its actions on the clotting mechanism are multiple and complicated, but the end result is a prolongation of clotting time. The anticoagulant effect of heparin is seen within a minute or two of injection, but passes off within a few hours.

Therapeutics. Heparin is often used at the beginning of anticoagulant treatment because its effects are so rapid. It may be given by continuous intravenous infusion or by intermittent subcutaneous injection.

Infusion is best given via a syringe pump at the rate of 25 000–30 000 units in 24 hours following an initial bolus of 5000 units. If a pump is not available the heparin can be added to 1 litre of saline or 5% dextrose and given as an infusion. Whichever method is used the infusion rate must be carefully controlled.

The rate of infusion is monitored by measuring the *kaolin cephalin time or activated partial thromboplastin time (APTT)* 6 hours after starting infusion and then at least once daily and these should be kept between 1.5 and 2.5 times the control value.

When used to *prevent* thrombosis, heparin is given in doses of 5000 units in 0.2 ml subcutaneously twice daily. It is injected into the subcutaneous tissue of the abdominal wall via a fine needle (gauge 25, length 16 mm). An inch of skin should be picked up at the site of injection and the needle inserted perpendicularly to its full length. Local pressure is applied for 5 minutes after injection to prevent excessive bruising. Cleansing the skin before injection with isopropyl alcohol (a vasodilator) increases the chance of haematoma formation.

Adverse effects. The only common adverse effect from heparin is bleeding due to overdose. As with all anticoagulants this often first appears as haematuria, but may occur from any site. The treatment is to stop the heparin. Prolonged use may lead to osteoporosis. Very rarely, severe thrombocytopenia develops and a platelet count should be carried out if the patient receives heparin for more than 5 days.

Protamine sulphate, which reverses the action of heparin, can be given intravenously. Protamine sulphate may cause a fall in blood pressure. If blood loss is excessive, transfusion may be necessary.

Low molecular weight heparins. Heparin is a large molecule that can be broken down into a number of fragments which also have anticoagulant properties and are known as low molecular weight heparins. Their anticoagulant action is very similar to that of unfractionated heparin but is prolonged and is more consistent than that of unfractionated heparin; thus, continuous laboratory monitoring may not be required. Low molecular weight heparins are a little better than ordinary low-dose heparin in preventing venous thrombosis complicating surgery, particularly hip and knee replacement, and, given subcutaneously, they are certainly as effective as unfractionated heparin, given intravenously, in the prevention and treatment of venous thrombosis and pulmonary embolism. They have also been used, with success, in unstable angina. As they do not cross the placental barrier, they can be used during pregnancy.

Low molecular weight heparins are given once or twice daily by subcutaneous injection and the dose can be calculated from the weight of the patient. Lower doses are used for prevention of thrombosis.

Those available at present include **dalteparin, enoxaparin, tinzaparin** and **certoparin**. It seems probable they will replace unfractionated heparin in certain circumstances but they are considerably more expensive.

Adverse effects. Bleeding can occur but osteoporosis and thrombocytopenia are less common than with unfractionated heparin.

Hirudin

Hirudin was originally obtained from leeches and has been recognized as an anticoagulant for many years. It can now be made by recombinant methods. It differs from heparin in its mode of action, being a specific inhibitor of thrombin. It is given by intravenous injection or infusion and, although experience is still limited, it appears to be as effective as low molecular weight heparin, although bleeding may be a problem. Similar substances will probably be introduced in the next few years and then their place in anticoagulant therapy will become better defined.

The coumarin group

There are two substances in this group which are used in anticoagulant treatment: **warfarin** and **phenindione**. Their mode of action is similar and they will therefore be considered together.

They are effective by mouth and prevent vitamin K from taking part in the formation of various clotting factors in the liver. Patients with liver disease are thus more sensitive to their actions.

Therapeutics. This group of drugs is given orally. It is very important that strict accuracy is observed in the timing of doses. The effectiveness of the drug in interfering with coagulation is measured by prothrombin time estimations.

Contraindications include active peptic ulcer, severe liver disease and renal failure.

Warfarin. The initial dose of warfarin is 10 mg given at the same time daily, for 2 days. Various factors such as old age, poor nutrition, liver disease, heart failure, previous surgery and concurrent drugs will increase the patient's sensitivity to warfarin and require smaller dosage.

The prothrombin time should be measured before starting treatment, then daily, and the dose adjusted until the INR (see below) is stabilized. The ratio:

$$\frac{\text{Patient's prothrombin time}}{\text{Normal prothrombin time}}$$

is known as the *International Normalized Ratio* (INR) and the dose is adjusted to keep this between 2.0 and 3.5 (depending on the clinical situation), which gives effective anticoagulation with minimal risk of bleeding. The daily dose for most patients lies between 3 and 6 mg. The initial stages of anticoagulation are carried out in hospital, but thereafter they are controlled on an outpatient basis and only monthly measurements of prothrombin time may be required.

Phenindione is shorter acting and now rarely used.

Adverse effects. Overdosage is the most important side-effect of the coumarin group of drugs and may lead to haemorrhage from any site. An INR of above 5 suggests a risk of bleeding. It is best treated by withdrawal of the drug. If necessary the effect of the anticoagulant can be reversed rapidly by an infusion of fresh frozen plasma. Alternatively, phytomenadione (vitamin K) intravenously can be given, but takes about 12 hours to become effective. Larger doses of phytomenadione interfere with further anticoagulation for some days. Rarely, transfusion with fresh blood is required if blood loss has been excessive.

In addition, skin rashes, drug fever and jaundice can occur rarely with phenindione.

Use in pregnancy. Warfarin crosses the placenta and may cause fetal abnormalities if given in the first 3 months of pregnancy. If anticoagulation is required during pregnancy, either heparin can be used throughout or heparin used up to 16 weeks, warfarin from 16 to 36 weeks and heparin until delivery. Pre-filled syringes of heparin calcium containing 5000 units are available for self-injection by pregnant women at home.

Interactions of oral anticoagulants with other drugs are important because even a small increase or decrease in their effectiveness may

---

Special points for patient education

1. The dose of anticoagulants is critical—the correct dose must be taken at the correct time.

2. Overdosage is dangerous—any evidence of bruising or bleeding must be reported immediately. In hospital, the urine should be tested daily for blood.

3. As far as possible patients should not alter their lifestyle, but even one night of heavy drinking may alter the efficacy of oral anticoagulants.

4. There are many interactions with other drugs. These (even those obtained over the counter) should not be taken without medical advice.

5. All patients on oral anticoagulants should carry a card and attend regularly for estimations of prothrombin time.

render them dangerous or useless. Warfarin activity is increased by antibiotics, aspirin, alcohol, cimetidine, dipyridamole and phenytoin and decreased by barbiturates. This list is by no means complete and, if possible, the use of other drugs with anticoagulants should be avoided. If the drug regimen has to be changed, the prothrombin time must be monitored carefully.

PREVENTION OF VENOUS THROMBOSIS

Patients *immobilized in bed* as a result of surgery, severe illness or trauma are at risk of venous thrombosis and pulmonary embolism. Overall about 20% of untreated postoperative patients develop a thrombosis and about 1% have a fatal pulmonary embolus. These risks can be considerably reduced by giving 5000 IU of heparin subcutaneously, twice daily or low molecular weight heparin once daily (see earlier) over the operative and postoperative period. With correct dosage it is possible to achieve thrombus prevention without undue bleeding at operation.

The risk of thrombosis continues for several weeks and although it is usual to stop heparin on discharge from hospital, the possibility of continuing prophylaxis as an outpatient should be considered. The use of full-length anti-embolism stockings further reduces the risk.

Patients with *prosthetic heart valves* require full anticoagulation with warfarin to prevent thrombosis on the valve.

In patients with *established atrial fibrillation* long-term anticoagulation with warfarin is effective in preventing emboli, and aspirin, taken regularly, confers some benefit.

THE TREATMENT OF VENOUS THROMBOSIS/PULMONARY EMBOLUS

Patients in whom immediate anticoagulant treatment is required should be started on heparin after a baseline APTT and *prothrombin time* have been obtained. It is usually given by intravenous infusion as detailed earlier. Some authorities consider twice daily subcutaneous injection to be equally effective. At the same time the patient is started on oral warfarin, the dose being adjusted to produce the required prothrombin time which, initially, is measured daily. When this is achieved the heparin is stopped.

If there is less urgency, treatment should be started with warfarin.

The duration of treatment depends on circumstances, but should be continued (usually on an outpatient basis) for at least 3 months and in some patients (e.g. with recurrent episodes) up to a year or longer.

ATHEROMA AND ARTERIAL THROMBOSIS

This arises in a rather different way from venous thrombosis. With increasing age the lining (endothelium) of the arterial wall may become damaged by the flow and eddying of blood, stress and strains due to raised blood pressure, high levels of circulating cholesterol and possibly other factors such as irritants from tobacco smoke. This leads to the patchy accumulation of cholesterol-containing lipoproteins and macrophage cells under the arterial endothelium, together with the deposition of platelets. Ultimately, the patch may break down leaving a rough area (*atheromatous plaque*) on which a thrombus may form and block the artery. Atheroma is widely distributed throughout the vascular system, but it particularly affects the coronary arteries causing ischaemic heart disease, the carotid and cerebral arteries causing strokes, and the legs causing claudication.

ISCHAEMIC HEART DISEASE

Advancing age coupled with risk factors such as high blood pressure, smoking and raised plasma cholesterol levels lead to narrowing of the coronary arteries by atheroma. If severe, this interferes with the blood supply to the heart muscle. The coronary blood flow is usually adequate when the patient is at rest, but with

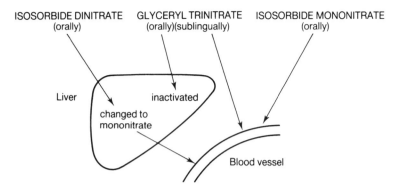

Figure 6.2 The absorption and metabolism of some commonly used nitrates.

effort, the increased demands of the heart muscle for oxygen cannot be met by the narrowed coronary arteries. This results in chest pain which characteristically comes on with effort and is relieved by rest (*angina of effort, angina pectoris*). In a few patients the coronary artery may also be narrowed by spasm, which can also give rise to chest pain.

If a thrombus forms on a plaque of atheroma (*coronary thrombosis*) the blood supply to the area of heart muscle supplied by that artery is cut off and the muscle dies (*myocardial infarct*).

Drugs used in angina of effort

Several groups of drugs relieve the symptoms of angina, but they do not reverse the underlying atheroma.

The nitrates

These drugs act directly on the plain muscle of the body causing it to relax. This action is particularly marked on the walls of blood vessels. It is due to the release of *nitric oxide* which acts as a vasodilator. Nitrates relieve the pain of angina in two ways:

1. By venodilation, which is their main action. This reduces the venous return of blood to the heart and thus reduces the heart work and lowers the demand for oxygen.

2. By dilating the coronary arteries, particularly if in spasm, so that the blood flow through these arteries is increased.

Some drugs in the nitrate group have powerful, but short-lived, actions; others act less powerfully, but over a longer period (Fig. 6.2).

Glyceryl trinitrate is an oily liquid. It is prepared as tablets by mixing with an absorbent base. It is taken orally and sucked, the drug being absorbed from the mucous membrane of the mouth. If swallowed whole it is not effective because the drug is rapidly destroyed as it passes through the liver. Its effects start within a minute and last for 15–20 minutes. It causes a marked general vasodilatation with a fall in blood pressure. The tablets lose potency and should not be kept for more than 2 months, and they should be stored in a glass container and not exposed to light or cotton wool.

A very useful alternative is to give glyceryl trinitrate via a *metered aerosol*; this acts rapidly. Each dose contains 400 micrograms, which is sprayed under the tongue and the mouth is then closed.

Glyceryl trinitrate is also absorbed through the skin and *impregnated patches* are available for application. They release the drug slowly over 24 hours, thus producing a prolonged effect. They have not proved particularly useful as it is difficult to control dosage, headaches can be troublesome and tolerance of the drug's action may develop. If this is suspected, the patches should be removed several times each day.

Glyceryl trinitrate can be given by intravenous infusion. This approach is reserved for patients with severe chest pain usually following a cardiac infarct, when it may relieve the pain and

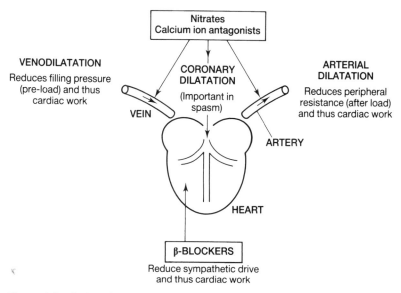

Figure 6.3   Action of drugs used in angina.

also improve any complicating heart failure. It is best given in saline or 5% glucose by a syringe pump. PVC containers (Viaflex and Steriflex) must not be used.

Isosorbide dinitrate is similar to glyceryl trinitrate. It is broken down in the liver to isosorbide mononitrate which is the active agent. It is available in several forms.

Isosorbide mononitrate is the active breakdown product of isosorbide dinitrate and is available for clinical use. It is given twice daily as its action is quite prolonged. The dinitrate is available for intravenous use.

Therapeutics. The main use of nitrates is in the treatment of angina of effort (Fig. 6.3). They can be used in several ways to treat angina. They may be taken intermittently to relieve the pain in an attack or, better, taken *before* performing some action which the patient knows from experience will cause pain. Glyceryl trinitrate is the best drug for this purpose.

One tablet (300 or 500 micrograms) is sucked and the dose may be repeated as frequently as is required. In patients who have repeated attacks, a long-acting nitrate such as sustained-release isosorbide dinitrate or isosorbide mononitrate can be given *regularly* to prevent attacks or diminish their severity.

In patients with severe angina or myocardial infarction, glyceryl trinitrate or isosorbide dinitrate may be given by intravenous infusion.

Adverse effects. In addition to flushing, headaches and palpitations these drugs may cause a fall in blood pressure which can be particularly troublesome with long-acting preparations when the patient may feel faint. Rarely, large doses cause methaemoglobinaemias leading to a cyanotic appearance.

Tolerance to the action of nitrates occurs with long-acting preparations or frequent dosage, but sensitivity is rapidly restored if the drug is stopped for a few hours. Intravenous infusions should not be given for more than 36 hours without a break. The last dose of sustained-release or long-acting preparations should be taken with the evening meal and the patch removed overnight unless nocturnal angina is a problem. Glyceryl trinitrate is unlikely to produce tolerance as it is so short-acting.

β blockers (see p. 48)

β blockers have proved very useful in treating

Table 6.1 Duration of action of nitrates

	Onset of effect	Duration of effect
Glyceryl trinitrate		
(sucked or chewed)	2 minutes	30 minutes
(patch)	1–2 hours	up to 24 hours
Isosorbide mononitrate		
(swallowed)	20 minutes	10 hours
Isosorbide dinitrate		
(chewed)	2 minutes	2 hours
(swallowed)	20 minutes	5 hours
(modified release)	20 minutes	12 hours

angina of effort. The rise in heart rate and heart work which occurs on exercise is partially brought about by the activity of the sympathetic nervous system. By blocking this stimulating effect the β blockers protect the heart from overactivity and prevent the development of anginal pain.

Therapeutics. Most β blockers have been used successfully in treating angina of effort and there is no evidence that any one drug is to be preferred. The usual method of giving these drugs is to start with a small dose and increase it until a satisfactory control of symptoms is obtained. The drug is given *regularly to prevent pain* rather than to treat attacks.

Nifedipine, verapamil and diltiazem
(see p. 69)

These drugs decrease cardiac work by dilating the peripheral blood vessels and this lowers resistance to blood flow. In addition, they dilate the coronary blood vessels; therefore they are useful in treating angina, particularly if it is believed that coronary spasm is playing a part in producing the symptom. It has been suggested that the use of the short-acting preparation of nifedipine in patients with coronary artery disease is associated with increased mortality. At the time of writing this view is being contested and the final answer is awaited.

Therapeutics. They are taken regularly to prevent angina. Nifedipine slow release (Adalat retard) is given twice daily; and verapamil and diltiazem, three times daily.

Nicorandil

This is a new class of drug for the treatment of angina. It has a similar action to the nitrates—dilating blood vessels—but, in addition, has a further dilating action similar to that of the calcium channel blockers. Whether it is an improvement on drugs already available is not yet determined.

Adverse effects include headache, flushing and nausea.

Unstable angina

Sometimes angina is not clearly related to effort but occurs irregularly and includes attacks at rest. This indicates that a plaque of atheroma on the wall of a coronary artery is becoming detached and may herald a myocardial infarct. Aspirin 300 mg followed by 150 mg daily, to prevent the formation of a platelet thrombus on the unstable plaque, is the most important part of treatment. Glyceryl trinitrate relieves pain

---

Special points for patient education

Patients with angina can learn to avoid or treat their attacks.

1. If possible, they should avoid situations known to precipitate attacks, e.g. undue exertion, heavy meals.

2. They should differentiate between drugs which are used intermittently to treat an attack or taken immediately before exertion to prevent one, and those which are taken regularly as a prophylactic measure.

3. They should be aware of the main adverse effects they may encounter and it is helpful if the first dose of glyceryl trinitrate is taken under supervision so that patients may become familiar with the side-effects.

4. Patients may ask if the drugs will become less effective with continued use. This is unlikely with glyceryl trinitrate, but not for the longer-acting nitrates (see text). Tolerance does not occur with β blockers or calcium antagonists.

5. Patients should be told to call their doctor if an attack is prolonged and fails to respond to glyceryl trinitrate.

6. Patients should be encouraged to stop smoking, reduce weight (if obese) and their plasma cholesterol should be lowered (if raised). Provided there are no contraindications, aspirin 75 mg daily should be given to prevent thrombus formation.

and β blockers (best given intravenously at first) reduce the risk of a myocardial infarct. Heparin is also used and treatment should not be delayed.

Drugs used in the treatment of coronary thrombosis

When a thrombus forms on an atheromatous plaque, it may block the artery and cut off the blood supply to the relevant area of myocardium, causing an infarct (death) of that segment of muscle.

This is one of the most common medical emergencies. Except for a few elderly patients with minimal infarction, patients are nursed in hospital and usually spend the first 48 hours in a special unit because this is the period when dangerous complications such as arrhythmias may occur. Treatment includes:

1. Relief of pain, which may be severe. Diamorphine 2.5–5.0 mg intravenously is the best analgesic and to prevent opioid-induced vomiting it should be combined with metoclopramide or prochlorperazine.

2. Dissolving the thrombus. The early use of thrombolytic drugs (see later) reduces the mortality by 25–30 deaths per 1000 patients. It is very important to start this treatment as soon as possible after the onset of symptoms, certainly within 12 hours. Streptokinase is probably as effective as other thrombolytic drugs and a good deal cheaper. If the patient has received streptokinase within the preceding year alteplase should be used.

3. Preventing further platelet thrombus formation (see later) is achieved by giving aspirin 300 mg, chewed and swallowed, as early as possible after the onset of symptoms, followed by 150 mg orally daily.

4. Preventing arrhythmias. There is no really satisfactory solution to this problem. Plasma potassium must be kept at about 4.5 mmol/litre. Otherwise arrhythmias are treated in the usual ways (see p. 62) and it is essential to have a defibrillator immediately available.

Aftercare

Most patients are discharged home within 1 week so aftercare is important to help them to return to a normal life while minimizing the chances of a further episode. This should include:

1. Reassurance and support—many patients are anxious and have lost confidence.
2. Patients should give up smoking.
3. Weight should be reduced to the ideal level.
4. The plasma cholesterol concentration should be reduced if this is raised above 5.5 mmol/litre. This is achieved most effectively with *statins*.
5. Further studies should be arranged to determine whether a coronary bypass operation would be beneficial.
6. Heart failure, if present, can be treated with ACE inhibitors.

Drugs to prevent recurrence

1. Provided there is no contraindication, patients should receive aspirin daily to minimize platelet thrombus formation.
2. There is some evidence that β blockers improve the long-term prognosis, but they should be avoided in patients with heart failure.

FIBRINOLYTIC DRUGS (Fig. 6.4)

Streptokinase is a streptococcal exotoxin. It reacts with a plasma globulin—plasminogen—liberating plasmin which breaks down fibrin. Following a thrombosis intravenous streptokinase thus breaks down fibrin within the clot forming soluble fibrin degradation products. Circulating plasmin, however, is rapidly neutralized by antiplasmins.

Therapeutic use. Streptokinase has been used for many years to treat venous thrombosis. It appeared to have no advantage over the anticoagulants described earlier and was more difficult to use as it was necessary to neutralize circulating antistreptokinase from previous streptococcal infections before plasminogen was activated.

At present its most important use is in lysing the thrombus in coronary thrombosis. For this purpose 1.5 million units of streptokinase are

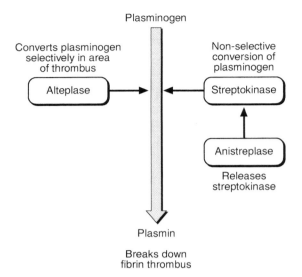

Figure 6.4 The action of thrombolytic drugs.

infused over 1 hour. This may be preceded by chlorphenamine 10 mg and hydrocortisone 100 mg to reduce allergic reactions. This is combined with 300 mg of oral aspirin, which should be chewed before swallowing, and followed by 150 mg daily.

Adverse effects. The main risk with streptokinase is bleeding and this is particularly liable to occur at sites of recent trauma or invasive vascular procedures, which must be avoided if possible. It is contraindicated in those in whom it might precipitate bleeding (e.g. patients with peptic ulcers, oesophageal varices, severe hypertension or recent head injuries).

Allergies are common and include fever, bronchospasm and rashes.

It should not be used if the patient has had previous streptokinase within the last 12 months.

Hypotension can occur and the blood pressure should be monitored.

Other plasminogen activators are:

Alteplase (tissue plasminogen activator) directly converts plasminogen to plasmin and its action is largely confined to the site of the thrombus. It is not neutralized by circulating streptococcal antibodies; therefore it can be used in patients who have had streptokinase or a streptococcal infection. It is, however, considerably more ex-

pensive than streptokinase. The dose is 100 mg i.v. given in divided doses over 1.5 hours. Alteplase may be followed by heparin to prevent re-occlusion.

Anistreplase is a plasminogen–streptokinase complex which liberates streptokinase and can be given as a single intravenous injection of 30 units over 5 minutes. It is also expensive.

On the present evidence streptokinase appears to be at least as effective for patients requiring thrombolytic treatment as the alternative plasminogen activators and is a lot cheaper. Alteplase should be used in those with circulating streptococcal antibodies. Anistreplase, which is easy to administer (no infusion required), may have a place for emergency treatment outside hospital where facilities are limited.

Nursing points

When giving thrombolytic drugs:
  1. Avoid intramuscular injections.
  2. Avoid subclavian catheters for central venous lines.
  3. Use indwelling venous or arterial catheters for access.
  4. Look out for bleeding.
  5. There are several contraindications to the use of thrombolytic drugs. Check that they have been considered and excluded.

Strokes

Strokes are an important cause of death and disability. Most of them (80%) are ischaemic, due to thrombi developing on atheroma, or emboli from atrial fibrillation blocking a branch of the cerebral circulation; the rest are due to haemorrhage.

The use of fibrinolytic agents or anticoagulants *immediately after an ischaemic stroke* to dissolve the obstruction would seem reasonable but the results of trials are conflicitng, and there is the ever-present danger of causing a bleed.

Preventative measures can considerably reduce their incidence or prevent recurrence and include:

a. Lowering a raised blood pressure, which should not exceed 140/85, if possible.

b. Regularly using antiplatelet agents (e.g. low-dose aspirin), which should be started 6 weeks after a stroke or a transient ischaemic attack.

c. Lowering a raised blood cholesterol with statins.

d. Using anticoagulants in patients with atrial fibrillation, to prevent emboli.

e. Stopping smoking.

f. Taking adequate exercise.

DRUGS AND PLATELET CLUMPING

Arterial thrombosis such as occurs in coronary thrombosis and strokes is partly due to an aggregation of platelets which ultimately forms small plugs in blood vessels. Certain drugs have been shown to reduce platelet 'stickiness' so that aggregation is less likely to occur. These drugs are undergoing extensive trials to see whether it is possible to prevent thrombotic disease. Among those which may be useful are *aspirin* (see p. 124) and *dipyridamole*.

Aspirin, by inhibiting the production of thromboxane in platelets, prevents them adhering to each other and to atheromatous plaques and so forming or extending a thrombus.

The uses of aspirin in vascular disease so far determined, *provided there is no contraindication*, are:

1. In acute coronary thrombosis—combined with streptokinase.

2. Taken regularly following a coronary thrombosis to prevent recurrence.

3. Taken regularly following transient ischaemic attacks or strokes to prevent recurrence.

4. In angina of effort to prevent vascular episodes.

5. In unstable angina to prevent progress to myocardial infarction.

6. In patients with atrial fibrillation, aspirin has some effect in reducing the formation of emboli.

It may also have a place in preventing eclampsia in pregnancy and in slowing the progress of diabetic retinopathy.

There is as yet no good evidence that regular aspirin prevents vascular disease in healthy (low-risk) people. There is a slight chance of gastric bleeding, which is dose-related, and 75 mg daily is adequate in most cases. There is no increased risk of cerebral haemorrhage.

Dipyridamole, like aspirin, prevents platelet clumping. It is not very effective when given alone, but may be combined with aspirin or warfarin. The dose is 300–600 mg daily.

Glycoprotein 11b/111a receptor antagonists. The final step in the clumping of platelets is the deposition of fibrin on the platelet surface, leading to the formation of a thrombus and is due to the activation of a receptor on the surface of the platelet. Drugs are now available which can block this receptor and thus prevent thrombus formation.

Abciximab is given by intravenous infusion. Evidence suggests that, when combined with aspirin and heparin, it improves the outcome in unstable angina and after coronary angioplasty.

Clopidogrel is similar and is given orally.

Fish oil. Eskimos have a low incidence of coronary thrombosis and this appears to be related to their large consumption of fish. The fatty acids in fish differ from those of meat and reduce the production in the body of prostaglandins (which promote thrombosis and inflammation) and increase that of prostacyclin (which is anti-inflammatory). The role of fish oil in preventing thrombotic disease and also rheumatoid arthritis and psoriasis is being studied and the results are encouraging.

THE HYPERLIPIDAEMIAS AND ATHEROMA

The hyperlipidaemias are a group of disorders of metabolism in which there are increased amounts of various lipoproteins in the blood. Lipoproteins are substances which are composed of fats and proteins and are produced by the liver. The concentration of blood lipoproteins is determined partly by the dietary intake of fats and partly by metabolic processes within the body. It is therefore possible to lower the lipoprotein levels either by decreasing the intake or absorption of fats or by changing the metabolism.

The most important lipid in lipoproteins is cholesterol and there is strong evidence that a high level of cholesterol in the blood, especially in the form of low-density lipoproteins (LDL), is associated with an increased risk of atheroma and coronary thrombosis.

Approximate relationship between blood cholesterol levels and coronary thrombosis:

Blood cholesterol level in mmol/litre	Coronary deaths/1000
4.5	5
6.0	8
7.0	12

It therefore seems reasonable to lower the blood cholesterol concentration and thereby reduce the risk of coronary artery disease. Reducing raised blood cholesterol levels in patients following myocardial infarction improves their prognosis.

There is also increasing evidence that even in apparently healthy subjects with raised blood cholesterol, lowering the level reduces the risk of coronary disease. It has been suggested that lowering cholesterol levels, particularly in younger men, by 10% would reduce the incidence of coronary disease by 20–50%. The benefit would be increased if other risk factors (e.g. smoking and hypertension) were also controlled.

Mild hyperlipidaemia (plasma cholesterol 5.2–6.5 mmol/litre) is very common in the adult population of the UK and the problem is largely one of health education and changing people's lifestyle rather than using drugs.

There are several ways of lowering plasma cholesterol levels:

1. Diet and weight reduction. A decrease in the total fat intake and the proportion of saturated (animal) fat to unsaturated (fish and vegetable) fat will reduce plasma cholesterol, but requires adherence to a strict diet. Attempts to lower blood cholesterol, using dietary advice alone, are disappointing and only achieve a 3–6% reduction with minimal effect on the risks of coronary disease.

Until recently, attention had been focused on lowering plasma cholesterol levels by limiting saturated fat intake. It is now realized that other dietary factors are involved: antioxidants (see below), fruit and vegetables, nuts and alcohol (especially red wine) can all play a part in preventing atheroma.

2. Drugs.
   a. Agents which **combine with bile acids and cholesterol** in the gut thus preventing their absorption and increasing faecal excretion.
   They produce a fall in plasma cholesterol but, being rather gritty powders, are unpleasant to take. They are usually dispersed in fruit juice and given just before meals. They may cause abdominal discomfort and diarrhoea.
   • Colestyramine A
   • Colestipol.
   b. **Fibrates** alter the metabolism of lipoproteins, so lower blood cholesterol and triglycerides, and have been shown to reduce the risk of coronary disease. They are given orally:
   • Bezafibrate
   • Gemfibrozil.
   They can cause headaches, fatigue, rashes and dyspepsia and muscle pain. They should not be given to alcoholics.
   c. **Statins** block the synthesis of cholesterol in the liver and thus lower the blood level.
   • Simvastin, 10–40 mg at night
   • Pravastatin, 10–40 mg at night
   • Atorvastatin
   • Fluvastatin
   • Cerivastatin.
   They are given at night because cholesterol synthesis is greatest at this time.
   In general they appear to be most useful drugs for lowering blood cholestrol.

Adverse effects. Liver disturbances can occur, and regular liver function tests should be carried out for the first year of treatment.

Rarely, severe muscle pain and damage develops.

Antioxidants These substances, which are found in green vegetables, carrots and fruit and include vitamin E, are thought to reduce the ability of LDL to cause atheroma and are also believed to reduce the incidence of some types of cancer. Whether this is true is still debated, but they should form part of a healthy diet.

Management of raised plasma cholesterol

Patients with a modestly raised plasma cholesterol, found on routine screening and who are symptom-free, will need some encouragement to stick to a strict low-fat diet, as it may seem very unexciting; yet, too much pressure may induce anxiety. In these circumstances, the best advice is to avoid animal fats as far as possible, use vegetable oils, develop a taste for oily fish, increase the intake of fruit and vegetables and, if appropriate, enjoy a modest wine consumption.

If however, the subject has a blood cholesterol in the higher ranges, has a bad family history or already has symptoms of atheromatous disease (usually coronary thrombosis), there is a clear advantage in reducing the blood cholesterol, and this is achieved most effectively by using *statins*. Widespread use of these expensive drugs would add considerably to the NHS drug bill, and the Standing Medical Advisory Committee has issued guidelines detailing the degree of risk of a coronary event which justifies their use. In addition, other risk factors must be addressed: in particular, smoking, hypertension, obesity and lack of exercise.

Other rare and more complex hyperlipidaemias may require different management, usually by a specialized unit.

Nursing points

Hyperlipidaemia may be due not only to an inherited disposition and dietary indiscretion, but to myxoedema, diabetes, nephrotic syndrome and alcohol abuse.

FURTHER READING

Antiplatelet Trialists' Collaboration 1994 Collaborative overview of randomised trials of antiplatelet therapy. British Medical Journal 308: 81

Editorial 1992 Preventing and treating deep vein thrombosis. Drug and Therapeutics Bulletin 33: 129

Editorial 1992 How to anticoagulate. Drug and Therapeutics Bulletin 30: 77

Editorial 1995 Fish oils and cardiovascular disease. British Medical Journal 310: 819

Editorial 1995 Nicorandil for angina. Drug and Therapeutics Bulletin 33: 12: 89

Editorial 1996 Evidence-based guidelines for the primary care of stable angina. British Medical Journal 312: 827

Editorial 1996 The management of hyperlipidaemias. Drugs and Therapeutics Bulletin 14: 89

Editorial 1997 The emerging role of statins in the prevention of coronary heart disease. British Medical Journal 315: 1554

Editorial 1997 Managing established coronary disease. British Medical Journal 315: 69

Editorial 1997 Antithrombotic agents and thromboembolic disease. New England Journal of Medicine 337: 1383

Editorial 1997 Low molecular weight heparins. New England Journal of Medicine 337: 688

Editorial 1998 Low molecular weight heparins for venous thromboembolism. Drug and Therapeutics Bulletin 36(4): 25

Furberg C D et al 1995 Dose related increase in mortality in patients with coronary heart disease. Circulation 92: 1329

Gershlick A H, More R S 1998 Treatment of myocardial infarction. British Medical Journal 316: 280

ISIS 3 1992 A comparison of thrombolytic régimes. Lancet 339: 753

Law M R et al 1994 The cholesterol papers. British Medical Journal 308: 363

Lensing A W A et al 1999 Deep-vein thrombosis. Lancet 353: 479

Manson J E 1992 Primary prevention of myocardial infarction. New England Journal of Medicine 326: 1406

McMurray J, Rankin A 1994 Treatment of myocardial infarction, unstable angina and angina pectoris. British Medical Journal 309: 1343

O'Connor P et al 1990 Lipid lowering drugs. British Medical Journal 300: 667

Opie L H, Messerti F H 1995 Nifedipene and mortality. Circulation 92: 1068

Parker J D, Parker J O 1998 Nitrate therapy for stable angina pectoris. New England Journal of Medicine 338: 520

Tang J L et al 1998 Systematic review of dietary intervention to lower blood total cholesterol. British Medical Journal 316: 1213

Turner-Boutle M 1998 Cholesterol and coronary heart disease. Nursing Times 94(15): 46

Weinmann E E, Salzman E W 1994 Deep vein thrombosis. New England Journal of Medicine 331: 1630

Weston C F M, Penny W J, Julian D G 1994 Guidelines for the early management of patients with myocardial infarction. British Medical Journal 308: 767

Wolf P A 1998 Prevention of strokes. Lancet 352 (Supplement III): 15

7

Drugs affecting the alimentary tract

THE MOUTH

DISORDERS OF SALIVATION

A proper flow of saliva is necessary to keep the mouth fresh and free from infection. Salivary flow will be diminished in fever and dehydration and also by certain drugs, notably those of the phenothiazine group and the tricyclic antidepressants. Severe oral infection may supervene if salivary flow is markedly decreased and was a frequent complication in very ill patients in former times when dehydration was not adequately corrected and measures to ensure oral hygiene not practised. Patients receiving cytotoxic drugs are especially at risk as their resistance to infection is lowered and some cytotoxic drugs cause ulceration of the mouth.

Prevention of oral infection

1. Before major surgery or any other procedure with a special risk of oral infection, the mouth should be inspected and infected gums or teeth treated. The help of a dentist or dental hygienist may be needed.

2. Dehydration must be avoided.

3. Mouthwashes play a useful part in preventing infection and making the patient more comfortable.

Mouthwash solution tablets contain thymol, a mild antiseptic, and are adequate for most patients. One tablet is dissolved in a glass of warm water and used three or four times daily.

For patients at special risk various regimens can be used.

Chlorhexidine gluconate, a more powerful antiseptic, is used in a 0.2% solution (Corsodyl). The mouth is rinsed out two to three times daily with 10 ml for about 1 minute. The tongue and teeth may be stained brown, but this can be largely avoided by brushing the teeth *before* use. Chlorhexidine 1% dental gel is useful for children and handicapped patients. Mouthwash solution can be used every 2 hours in between.

If a dry mouth is a special problem, various artificial salivas are available, instead of or as well as mouthwash solutions. These include Glandosane and Luborant.

In unconscious patients the mouth should be cleaned regularly. *Sodium bicarbonate* one-quarter teaspoonful in 50 ml is particularly valuable in clearing mucus.

Hydrogen peroxide is used in some hospitals to remove debris from ulcers, etc. A 20 volume solution (6%) is diluted, one part in four parts warm water, and used two or three times daily.

In seriously ill patients the care of the mouth is a particularly important aspect of nursing care. Hospitals using different regimens and nurses will have to draw their own conclusions as to the most effective.

Nursing point

In oral infection, prevention is better than cure and recognition that it is a potential problem is important as it can cause considerable discomfort.

Oral infections

In spite of care some patients will develop infections in the mouth, particularly those receiving cytotoxic drugs or at special risk. The main infections are:

Candida. This is common and is best treated by *nystatin*, an antifungal antibiotic (see p. 234) which is not absorbed from the intestine. Pastilles (100 000 units of nystatin) are dissolved in the mouth four times daily after food; or a suspension can be used. Some patients find the taste unpleasant. Treatment should be continued for 48 hours after symptoms have resolved. An alternative is to use *amphotericin*, another antifungal antibiotic, as lozenges, four to eight times daily.

In young children *miconazole* gel smeared round the mouth is easier, but expensive.

Dentures must be removed during treatment and should be soaked in 1% *sodium hypochlorite* solution overnight and rinsed before being replaced.

Oral herpes simplex. *Aciclovir* suspension 200 mg five times daily for 5 days is used.

Herpes labialis (cold sores) must be treated when symptoms (local burning) just develop. There is no ideal remedy. Aciclovir 5% cream, corticosteroid cream or ice cubes applied locally have all been tried with some success.

Nonspecific stomatitis with/without ulceration. Dehydration, if present, should be corrected.

Chlorhexidine mouthwashes as above. *Hydrogen peroxide* can be used to cleanse ulcers.

Benzydamine mouthwash, which acts as a local anaesthetic, is extremely effective in relieving the discomfort of oral ulceration. The mouth should be rinsed out every 2–3 hours with the undiluted solution. If this causes stinging a 50:50 diluted solution should be used.

Choline salicylate (Bonjela) is a mild local anaesthetic in gel form which may be applied before meals and at night.

Aphthous ulceration. These small, painful, recurrent oral ulcers are common in healthy people. The cause is unknown and treatment only partly effective. *Hydrocortisone pellets* (2.5 mg) dissolved in the mouth four times daily or *tetracycline* mouthwashes are used.

Infections of the pharynx and tonsils are very common and are usually viral. Most of them require no specific treatment as recovery is rapid. Many people use gargles, although there is little evidence that they do any good. *Thymol glycerine*, a mild antiseptic, is popular and does no harm. *Soluble aspirin* is also used as a gargle. It is doubtful whether it has any effective local action but when swallowed will rapidly produce its systemic analgesic and anti-inflammatory effect.

Serious throat infections require the use of the appropriate antibiotic given systemically and there is little indication for the local use of antibiotics in these circumstances.

THE OESOPHAGUS

Inflammation may occur at the lower end of the oesophagus; it is usually due to reflux of acid from the stomach and can be relieved by antacids. Preparations are available which combine an antacid with a local anaesthetic and these are particularly valuable in relieving the pain of swallowing.

Gaviscon and Gastrocote are combinations of an antacid with alginates which float on the gastric contents. If reflux occurs they protect the mucosa of the lower oesophagus.

Mucaine contains the antacids aluminium hydroxide and magnesium hydroxide with oxethazaine, a local anaesthetic which, it is claimed, relieves the pain arising from the inflamed oesophagus.

If reflux is severe and persistent, more active treatment is used. This requires reducing gastric acidity and increasing the motility of the lower oesophagus.

H$_2$ blockers can be combined with antacids, but are less effective than in the treatment of peptic ulcers.

Proton pump inhibitors (see p. 96), which abolish gastric acid secretion almost entirely, are more effective and are used in severe cases of reflux oesophagitis.

Drugs that stimulate oesophageal motility and thus keep the oesophagus empty are also useful. **Metoclopramide** (see p. 107) is the first choice, but adverse effects may preclude its use. Alternatives are **domperidone** or **cisapride**, which are free from central adverse effects, although cisapride has a number of potentially dangerous interactions with other drugs. Finally, nondrug measures such as weight loss in the obese, elevation of the bedhead and stopping smoking are advised.

THE STOMACH

The stomach is a hollow organ receiving food from the oesophagus and passing it on, after a variable interval, to the intestines. It is concerned with the mechanical breaking down of the food to render it more easily digested and more easily absorbed. Its muscular walls are capable of powerful waves of peristalsis which mix and macerate the food. The mucosa lining the stomach secretes hydrochloric acid and pepsin, which together initiate the digestion of proteins.

ANTACIDS

Antacids were once widely used in the treatment of peptic ulcers and other forms of dyspepsia. They act by reducing the acidity in the stomach and they also reduce pepsin activity. They are very effective at temporarily relieving the pain from an ulcer, but, unless used intensively, do not accelerate healing. They are also used in various minor gastric upsets; whether they do any good in these circumstances is open to doubt, but they are useful placebos. Magnesium or aluminium salts are the most popular. Magnesium is available as magnesium oxide, hydroxide or trisilicate.

Magnesium trisilicate is a white, gritty powder usually prescribed as the mixture which contains sodium bicarbonate and magnesium carbonate as well. Taken in the usual dose of 10 ml it is effective for about 40 minutes. If, however, it is taken 1 hour after food it assists the neutralizing effect of food and its action may be considerably longer. Magnesium salts are very poorly absorbed from the gut and cause diarrhoea.

Aluminium hydroxide is a white powder, insoluble in water and usually given as a mixture or a tablet which is sucked to prolong its effect. In addition to reducing gastric acidity, aluminium salts inactivate gastric pepsin. This antacid is slightly astringent and can cause constipation. The usual dose is 10 ml or one tablet.

The frequency of dosage of antacids is important. They are usually given 1 hour after meals throughout the day and on retiring. This produces a moderate reduction in acidity and keep symptoms at bay; however, to accelerate healing larger than usual doses must be given more often.

Antacid mixtures. There are many antacid mixtures available. They contain a variety of antacids sometimes combined with substances which protect the mucosa, anticholinergics or local anaesthetics. Generally they have little advantage except in special circumstances (see under Gaviscon and Mucaine) and are usually more expensive.

Antacids in renal failure and other disorders

Although the amount of magnesium or aluminium absorbed is very small and harmless in patients with normal renal function, accumulation can occur in patients with renal failure.

Some antacids contain fairly large amounts of sodium and cause fluid retention and oedema in patients with cardiac, renal or hepatic failure; also in pregnant women and in infants under 6 months.

Interactions. Antacids may interfere with the absorption of digoxin, tetracycline, iron salts, indomethacin and isoniazid.

MANAGEMENT OF PEPTIC ULCERS
(Fig. 7.1)

Peptic ulcers may be either in the stomach (gastric) or the duodenum (duodenal). Their symptoms are rather similar. Hydrochloric acid, which is produced to excess in duodenal but not in gastric ulcers, is responsible for the pain and, for many years, the use of antacids was the mainstay of treatment. The whole approach to the healing of ulcers has changed with the discovery that infection of the stomach lining by the organism *Helicobacter pylori* is a major cause of them.

Infection of the lower part of the stomach (the antrum) increases acid production. This passes to the duodenum and the combined effect of acidity and damage to the mucosa gives rise to duodenal ulceration and prevents healing. Infection of the body of the stomach is a frequent cause of gastric ulcers and may also lead to gastritis and gastric carcinoma. Eradication of this infection results in healing of the ulcer.

Other factors may be involved, the most important being the resistance of the lining of the stomach, acid and pepsin. Prostaglandin E_2, which is formed in the stomach, reduces acidity and helps in the secretion of a layer of mucus which coats and protects the gastric lining. If the production of prostaglandin E_2 is inhibited by NSAIDs (see p. 124), the protection is lost and ulcers are liable to develop.

Nursing point

In patients with peptic ulcers, always enquire about the use of NSAIDs.

The treatment of peptic ulcers is therefore:

1. To reduce acidity, which relieves pain and also helps the healing process.
2. To eradicate *H. pylori* infection.
3. To avoid using NSAIDs.

Although antacids were used formerly, reduction of acidity is now achieved by suppressing acid secretion which is a complex process. There are two ways in which it can be provoked (Fig. 7.1):

1. Stimulation of the vagus nerve leads to the release of *acetylcholine* and thus to increased secretion of acid. In the intact individual this is brought about by the thought, sight or smell of appetizing food. Adequate acid and pepsin are thereby produced to start the digestion of food when it arrives in the stomach. In patients with ulcers, the acid causes the typical pain, particularly if the hoped-for food is delayed.
2. Distension of the stomach (for instance by food) causes the production of the hormone *gastrin* and this in turn stimulates the stomach to produce acid.

The common factor in acid production by both these mechanisms is the release in the stomach wall of *histamine*, from cells called

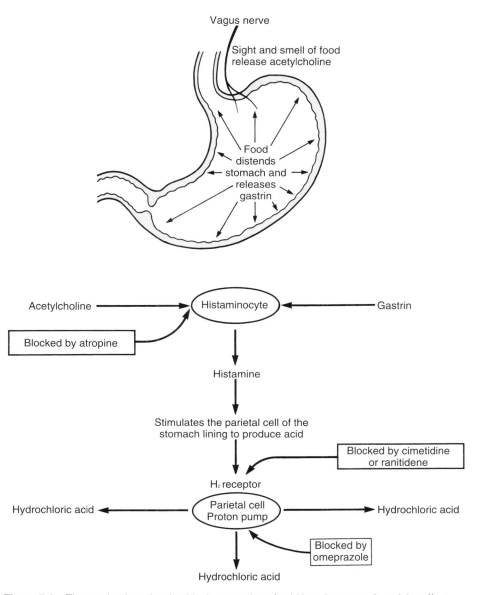

Figure 7.1 The mechanisms involved in the secretion of acid into the stomach and the effect and site of action of H_2 blockers.

histaminocytes, which, by stimulating the *proton pump* in the parietal cells, causes the release of acid in the stomach. The effect of histamine on the stomach is mediated by H_2 *receptors*; in addition, it has effects at other sites including the bronchial muscle and on blood vessels, which are mediated by H_1 *receptors*.

Gastric acid secretion is reduced in two ways:

1. By blocking the action of histamine at the H_2 receptors.
2. By inhibiting the proton pump.

1. Histamine receptor (H_2) blockers—cimetidine, famotidine, ranitidine and nizatidine. These drugs block the action of histamine on receptors in the stomach wall and thus reduce the excretion of acid by about 70%.

Therapeutics. They are given orally.

Cimetidine — 800 mg at night (or 400 mg twice daily) for 6 weeks and then 400 mg at night if necessary.

Ranitidine — 300 mg at night (or 150 mg twice daily) for 6 weeks, then 150 mg at night if necessary.

Famotidine — 40 mg at night for 6 weeks and then 20 mg at night if necessary.

Nizatidine — 300 mg at night for 6 weeks, then 150 mg at night if necessary.

This reduces acid secretion over most of the night and day. Ulcer symptoms usually disappear within a week and about 85% of duodenal ulcers heal in a month; gastric ulcers may take rather longer. Unfortunately, about half the patients will develop a recurrence of symptoms after treatment is stopped.

H_2 blockers can also be used in reflux oesophagitis (see earlier) or to prevent the development of ulcers in patients under severe stress. Injections of cimetidine and ranitidine are available.

There is little to choose between these drugs; cimetidine and ranitidine have been in use the longest. Adverse effects are a little more troublesome with cimetidine.

Adverse effects are rare but with cimetidine include gynaecomastia, impotence due to interfering with the action of normally occurring androgens and confusional states in elderly patients. Cimetidine *interacts* with various drugs by interfering with their metabolism in the liver. Drugs whose action may be prolonged are:

Phenytoin	Morphine
Warfarin	Methadone
Theophylline	Labetalol
Propranolol	Diazepam
Metoprolol	

These effects have not been reported with the other H_2 blockers.

2. Proton pump inhibitors—these drugs inhibit gastric acid secretion more powerfully than H_2 blockers. They are used to treat peptic ulcers in patients who have not responded to H_2 blockers, and are combined with antibiotics to eliminate *H. pylori*. They are also used in reflux oesophagitis and in the rare Zollinger–Ellison syndrome in which there is gross oversecretion of acid. They are given orally.

Omeprazole 20–40 mg daily
Lansoprazole 30 mg daily
Pantoprazole.

Adverse effects include headache, nausea, diarrhoea and rashes.

In addition to reducing acid, ulcer healing can be encouraged by drugs which protect the ulcer and increase the resistance of the gastric and duodenal lining to acid.

Tripotassium dicitratobismuthate (bismuth chelate: De-Nol) is a bismuth-containing compound. It is believed to relieve the symptoms of peptic ulcers by causing coagulation at the base of the ulcer and thus protecting it and promoting healing. It also has some action against *H. pylori*.

This solution has an unpleasant taste and most patients prefer tablets (De-Noltab) which are washed down with water. The tongue and stools may appear black and it should *not* be combined with antacids. Treatment is usually continued for 4 weeks and may be repeated after a month.

Sucralfate is a compound of aluminium and sucrose which coats the base of an ulcer, protecting it from pepsin and allowing healing to take place.

Prostaglandins (p. 206) exert some protective effect on the gastric mucosa and this is the reason why drugs which inhibit prostaglandin production (e.g. NSAIDs) can cause peptic ulcers. *Misoprostol* which is related to prostaglandin has been shown to reduce the risk of gastric ulcers in patients at special risk (e.g. the elderly, those with a history of ulcers) who are taking NSAIDs.

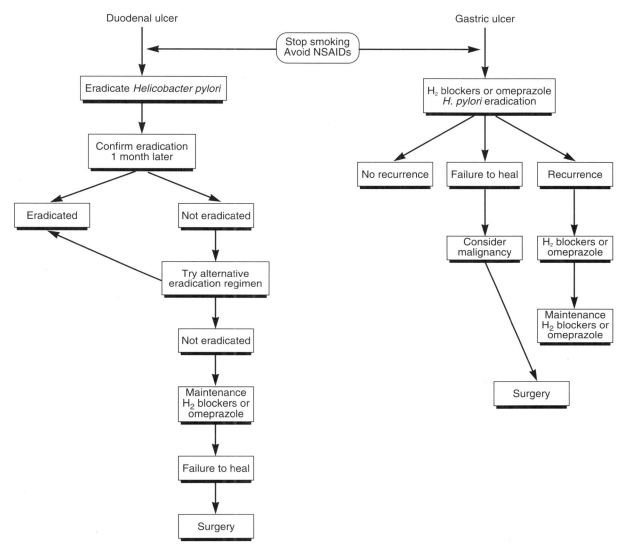

Figure 7.2 Flow diagram of the management of duodenal and gastric ulcers.

Treatment of peptic ulcers (Fig. 7.2)

Reducing acidity and protecting the ulcer from acid will relieve the pain of duodenal ulcer and will heal the majority of ulcers, but relapse within a year is very common (75%) unless the associated *H. pylori* infection is eradicated. This is achieved by reducing acid secretion (usually by a proton pump inhibitor) and using a combination of antibacterials (see below). This will cure the majority of patients but a few will require further treatment.

For gastric ulcers the initial treatment may be either with H_2 blockers or the eradication of infection, if present. After the treatment of gastric ulcers, repeat endoscopy is essential to eliminate the possibility that the ulcer may be malignant. Ulcers due to NSAIDs usually respond to an H_2 blocker or omeprazole. If a patient who is at a high risk of developing an ulcer (elderly, previous history of an ulcer, high dose NSAID) requires an NSAID, then omeprazole may be co-prescribed.

Eradication of *Helicobacter pylori*

Various drug combinations which are effective include:

Triple therapy
Omeprazole + metronidazole + amoxycillin (1 week) This is effective and fairly cheap.

Omeprazole + clarithromycin + metronidazole (1 week)
Omeprazole + clarithromycin + amoxycillin (1 week) This is effective but more expensive.

Ranitidine + amoxycillin + metronidazole (2 weeks) This is cheaper but takes longer.

Diarrhoea may complicate all these treatments.

Non-ulcer dyspepsia

This too may be associated with *H. pylori* infection but the link is less clear-cut. Patients should be screened for infection and the older age group also endoscoped to exclude cancer.

In those with evidence of infection, eradication (as above) can sometimes produce an improvement, though it may be delayed for some

months. Those without infection are usually treated with antacids or H_2 blockers.

CARMINATIVES

Carminatives are substances which when taken by mouth produce a feeling of warmth in the stomach. They cause relaxation of the cardiac sphincter and allow the 'belching up' of wind and may thus relieve gastric distension. Examples in common use are the oils of ginger and peppermint.

THE INTESTINES

After food has been partially digested in the stomach, it passes into the small intestine where digestion of proteins, carbohydrates and fats is completed and absorption occurs.

The passage of food through the small intestine takes about 12–24 hours and the residue then enters the colon where further absorption, largely of water, takes place and the intestinal contents become semi-solid. The filling of the rectum produces the characteristic sensation of the 'call to stool' and the bowels are then emptied by a complicated mechanism, partially voluntary and partially involuntary.

The passage of food through the intestines is brought about by peristalsis, which consists of a wave of contraction preceded by a wave of relaxation. Parasympathetic stimulation increases peristaltic activity and sympathetic stimulation decreases it.

DRUGS IN CHRONIC INFLAMMATORY BOWEL DISEASE
Crohn's disease and ulcerative colitis

These are chronic diseases which are inclined to run a relapsing course. Crohn's disease may affect any part of the gastrointestinal tract, but commonly affects the small bowel and colo-rectum. Ulcerative colitis is confined to the colon and rectum. The cause of these diseases is not known.

Special points in patient education for those with peptic ulcers

1. Bed rest helps to heal ulcers but is rarely practical for those who work or look after young families.
2. Special diets are no longer popular. Patients should be advised to take regular meals (not too widely spaced), avoiding irritating foods and alcohol.
3. Patients should stop smoking.
4. NSAIDs (including aspirin) make ulcer bleeding and perforation more likely, particularly in elderly patients. Steroids in high doses may cause ulcers to develop and make their complications more dangerous. Both drugs should be avoided if possible in patients with a history of peptic ulcers.

The usual pattern of treatment is to bring the acute attack under control and then keep the patient in remission. In addition to the use of drugs, other aspects of management include the maintenance of nutrition and electrolyte balance, correcting anaemia (if present) and surgery on occasions to deal with complications or intractable disease.

Corticosteroids are used to induce remission in both disorders. Prednisolone, orally, is given until the disease remits, then it is reduced stepwise. Budenoside (Entocort) is a retarded-release steroid which may have a more marked local action in the terminal small intestine and is preferred by some. In mild ulcerative colitis, if it is confined to the descending colon, prednisolone enemas may be used instead.

Sulfasalazine can then be started to keep the patient in remission. It is a combination of 5-aminosalicyclic acid and sulphapyridine and is broken down in the bowel to release 5-aminosalicyclic acid, which is the active component. Its action is largely anti-inflammatory. It is effective in maintaining a remission in ulcerative colitis and in colonic Crohn's disease.

Adverse effects include headache, nausea, rashes and, rarely, blood disorders. Male fertility may be temporarily reduced.

Mesalazine (5-aminosalicyclic acid) is also available and has fewer side-effects than sulfasalazine, but is more expensive. Mesalazine enemas can be used to treat distal colitis. *Asacol* is a delayed-release preparation, useful in distal disease.

Patient education In view of the risk of a suppressed blood count, patients taking sulfasalazine or mesalazine should be warned to report sore throat, fever, bruising or bleeding immediately.

Azathioprine, which suppresses immunity, is sometimes used combined with steroids so that the steroid dose can be reduced.

In addition to the drugs detailed above, an *elemental diet* which contains the essential constituents for nutrition (e.g. carbohydrates, amino acids, fats and vitamins in pure form) given for 2 weeks has a specific therapeutic effect in Crohn's disease, but not in ulcerative colitis.

PURGATIVES

Purgatives may be defined as drugs which loosen the bowel. They are widely used and a great deal of their use is unnecessary and may even be dangerous. The bowel habit of individuals varies considerably and many people require to have their bowels open less frequently than is usually considered 'normal'. There is nothing to be gained by these people trying to attain a more frequent bowel action by means of purgatives.

Even more dangerous is the indiscriminate use of purgatives for all types of abdominal pain. In many acute abdominal diseases the use of such drugs aggravates the condition, a classical example being the rupture of an acutely inflamed appendix following a purgative. Purgatives should never be given to patients with undiagnosed abdominal pain.

There are a large number of purgatives which may be classified:

1. *Bulk purgatives*. High residue foods; bran; ispaghula (Isogel).
2. *Stool softeners*. Docusate sodium.
3. *Osmotic purges*. Magnesium sulphate, lactulose.
4. *Stimulant purges*. Anthracenes; bisacodyl.

The bulk purges increase the contents of the bowel and thus stimulate peristalsis. The emollient purges aid the passage of faecal material by their lubricating action. The stimulant purges increase peristalsis and thus the intestinal contents pass more rapidly through the bowel and remain more fluid.

Bulk purges

High residue foods contain a high proportion of cellulose which is not digested or absorbed and thus increases the bulk of the intestinal contents. Common examples are green vegetables, fruit and wholemeal bread. **Bran**, which is a by-product of milling, contains about 30% fibre made up of celluloses, pectins and lignins, substances which are not absorbed from the intestine and which swell as they take up water and thus increase the bulk of the faeces. The initial dose is one tablespoonful, combined with fluid, daily and this is increased at weekly intervals until a satisfactory result is achieved. The main side-effect is wind.

Methylcellulose is available in a number of preparations either as granules or tablets. It is an effective bulk purge.

Ispaghula husk is of plant origin and swells on contact with water, thus acting as a bulk purge. It is available as Isogel and Regulan and other preparations.

Combine both with plenty of water.

Bulk purges depend on the ability of the colon to respond to distension and may not be effective in elderly patients.

Stool softeners

Liquid paraffin may cause leaking via the anal sphincter; lipoid pneumonia (if inhaled) may occur in the very young and very old, and it may interfere with the absorption of vitamins A, D and K. It should not therefore be used for long periods.

Docusate sodium is available as tablets or syrup. The dose is 100 mg three times daily, increasing to 200 mg three times daily, if necessary. It acts by softening the stools and this may be sufficient to relieve constipation, particularly if a painful condition such as piles or anal fissure is interfering with bowel evacuation. It may be combined with a stimulant laxative as it takes two or three days to be effective.

It can also be used as a micro-enema in the management of faecal impaction, when 90 or 120 mg of docusate in solution is injected into the rectum.

Osmotic purges

Saline purges. The most commonly used saline purge is **magnesium sulphate** (Epsom salts). It is poorly absorbed from the intestinal tract. Originally it was thought to make the intestinal contents more fluid, but it is now considered that its purgative effect is a response to magnesium ions reaching the intestine.

A saline purge should be given on an empty stomach (before breakfast is a good time) so that it passes rapidly through the stomach and into the intestine. If it is held up in the stomach, it may not be effective. It is given dissolved in water and the concentration should not exceed 8 g of magnesium sulphate to 120 ml of water as a more concentrated dose may cause closure of the pyloric sphincter and delay the drug leaving the stomach. These drugs are usually effective within 1–2 hours.

Therapeutics. Magnesium sulphate 8 g in 150 ml of water before breakfast.

Fruit salts usually contain some sodium bicarbonate and tartaric acid. When these are mixed with water, sodium tartrate is formed with the liberation of carbon dioxide. The sodium tartrate acts as a mild purge.

Lactulose is a sugar which is broken down by bacteria in the large bowel with the production of various acids. These act as osmotic purgatives rendering the bowel contents more fluid, and as mild irritants, both of which produce a laxative effect. In liquid form, lactulose is given in doses of 15–20 ml twice daily, or as a powder, which can be mixed with food or water. It takes several days to act and may cause a certain amount of flatulence and distension. For these reasons it is not a particularly good purgative, but is sometimes used in the long-term treatment of constipated elderly patients and for those receiving opioids for intractable pain when constipation may be a problem. It also has a limited use in patients with severe liver disease to reduce the absorption of toxic substances from the bowel.

Stimulant purges

The anthracene group of purges all contain the anthraquinone, *emodin*, which is the chief active constituent of the group; the varying properties of the anthracene purges depend on the ease with which this active constituent is released. After liberation in the intestine, emodin is absorbed into the bloodstream and acts on the large intestine, causing increased peristalsis. All members of this group of drugs therefore take about 8–12 hours to act and are *best given at bedtime*. They may occasionally cause griping and should be avoided during pregnancy.

The commonly used anthracene purges are:

Senna is usually prescribed as **Senokot**. This is a proprietary preparation which contains the purified principles called sennoside A and sennoside B. It is highly satisfactory and can be used either as granules, tablets or syrup. The dose is 2–4 tablets, 1–2 teaspoonfuls of granules or 10–20 ml of syrup.

Bisacodyl is a preparation which stimulates activity of the colon when it comes in contact with the wall of the bowel. It can be used either orally in doses of 1–3 tablets (5–15 mg) or as a suppository.

Co-danthramer is a mixture of a stool softener and a stimulant purge (dantron). Unfortunately, it has been shown to produce tumours in rodents with high and prolonged dosage, although there is no evidence that this occurs in humans. Its use is therefore restricted to elderly patients with obstinate constipation or those whose constipation is due to opioid analgesics (e.g. terminally ill patients).

Sodium picosulphate is a very powerful bowel stimulant used for preparation before surgery or radiology and not for the long-term treatment of constipation.

Laxative abuse

Some patients become dependent on laxatives because they believe that these drugs wash away poisons from the body. If carried to extremes this can lead to serious electrolyte depletion and damage the bowel with dilation of the colon.

THE TREATMENT OF CONSTIPATION

Before making a diagnosis of constipation it is important to realize that there is considerable natural variation in the frequency with which people open their bowels. The majority vary between twice daily and once every other day. Constipation has two main causes:

1. Delayed passage of faeces through the colon. This in turn may be due to:

a. Local lesions of the bowel

b. Disorders which interfere with bowel muscle function such as hypercalcaemia or myxoedema

c. Pregnancy

d. Old age

e. Depression

f. Weakness of the abdominal muscle

g. Low bulk diet

h. Various drugs including opioids, antidepressants and verapamil.

2. Neglect of the call to stool. This may occur for social reasons or may be due to illness, surgery or some painful lesion of the anus such as a fissure. As a result the rectum becomes used to distension of its walls by faeces and loses its ablity to contract and empty.

In patients who are ill and who have been constipated for a few days, 2–4 Senokot tablets at night followed by a glycerine suppository the next day are often sufficient.

In *chronic constipation* the object of treatment is to re-educate the intestines so that a normal bowel habit is restored. This can be achieved by increasing the bulk of the faeces either by a high fibre content in the diet, i.e. bran or similar substances, or by the use of bulk purgatives such as methylcellulose. A reasonably high fluid intake and exercise are also helpful. This should be combined with regular habits and may require the use of some purgative such as Senokot at night until a normal rhythm is regained.

Constipation is a common problem in the *elderly*, especially those who are institutionalized. It is due to poor diet, inadequate muscle tone and immobility. If faecal impaction occurs it can be relieved by a retention enema of docusate sodium followed by washouts. If this fails or rapid evacuation is required, manual removal may be necessary.

Long-term management needs dietary advice, as much exercise as is practicable, regular habits and the use of a laxative as required. Senna or bisacodyl are cheap and probably as effective as more expensive preparations.

Laxatives are also used before investigation of the intestinal tract.

Enemas and suppositories

The wall of the rectum contains nerve receptors which respond to pressure to produce the normal call to stool, but may also be stimulated by various substances which can be introduced into the rectum as suppositories or micro-enemas to initiate the evacuation of the bowel. Larger-volume enemas distend the rectum and lower bowel, causing contraction, and also have some wash-out effect.

Suppositories. Glycerol suppositories, one inserted moistened with water, are quite satisfactory. Other suppositories are available but, in general, offer no advantage.

Enemas. These may be used to soften the stool and include arachis oil or docusate sodium. To promote evacuation a phosphate enema, run into the rectum, is useful—for example, before sigmoidoscopy. An alternative is to use a micro-enema such as Micolette; 5 ml is given rectally and it acts as a colon stimulant.

Laxatives are also used to prepare the bowel before colonic surgery or colonoscopy. Various regimens are used, but essentially a low-residue diet is taken for a few days and one sachet of *sodium picosulphate* in water is given in the morning and one in the afternoon on the day before the procedure. Sodium picosulphate is a bowel stimulant which induces a thorough emptying of the bowel. Other similar preparations are available.

Enemas can also be used to treat conditions of

the bowel. In ulcerative colitis steroids (either prednisolone or hydrocortisone) can be introduced into the rectum and retained if possible for at least 1 hour. A certain amount of steroid is absorbed into the circulation and so both local and general therapeutic effects result.

INTESTINAL SEDATIVES

The peristaltic activity of the intestines may be diminished by several groups of drugs.

1. The *anticholinergic group* (p. 49) decrease gut tone by blocking the action of the parasympathetic nervous system. They are particularly useful in colon spasm. *Mebeverine* has a similar action but fewer side-effects.

2. The *opium group* (p. 117) actually increase gut tone but reduce peristalsis. They are useful in various forms of diarrhoea. The most widely used is *codeine phosphate* in doses of 10–60 mg every 4 hours.

3. *Co-phenotrope* (*Lomotil*) is a combination of atropine and diphenoxylate hydrochloride. The latter drug is related to the narcotic analgesics (see p. 113). It is widely used in controlling diarrhoea, but it must be remembered that it is dangerous in overdose, particularly in children, as it can cause depression of respiration.

Loperamide decreases large bowel motility. Toxicity is low and the usual adult dose is 4 mg initially followed by 2 mg three times daily. It is available for adults and older children without prescription.

Diarrhoea may cause *dehydration* and *electrolyte depletion*, particularly in children, and replacements may be required.

In severe depletion, intravenous replacement may be required, but for the majority of patients the oral route is satisfactory and preparations containing sodium, potassium, glucose and water in the optimum concentrations are available.

PANCREATIC SUPPLEMENTS

As a result of pancreatic disease (usually cystic fibrosis or chronic pancreatitis) the pancreatic enzymes may be deficient, leading to a failure to digest fat and protein, malabsorption and loose fatty stools (steatorrhoea). The missing enzymes may be given orally, but they are broken down by the acid in the stomach and thus rendered ineffective. This may be circumvented by combining the enzyme with an H_2 blocker to reduce gastric acidity or by using preparations which are coated to protect them against acid.

Available preparations include:

Pancrex, which is supplied as a powder, capsules or tablets and is given before meals (or feeds). The capsules should be broken and mixed with water or milk.

Creon capsules containing coated pellets which may be swallowed whole or opened and the pellets mixed with food. They must not, however, be chewed as they will lose their protective coating. The dose is very variable and is best judged by observing the nature of the stool.

Patient education

Maintain a reasonable fluid intake. Some high-strength pancreatic supplements have been associated with bowel strictures. The development of new abdominal symptoms should be reported.

GALLSTONES

Gallstones are a common finding, although they do not always cause symptoms. They are usually removed surgically either by open operation or by endoscopy. There are, however, drugs which dissolve cholesterol-rich gallstones and they are used to treat selected patients.

Chenodeoxycholic acid and ursodeoxycholic acid. Most gallstones are largely composed of cholesterol. These two drugs, which are bile salts, reduce the concentration of cholesterol in the bile and make it more soluble so that cholesterol-containing stones are slowly dissolved.

Therapeutic use. Only small stones are suitable for this treatment. The two drugs are often given together orally as a single dose at bedtime and it may take from 6 to 18 months for the stones to disappear. Relapse is liable to occur when the treatment is stopped. Because of the

relatively few patients suitable for this method of treatment and the lengthy supervision required, it has not become popular.

DRUGS AND THE LIVER

The liver plays an important part in the use of drugs.

1. Drugs pass through the liver either via the portal system after absorption from the intestine or, if the drug has been injected, via the systemic circulation. Many drugs are inactivated by the liver, being either broken down or combined with some substance which renders them inactive.

If the liver cells are damaged by disease or if the portal circulation partially bypasses the liver, as in cirrhosis, the elimination of drugs may be reduced and they will accumulate and produce toxic effects. It is therefore important to consider this possibility whenever drugs are given to patients with liver disease and to adjust the dose as necessary.

A comprehensive list of drugs to avoid or use with care is given in the *British National Formulary—Appendix 2.*

2. A few drugs can cause liver damage. This may be either dose-related or idiosyncratic, although the distinction is not always easy. The drugs involved include:

Paracetamol   Phenothiazines (Chlorpromazine)
Methotrexate   Isoniazid
Rifampicin   Pyrazinamide
               Halothane

Recovery usually occurs when the drug is stopped, but in a few (i.e. paracetamol overdose) the damage can be severe and fatal.

3. Drugs can be used to treat diseases of the liver.

Chronic viral hepatitis

Viral hepatitis B and C present a serious and widespread health hazard which is likely to increase. Hepatitis B virus is transmitted by intravenous drug abuse, sexual promiscuity and blood or blood products. The majority of patients clear the virus and make a complete recovery but in about 5% the infection continues and becomes chronic active hepatitis. Hepatitis C infection is also associated with intravenous drug abuse and the injection of blood and blood products. In about 30% of infected subjects the disease progresses as a very slow and indolent hepatitis. Some of these patients will remain as asymptomatic carriers of the virus, but some may develop cirrhosis and, a few, a hepatic carcinoma.

The only specific treatment available at present is with interferons (see also p. 238). These drugs stimulate immunity and also have an antiviral action. The course of treatment is prolonged but in about 50% of those with hepatitis B and 25% of those with hepatitis C, the progress of the disease is halted. Interferons may be combined with other antiviral agents.

For those exposed to the risk of infection with the hepatitis B virus a vaccine is available and there is also a specific hepatitis B immunoglobin when rapid protection is required (see p. 250).

FURTHER READING

Allbright A 1984 Oral care of cancer chemotherapy patients. Nursing Times 80(21): 40

Amin D 1997 Clinical use of laxatives in general practice. Prescriber, September 1997

Butler M 1998 Laxatives and rectal preparations. Nursing Times 94: 56

Di Bisceglie A M 1998 Hepatitis C. Lancet 351: 351

Editorial 1995 Interferon and hepatitis C. New England Journal of Medicine 332: 1509

Forbes G M et al 1994 Duodenal ulcer treated by *Helicobacter pylori* eradication — seven year follow-up. Lancet 343: 258

Forgacs I 1995 Clinical gastro-enterology. British Medical Journal 310: 113

Gorbach S L 1997 Treating diarrhoea. British Medical Journal 314: 1776

Hanauer S B 1996 Inflammatory bowel disease. New England Journal of Medicine 334: 848

Hopkins S 1992 Drugs update: undermining ulcers. Nursing Times 88(16): 62

Langman M J S 1991 Omeprazole. British Medical Journal 303: 481

McCarthy M, Wilkinson M L 1999 Recent advances in hepatology. British Medical Journal 318: 1256

Pope C E 1994 Acid-reflux disorders. New England Journal of Medicine 331: 656

Sladen G 1995 The place of laxatives in managing constipation. Prescriber 6(4): 56

Tsai H H 1997 *Helicobacter pylori* for the general physician. Journal of the Royal College of Physicians, London 31: 478

Walsh J H, Peterson W L 1995 The treatment of *Helicobacter pylori* in the management of peptic ulcer disease. New England Journal of Medicine 333: 984

8

Emetics and anti-emetics. Cough remedies. Respiratory stimulants

EMETICS

Vomiting is a complex series of actions involving the stomach, oesophagus and pharynx with the voluntary muscles of the chest and abdomen and resulting in the ejection of food from the stomach. These actions are coordinated by a *vomiting centre* in the medulla. This centre can be stimulated directly from the labyrinth of the ear in such conditions as seasickness or vertigo, by gastric irritation or distension or even by mental activity (i.e. sick with fright). It can also be stimulated via the *chemoreceptor trigger zone* (CTZ) which lies close to the vomiting centre in the brain stem and which is stimulated by a number of circulating substances including certain drugs (see Fig. 8.1). Finally, there are receptors which are stimulated by 5-hydroxytryptamine (5-HT) found in both the peripheral and central connections of the vagus nerve close to the CTZ. Circulating cytotoxic drugs (particularly cisplatin) release 5-HT and activate these receptors and, ultimately, the vomiting centre. Before the act of vomiting occurs, stimulation of the vomiting centre produces a sensation known as nausea, which is often associated with increased secretion by the salivary and bronchial glands.

Emetics or drugs which provoke vomiting are rarely used in medical practice except in poisoning. They may be divided into two types, reflex emetics and central emetics.

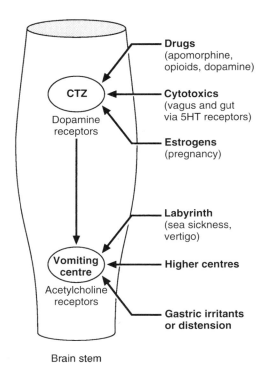

Figure 8.1   Drugs and other factors stimulating the CTZ and vomiting centre.

REFLEX EMETICS

This group of drugs produces vomiting by irritating the stomach. The only one in common use is *ipecacuanha*, which is dispensed as *Ipecacuanha emetic mixture* (paediatric) and the dose is:

Young children	10 ml
Older children	15 ml
Adults	30 ml

It should be followed by 200 ml of water and vomiting should occur in 15–30 minutes. It may be used as a first-aid treatment for overdose provided that:

1. The patient is fully conscious
2. Overdose is not of corrosive substances or petroleum products when inhalation could be fatal.

Ipecacuanha can be used up to 1 hour after ingestion of poison and longer for some substances, such as tricylic antidepressants and salicylates, when gastric emptying is delayed. It

is not so effective as a stomach washout, but is particularly useful in children when the upset of lavage should be avoided if possible and in removing such objects as berries which cannot be washed out of the stomach. In general, the use of emetics in poisoning is decreasing, because there is little evidence, even if used soon after ingestion of poison, that they usefully reduce absorption.

CENTRAL EMETICS

Apomorphine stimulates dopamine receptors in the CTZ. It is closely related to morphine but has none of its analgesic effect. It has, however, a very powerful emetic action and also produces some cerebral depression. It was formerly used as an emetic but because of its depressing action **it should not be used in treating patients who have taken an overdose**. At present its use is confined to patients with resistant Parkinson's disease (see p. 173).

ANTI-EMETICS

It is believed that acetylcholine, histamine, dopamine and 5-HT act as intermediate transmitters in the CTZ and vomiting centre. By blocking the action of these substances it is possible to prevent or diminish vomiting (Table 8.1).

Acetylcholine antagonists

Hyoscine blocks the action of acetylcholine on the vomiting centre and is useful for the short-term control of motion sickness. The usual dose for this purpose is 300 micrograms orally. It is also available as a transdermal preparation, a patch being applied behind the ear for maximum absorption, 6 hours before starting a journey. Drowsiness and blurring of vision, due to paralysis of ocular accommodation, can occur.

Antihistamines

Most of the antihistamine group of drugs have some acetylcholine blocking action and are effective anti-emetics. Among the most useful are **cyclizine** in doses of up to 50 mg three times

Table 8.1 The management of vomiting. There are several causes of vomiting and specific drugs are effective for different types

Types of vomiting	Effective drug	Comment
Vomiting of pregnancy	Promethazine, sometimes combined with pyridoxine	Dietary management if possible. Keep drugs to a minimum in early pregnancy owing to risk of fetal deformity. Promethazine appears to be safe
Motion sickness	Hyoscine	Dry mouth. Blurred vision. Some sedation. Short journey
	Cinnarizine	Preferred for longer journey
Vertigo	Prochlorperazine Cinnarizine Betahistine	
Opioids	Prochlorperazine Metoclopramide Chlorpromazine Haloperidol	Less sedating. Long-acting
Cytotoxic drugs	Prochlorperazine	Sedative
	Domperidone	Not sedative
	Metoclopramide	High doses required
	Ondansetron	
	Cannabinoids	
	Benzodiazepines	Particularly if
	Dexamethasone	anxiety is a factor
Migraine	Metoclopramide	
Postanaesthetic (often opioid)	Prochlorperazine Haloperidol	

daily and **promethazine** which occasionally has a place in *severe* vomiting of pregnancy, the starting dose being 25 mg.

Cinnarizine is an anti-emetic which has found particular favour among yachtsmen and others at risk from seasickness, but it can also be used in other types of vomiting, especially that associated with Ménière's disease. The dose is 30 mg 2 hours before sailing and then 15 mg every 8 hours. Sedation is not usually a problem.

Dopamine antagonists

Several of the phenothiazine drugs (see p. 154) are powerful anti-emetics due to blocking the effects of dopamine on the CTZ. Among those used are:

Prochlorperazine suppresses opioid-induced vomiting. It can be given orally or by intramuscular, but not subcutaneous, injection. If given intravenously, it must be well diluted before use.

Chlorpromazine is similar.

Haloperidol is similar but is longer acting and less sedating.

Levomepromazine is used, particularly in terminal care, to control vomiting and reduce agitation.

Domperidone is less sedative than chlorpromazine and less liable to produce dystonic reactions than metoclopramide (see later) because its action on the nervous system is confined to the CTZ. It also enhances gastric emptying. Unfortunately, only about 15% of the oral dose reaches the circulation and a parenteral preparation is not available. It can be used to suppress vomiting with long-term opioid treatment, levodopa and with the mildly emetic cytotoxic drugs. The dose is 10–20 mg every 4–8 hours orally or 30–60 mg as a suppository.

Metoclopramide increases gastric tone and dilates the duodenum. This causes the stomach to empty more quickly. In addition, it has some central action on the vomiting centre. It is a fairly effective anti-emetic in doses of 10 mg three times daily by mouth or 10 mg by intramuscular injection. It is used in postoperative and opioid-induced vomiting and in migraine. In very large doses it also blocks 5-HT receptors and is used to prevent vomiting due to cytotoxic drugs.

Adverse effects. These are rare but, even with normal doses, patients may develop spasm of the facial and neck muscles. This is more common in young people. They pass off within a few hours of stopping the drug and can be controlled by diazepam. Prolonged use has been reported as causing tardive dyskinesia (see p. 156).

5-HT antagonists

Ondansetron and granisetron probably block the 5-HT receptors associated with the central connections of the vagus nerve in the brain stem in close proximity to the CTZ. They are used to prevent vomiting in patients receiving highly emetic cytotoxic drugs, such as cisplatin, which release 5-HT. The usual dose of ondansetron is 8 mg orally 2 hours before treatment, but with the more emetic drugs, 8 mg intravenously before treatment, followed by 8 mg orally every 12 hours.

Others

Cannabinoids are derivatives of *Cannabis indica* (marijuana); they have an anti-emetic action and have been used with some success in controlling vomiting in patients receiving cytotoxic drugs. They also produce some sedation and occasionally confusion. Cannabis cannot be prescribed at present but **nabilone**, a derivative, is available.

Betahistine. This drug differs from other anti-emetics in that its use is confined to Ménière's disease in which vertigo and vomiting are due to a disturbance in the labyrinth of the inner ear. It is believed to lower pressure in the inner ear and thus relieve symptoms. The dose is 16 mg two or three times daily.

Dexamethasone has proved useful as an anti-emetic during cancer chemotherapy.

Benzodiazepines may be used in combination with other anti-emetics. It seems probable that they have no specific anti-emetic effect, but are useful in relieving anxiety.

Nursing points

As a general rule anti-emetics are best if given at least half an hour before the emetic stimulus. Prevention is easier than cure.

COUGH REMEDIES

EXPECTORANTS AND COUGH MIXTURES

The cough is a reflex. The stimulus may arise from inflammation or foreign material in the pharynx, larynx, trachea or bronchial tree. It may also be provoked by stimuli arising in the pleura. It is therefore advantageous to aid the removal of foreign material from the respiratory passages and this may be achieved by increasing the secretion of the bronchial glands and thus 'loosening' the sputum.

The bronchial glands are supplied by the vagus nerve and when nausea or vomiting occurs there is widespread vagal activity and a considerable increase in bronchial and salivary secretion. Expectorants are drugs which loosen the sputum and thus aid its ejection from the bronchial tree. They are nearly all emetics if given in large enough doses and the theory behind their use is that in smaller doses the emetic action is not provoked but the reflex stimulation of the bronchial glands remains.

There is no evidence that in the doses commonly prescribed expectorants have any useful action and in general their use should be discouraged. There are many excitingly coloured medicines with a powerful and sometimes unpleasant taste which can have a placebo effect and will no doubt continue to be used. Among the ingredients which may be found in such cough mixtures are ammonium chloride, ipecacuanha, guaiphenesin and squill, and many can be bought over the counter.

Certain compound preparations used for treating coughs do contain active drugs, but any benefit which follows their use is not due to an expectorant action.

Benylin preparations contain menthol, diphenhydramine hydrochloride and other substances in syrup. The benefit from this mixture is from the sedative effect of the diphenhydramine (antihistamine) and the soothing action of the syrup. It is useful to give a night's sleep to those with a troublesome cough when taken at bedtime.

Actifed (syrup or tablets) contains pseudoephedrine (vasoconstriction clears the nasal passages) and triprolidine (antihistamine).

Dimotapp (long-acting) contains phenylephrine and phenylpropanolamine (vasoconstriction clears the nasal passages) and brompheniramine (antihistamine).

There are many other mixtures of similar type

and efficiency. They are useful in the cold plus cough situation, but it must be remembered that those containing vasoconstrictors *must not be used by patients taking monoamine oxidase inhibitors* (see p. 163).

As a result of government action the antihistamine–decongestant preparations are no longer prescribable under the NHS, but are available on private prescription and many of them can be bought over the counter. The only way to obtain the drugs on the NHS is for the main ingredients to be prescribed separately.

INHALATIONS AND MUCOLYTIC AGENTS

In the past various drugs were inhaled, particularly in the treatment of chronic lung infections, although with the advent of antibiotics this treatment has been largely superseded. Steam itself is, however, a very good expectorant as it liquefies the sputum and thus enables it to be coughed up.

Benzoin tincture. This is one of the balsams which contains resins and volatile oils. When it is added to hot water, the volatile oil is given off and may be inhaled; it exerts a mildly soothing effect on the bronchial mucous membrane and is frequently used in acute bronchitis. *Menthol and eucalyptus* inhalation can be used in a similar way and produces a considerable outpouring from the bronchial glands and a transient vasoconstriction of the respiratory mucous membrane with clearing of the air passages.

Great care must be taken when young or elderly patients are inhaling these drugs that they do not spill the hot water over themselves or severe burns may occur.

Nursing point

Avoiding dehydration, giving hot drinks and efficient physiotherapy are more effective than medicines in 'clearing the chest'.

Pulmonary surfactants. Natural surfactants allow the surfaces of the pulmonary alveoli to separate so that the lungs can expand and function immediately after birth. In premature infants this factor may be lacking so the lungs do not function properly and respiratory distress syndrome develops. This is treated by mechanical ventilation and the inhalation via an endotracheal tube of **colfosceril palmitate**, a synthetic surfactant.

COUGH SUPPRESSANTS

Under certain circumstances it is advantageous to suppress a cough which is tiring the patient and serving no useful purpose. However, undue suppression of a cough can lead to sputum retention and cough suppressants should be used with care.

Demulcents

Coughs arising from irritation of the upper respiratory tract are helped by demulcents. **Simple linctus**, which is essentially flavoured syrup, in doses of 5.0 ml three to four times daily, is satisfactory but should be avoided in patients with diabetes as it contains sugar. A sugar-free substitute is available.

For many years the only really effective cough-depressing drugs were those derived from the opioid groups, which include **morphine, heroin** and **codeine**. These drugs were included in many cough mixtures and, by virtue of this action on the cough centre, were valuable antitussives.

The most popular of this group was codeine, which was included in **linctus codeine** (BPC). This linctus, although widely used, has been found by many doctors to be not very effective unless given in doses above those usually recommended, in which case it is often constipating.

Dose. Linctus codeine (BPC) 5–10 ml.

Pholcodine. This is closely related to codeine and depresses the cough centre. Weight for weight experimental results suggest it is more active than codeine, although the side-effects are probably similar. Its action lasts 4–6 hours. It is included in various mixtures including linctus pholcodine (BPC).

Dose. Linctus pholcodine (BPC) 10 ml.

In terminal care, morphine or diamorphine may be required to relieve a distressing cough.

Antihistamines

These have some antitussive effect, partly perhaps by a local antihistamine action, but more by their sedative effect on the nervous system.

RESPIRATORY FAILURE

Respiratory failure occurs when the lungs are unable to maintain an adequate exchange of oxygen and carbon dioxide. There are two types. In *type I* the balance between circulation and ventilation of the alveoli is disturbed. This results in a reduction of oxygen in the blood, but normal levels of carbon dioxide. It may occur in heart failure, pneumonia and shock lung. Oxygen may be given freely and the underlying disorder should be corrected if possible. *Type II* respiratory failure occurs in obstructive airways disease, usually associated with chronic bronchitis and emphysema. The essential abnormality is underventilation of the alveoli, resulting in a low blood oxygen concentration and a raised level of carbon dioxide.

Hypoxaemia can be relieved by the inhalation of oxygen, but this may lead to decreased respiration with a further fall in alveolar ventilation and an increased blood concentration of carbon dioxide which causes the patient to become disorientated and, finally, comatose. This situation can be avoided to some extent by giving low concentrations of oxygen (24–28%), which does not reduce alveolar ventilation. In addition, physiotherapy helps to remove retained bronchial secretions, antibiotics are used to treat complicating bronchial infections and bronchodilators relieve spasm.

Respiratory stimulants have a limited use in these circumstances. Given intravenously, they increase ventilation for a short period.

Nursing point

It is important to avoid sedatives which will further depress respiration and cause a deterioration in the patient's condition.

Doxapram is the most effective respiratory stimulant and is given by intravenous infusion at a rate of 1.4–4 mg/minute, the dose being adjusted depending on response. This treatment requires careful monitoring and every effort should be made to remove retained secretions in the respiratory tract by physiotherapy. In overdose, doxapram can cause convulsions.

FURTHER READING

Editorial 1991 Ondansetron vs dexamethasone for chemotherapy-induced emesis. Lancet 338: 478
Grunberg S M, Hesketh P J 1993 Control of chemotherapy-induced emesis. New England Journal of Medicine 329: 1790

Hawthorn J 1995 Understanding the management of nausea and vomiting. Blackwell, Oxford
Williams C 1994 Causes and management of nausea and vomiting. Nursing Times 90: 38

9

Analgesics

THE PERCEPTION OF PAIN (Fig. 9.1)

The central nervous system is constantly receiving nerve impulses arising in the body from the skin and internal organs. Under certain circumstances the brain interprets these as pain. There are a number of theories to explain how this occurs and the most popular today is the *'gate' (input control)* theory. This states that high-intensity stimulation activates a network of fine nerves at the periphery which terminate centrally in the posterior horn of the spinal cord. Here nerve impulses are relayed via the spinothalamic tract to the thalamus where they are felt as pain. There is then a further relay system to the cerebral cortex where discrimination and interpretation occur. The passage of nerve impulses through the relay 'gate' in the posterior horn is modified by:

1. Other impulses arising from the periphery. Low-intensity impulses damp down transmission and this explains why such methods as transcutaneous stimulation or counter-irritation applied to a painful area can relieve pain by 'closing the gate'. High-intensity impulses from an area of tissue damage as may occur after surgery facilitate transmission through the 'gate' and thus increase painful sensations. This may be reduced by blocking impulses from the area of damage by local anaesthesia or by giving an analgesic just before operation.

2. Nerve fibres arising in the brain and descending in the spinal cord terminate in the posterior horn and damp down transmission

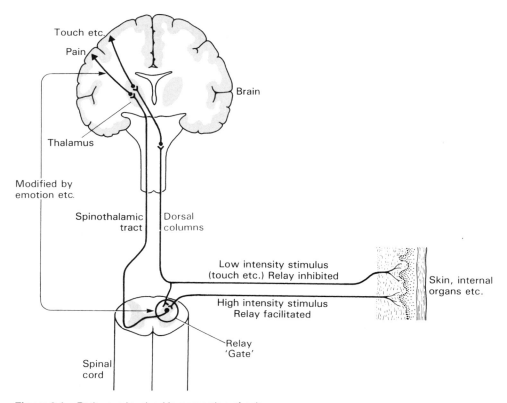

Figure 9.1 Pathways involved in perception of pain.

through the gate and thus decrease the sensation of pain.

It is common experience that distraction can make pain either better or worse. Patients who have been in pain often benefit when visitors arrive or cope better with their pain when they have something interesting to do: for example, read a good book or listen to the radio. This does not mean that the pain has not been genuine, but that it can be modified by environmental factors.

Analgesics are drugs which relieve pain. They are of great importance in the practice of medicine, as pain is a common and distressing feature of many diseases. It must be remembered, however, that pain has its uses, both as a warning of the presence of disease and also, by its nature, it may help in localization and diagnosis of the underlying cause.

Drugs which relieve pain may act at various sites along the pain pathways.

1. They may act on the brain and spinal cord and reduce the appreciation of pain. This is the major site of action of opioid analgesics.
2. They may suppress conduction in nerves carrying impulses from the painful area. This is where local anaesthetics act.
3. They may reduce inflammation and other causes of pain in the painful area. This is the site of action of the nonsteroidal anti-inflammatory drugs (NSAIDs).

Opioids*

Natural: opium; codeine.

Synthetic: diamorphine; methadone; levorphanol; meperidine; phenazocine; dextromoramide; dipipanone; dihydrocodeine, fentanyl.

---

*The term opioid is applied to any substance which has an opium-like action. These drugs are also called *narcotics*.

Nearly all the opioids are potentially **drugs of dependence** and this subject is discussed on page 307.

Minor analgesics

These include NSAIDs.

THE OPIOIDS

The mode of action of opioid analgesics

There are special receptors in the nervous system, particularly in the midbrain and posterior horn of the spinal cord. When these receptors are stimulated transmission of nerve impulses related to pain are inhibited and the appreciation of pain is suppressed. These receptors are stimulated by substances which occur naturally in the brain, called β endorphin and met-encephalin. It seems likely that they are part of a system in the brain which controls pain appreciation and may be involved in such phenomena as acupuncture.

Endorphins are released during physical exercise and may be responsible for the feeling of well-being that participation in sports so often engenders.

Opioid drugs also react with these receptors and thus relieve pain. This interaction can occur in three ways (see Fig. 9.2):

1. The receptor is stimulated—this happens with many opioids, e.g. morphine, diamorphine, meperidine—this is an *agonist* effect.

2. The receptor is partially stimulated and partially blocked—this occurs with buprenorphine and is a *partial agonist* effect (see p. 118).

3. The receptor is blocked—this occurs with naloxone and is an *antagonist* effect (see p. 118).

There are several types of opioid receptor in the nervous system but the most important are called **μ receptors** and are responsible for the analgesia, euphoria and respiratory depression seen with most opioid analgesics. Although the most important actions of the opioids occur in the central nervous system, there is now some evidence that they may also react with receptors on the peripheral nerves, which augments their analgesic action.

Opium

Opium is obtained from the unripe capsule of a poppy which grows throughout Asia Minor and the East. Crude opium is a brownish gum-like material and contains a number of substances; the most important are morphine, codeine and papaverine.

Morphine is the most powerful of these alkaloids and the actions of morphine and opium are similar and may be considered together.

Morphine

Morphine is given by mouth, by subcutaneous, intramuscular or intravenous injection or infusion via a syringe pump. After absorption morphine is combined in the liver to form several sub-

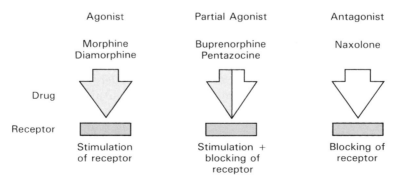

Figure 9.2 Mode of action of opioid agonists, antagonists and partial agonists.

stances, one of which (morphine-6-glucuronide) has powerful analgesic properties of its own. These substances are then excreted by the kidney. When given by *injection* it produces analgesia rapidly. When given *orally* as a *single* dose its effect is greatly reduced as about 75% of the dose is broken down by the liver before reaching the circulation. However, with *repeated* oral dosage it is very effective. This may be because morphine-6-glucuronide is slowly excreted and with repeated doses accumulates sufficiently to help to produce satisfactory analgesia. The analgesic effect of morphine usually lasts about 4 hours after injection but depends to some extent on the severity of the pain, the sensitivity of the patient to the drug, and the dose. Morphine will also cross the placental barrier and affect the fetus, a point of importance in obstetrics. Repeated doses of morphine may induce a state of tolerance to the drug so that increasing doses may be required to produce an effect. It is a *powerful drug of dependence*. The most important actions of morphine are on the central nervous system. They may be divided into depressing and stimulating effects.

Depressing effects:

1. Morphine depresses the appreciation of pain by the brain and thus acts as a powerful analgesic. It relieves all types of pain. If the pain is felt at all, it seems to have lost its unpleasant nature.

2. It is a euphoric and allays anxiety.

3. It depresses respiration.

4. It depresses the cough centre and thus damps down the cough reflex.

5. It is a mild hypnotic and may produce drowsiness and sleep.

Stimulating effects:

1. Morphine stimulates the CTZ in the brain stem (see p. 105), causing nausea and vomiting in about 30% of patients particularly if they are mobile.

2. The pupils of the eye are constricted due to an effect on the nucleus of the third nerve.

3. Morphine stimulates the vagus nerve. This action is particularly liable to be troublesome

when morphine is used for the pain of coronary thrombosis as it may cause undue slowing of the pulse and lowering of the blood pressure.

Other actions. Morphine decreases the peristaltic activity of the bowel and at the same time increases the tone, leading to constipation. It causes spasm of the sphincters, including the sphincter of Oddi at the lower end of the bile duct, and thus produces a rise in pressure in the biliary system. It also interferes with bladder function which may cause urinary retention, particularly after operation; it causes some histamine release, occasionally leading to brochoconstriction.

Therapeutics. Morphine is still one of the best analgesics for severe pain of a temporary nature such as occurs in surgical emergencies, in the postoperative period, following injury or after a coronary thrombosis, for not only does it relieve the pain but it also relieves the anxieties and miseries of the patient. It is very useful in controlling severe pain in terminal cancer (see p. 120) if given regularly. It is commonly used as a premedication, given half an hour before operation on account of its analgesic, euphoric and tranquillizing effects and because it reduces postoperative analgesic requirements.

Morphine is also useful in treating the dyspnoea of heart failure, particularly acute failure of the left ventricle with pulmonary oedema. Its mode of action under these circumstances is not clear, though it probably acts by its widespread sedative effect on the central nervous system and by dilating veins and relieving congestion of the lungs.

The dosage in severe pain or in acute left ventricular failure depends on many circumstances, including the age, weight and general health of the patient, but morphine 10–15 mg subcutaneously is the usual dose for an adult. Morphine can also be given slowly intravenously, the dose being 4–10 mg. The analgesic effect starts within 20 minutes of subcutaneous injection and 10 minutes of intravenous injection and peaks after about 1 hour.

Morphine in small doses can also be given by continuous subcutaneous infusion. This allows the dose to be modified as required and can be very useful in severe and fluctuating pain. However, this method needs careful titration of the dose in relation to the therapeutic effect and fixed dose regimens are not very successful (see p. 119).

It can be given orally for long-term control of pain as *Slow-Release tablets* which are only needed twice daily or as an *aqueous solution* containing either 10, 30 or 100 mg/5 ml or an *immediate release tablet* which must be given every 4 hours.

If vomiting is troublesome, morphine can be combined with the anti-emetic *prochlorperazine* 12.5 mg i.m. or in long-term oral treatment *haloperidol* 500 micrograms—3.0 mg orally twice daily may be preferred. Anti-emetics are usually only required for a few days.

Morphine, in smaller doses, is also included in some cough mixtures by virtue of its depressing action on the cough centre. It is used in mixtures usually containing bismuth or kaolin, in the treatment of diarrhoea.

Adverse effects are considered below.

Signs of overdosage. A patient who has received an overdose of morphine is drowsy or unconscious. The skin is cyanosed and sweating. The respirations are depressed and the pupils are pinpoint. The fatal dose is variable, but death usually occurs after a dose of 200 mg unless tolerance has been induced by repeated dosage.

Papaveretum (Omnopon) is a mixture of morphine and other opioids. Its actions are essentially those of morphine: 7.7 mg of papaveretum ≡ 5.0 mg of morphine. It is largely used perioperatively.

Diamorphine (heroin)

Diamorphine is obtained by modification of morphine. When given by injection it enters the nervous system more rapidly than morphine so that its action starts a little sooner. Thereafter it is quickly converted to morphine in the body. When given orally diamorphine is all converted to morphine in the liver before it enters the systemic circulation; therefore their actions are similar except that the effects of diamorphine are seen a little earlier after injection. It is more

Table 9.1 Equivalent doses of morphine and diamorphine if given regularly

Morphine orally 10 mg	=	Morphine subcutaneously 5.0 mg
Morphine orally 10 mg	=	Diamorphine subcutaneously 3.3 mg
Morphine orally 10 mg	=	Diamorphine orally 10 mg

soluble than morphine and this is useful when large doses are required by injection.

Although diamorphine is more popular than morphine among addicts, it is difficult to see a scientific reason for this and it may be for social or mythological reasons.

Therapeutics. Diamorphine can be used instead of morphine (Table 9.1). The dose is 5–10 mg by subcutaneous or intramuscular injection. For more rapid action it can be given intravenously in doses of 2.5–5.0 mg, and for the long-term control of pain, diamorphine elixir given orally should be used in doses sufficient to keep the patient free from pain. Its analgesic action lasts about 4 hours. If vomiting is troublesome it can be combined with *prochlorperazine* 12.5 mg intramuscularly.

Adverse effects of morphine and diamorphine are shown in Table 9.2. Other adverse effects of opioids are:

1. Bradycardia
2. Urinary retention
3. Dry mouth
4. Allergy
5. Dependence can develop rapidly when narcotics are used in a social context, but they very rarely present a problem when used therapeutically either in an acute painful situation or in terminal disease. However, their use in chronic painful, but non-fatal disorders, is asking for trouble.

Interactions. Opioids increase the effect of other central depressants, as do monoamine oxidase inhibitors, which are particularly dangerous with pethidine.

Certain patients are very sensitive to powerful opioids and a normal dose may produce signs of overdose. The most important of this group are patients whose respiratory centre is under stress, i.e. those with chronic bronchitis and emphysema,

Table 9.2 Adverse effect of morphine, diamorphine and other powerful opioids (Based on the Guys, St Thomas's and Lewisham Formulary)

Adverse effect	Approximate frequency (%)	Dose related	Tolerance	Comments
Constipation	100	No	No	Prophylactic laxative (e.g. Senokot) required
Nausea	30	Yes	Yes (5–7 days)	Prophylactic anti-emetic if needed Give oral or i.m. prochlorperazine or oral haloperidol
Sedation	30	Yes	Yes (3–4 days)	Usually mild. Wears off in 48 hours
Confusion, nightmares hallucinations (particularly at night)	1	No	No	Try reducing dose, then consider haloperidol 2–4 mg at night

and patients *during* an asthmatic attack. Patients with liver damage or impaired renal function suffer an exaggerated and prolonged response. Finally, the very old and the very young are especially sensitive and they should only be given a small dose until their sensitivity to the drug is known.

Methadone

Methadone is a synthetic opioid. Its analgesic action is as powerful as that of morphine, but it has little of morphine's euphoric and tranquillizing effect. Like morphine, it also has a depressing effect on the cough centre, but the effect on the respiratory centre is not so marked. It is a drug of dependence. It is rapidly and well absorbed after oral administration or subcutaneous injection and is less liable to produce vomiting than morphine. Its action is longer lasting than that of morphine and this can make repeated dosage difficult. It should not be given more than twice daily to avoid accumulation.

Therapeutics. Methadone may be used as a substitute for morphine in the treatment of pain, and in small doses is useful as a cough sedative.

It is also used orally as a substitute for morphine or diamorphine in the treatment of drug dependence. The usual dose is 5–10 mg orally or by injection. It is rarely required more frequently than every 12 hours in the management of opioid withdrawal.

Meperidine (Pethidine)

Meperidine is a synthetic substance, which is related chemically to atropine.

It is well absorbed after oral or subcutaneous administration. It is less powerful than morphine, but has less effect in therapeutic doses on the cough or respiratory centre. It causes some spasm of plain muscle of the bile ducts. It is not constipating. It does not cause constriction of the pupils and is therefore used in head injuries where observation of the pupil size may be important. Dependence can develop.

Therapeutics. Meperidine is used in the treatment of moderately severe pains, particularly those arising from viscera. For many years it was given to relieve the pain in the later stages of labour as it is short-acting, thus avoiding prolonged depression of the infant's respiration immediately after birth. There is now good evidence that, although it produces sedation, it is an ineffective analgesic in these circumstances and will probably be replaced by epidural analgesia or some other technique. The usual dose is 50–100 mg orally or by subcutaneous injection. Its action lasts 2–3 hours.

Fentanyl

This is one of a group of opioids which are very powerful and are short acting. They are used largely in the *intraoperative period* to help anaesthetic induction. Their use requires care as severe respiratory depression is a risk. Fentanyl can also be used as a patch, applied to dry, non-hairy skin, which allows slow absorption for up to 72 hours in the relief of terminal pain. Owing to its complex distribution in the body the action of fentanyl in these circumstances may continue for 24 hours after removal of the patch.

> **Nursing point**
>
> Increasing the doses of codeine or dihydrocodeine above those given here will not enhance the analgesic effect. Dihydrocodeine and probably codeine given alone are ineffective in postoperative dental pain.

> **Nursing point**
>
> Fever can increase absorption from patches and result in symptoms of overdose.

Codeine

Codeine is obtained from opium. It is given orally. It is a mild analgesic having only about one-seventh of the power of morphine (Table 9.3). Its most useful action is its depressing effect on the cough centre and it is about half as powerful as morphine in this respect. Like morphine, it also decreases peristalsis of the intestine.

Dependence on codeine is rare, but may occur.

Therapeutics. Codeine is widely used in various cough mixtures for its sedative effect on the cough centre. These cough mixtures usually also contain syrup, whose emollient action is useful in relieving coughs arising from the pharynx. The dose to suppress a cough is 15–30 mg.

Codeine will control diarrhoea, in doses of 15–60 mg every 6 hours. It is combined with aspirin or paracetamol as a mild analgesic, although there is some variation in its analgesic efficacy, due to differences in metabolism (see p. 126).

Dihydrocodeine is similar to codeine and is used as a mild analgesic. It causes constipation and occasionally dizziness and nausea. The dose is 30 mg orally or up to 50 mg by intramuscular injection.

Dextropropoxyphene is similar to methadone but is a much weaker analgesic. The usual dose is 30–65 mg orally and it is combined with para-cetamol as the compound tablet **Co-proxamol** (Distalgesic), which is useful in treating pain which does not respond to aspirin or para-cetamol alone. It is slightly addictive and like many drugs in this group it can cause vomiting. *Overdose* can be dangerous not only because the paracetamol in Distalgesic can cause liver damage, but because dextropropoxyphene can cause respiratory depression and collapse.

Table 9.3 Some other opioid analgesics and equivalent doses

Drug	Dose	Equivalent analgesic effect	Special features
Dextromoramide	5–20 mg orally	5 mg ≡ 15 mg oral diamorphine	Short acting (3 hours) Effective orally
Papaveretum (Omnopon)	7.7–15.4 mg orally or by injection	7.7 mg ≡ 5.0 mg morphine by injection	Contains alkaloids of opium. Action similar to morphine
Phenazocine	5 mg orally or sublingually	2.5 mg ≡ 10 mg oral diamorphine	Can be given sublingually if there are swallowing problems
Oxycodone	30 mg rectally	20 mg ≡ 10 mg diamorphine	Given as suppository analgesic effect lasts 8 hours (i.e. useful overnight)

Equivalent doses of opioids are only approximate. Much will depend on the circumstances in which the drug is given, previous drug history and individual responses.

PARTIAL AGONISTS

Opioid partial agonists (see p. 113) differ from opioid agonists such as morphine in some of their effects. They are powerful analgesics but are less addictive, less likely to depress respiration and are less euphoric.

Buprenorphine. This analgesic, although only a partial agonist, is as powerful as morphine. It can be given by injection or sublingually, but is not effective orally as it is broken down in the liver (large first pass effect). Its analgesic action lasts longer than that of morphine (6–8 hours) and it is less likely to depress respiration. The risk of dependence is low but it can occur.

Buprenorphine shows a 'ceiling effect' so that increasing the dose above the usual range will not improve its efficacy. Although it competes with powerful opioids such as morphine for receptor sites in the brain, in the therapeutic dose range buprenorphine only slightly reduces the analgesic action of other opioids when they are combined.

Therapeutics. Buprenorphine is used to treat moderate and severe pain. It can be given by injection in doses of 300–600 micrograms for postoperative pain, but it is slow to take effect. It is also given sublingually in doses of 200–400 micrograms every 6–8 hours for various forms of chronic pain.

Adverse effects. Buprenorphine sometimes causes troublesome vomiting which requires the drug to be stopped. Respiratory depression, although not so marked as with morphine, is only partly reversed by naloxone.

Meptazinol is similar. When given by injection it has a short action (2–3 hours) and is used in obstetrics where its rapid elimination by both mother and fetus is an advantage. It is also useful for breakthrough pain in the postoperative period. There is a large first pass effect so that only about 10% of the oral dose reaches the circulation and it is only used for moderate pain by this route. The dose is 75–100 mg i.m. or 200 mg orally.

Nalbuphine is similar. Its analgesic action only lasts about 4 hours and it can only be given by injection. It also shows a 'ceiling effect'.

Nefopam. This drug is a non-opioid analgesic. Unlike the narcotic group it does not depress the nervous system and does not appear to produce dependence. It is a fairly powerful analgesic, the usual dose being 30–60 mg three times daily orally. Further increase of dose does not increase efficacy (60 mg orally ≡ 20 mg by injection).

Adverse effects include sweating, tachycardia and nausea, particularly with larger doses, and difficulty with micturition. It should not be combined with MAOIs.

Tramadol is a relatively new analgesic. It is a weak opioid and, in addition, reduces pain appreciation by interfering with pain pathways through the spinal 'gate'. It can be given orally or systemically and is about as powerful as meperidine, its action lasting for about 6 hours. Its main use is to treat moderately severe pain, for example, postoperatively, although it can be used orally for chronic pain. Respiratory depression is not usually marked and its addiction potential is low.

Adverse effects include nausea and vomiting, dizziness and a dry mouth.

MORPHINE ANTAGONISTS

Several available substances antagonize the actions of morphine and other opioids. Generally they resemble morphine in their chemical structure and thus compete with it for receptor sites. Having occupied receptor sites, however, they produce little or no stimulation so that the actions of morphine are reversed (see Fig. 9.2). They are used to treat overdosage by opioids. The most widely used are:

Naloxone is pure antagonist having no stimulating actions. It reverses the effects of both natural and synthetic opioids, but with buprenorphine a larger dose may be required. It has no analgesic action. In the treatment of poisoning the initial dose is 800 micrograms intravenously or subcutaneously and it is very rapidly effective. It can also be used in doses of 100–200 micrograms to terminate the action of narcotic drugs in the postoperative period.

Its action is relatively short (about 1 hour) and

if used to reverse the effects of longer-acting opioids repeated doses may be needed.

Naltrexone is an orally active opioid antagonist used in special clinics in the treatment of opioid withdrawal.

ANALGESICS FOR ACUTE PAIN

Acute pain in hospital is frequently generated by surgery, but may occur as a result of trauma or as part of a medical illness such as myocardial infarction or some form of colic.

Attitudes to pain relief on the part of both nurses and doctors are still inclined to be complacent, especially towards pain after surgery. Patients needing opioids for the treatment of acute pain are too easily labelled as addicts and yet dependence, and respiratory depression, are rarely associated with the treatment of acute pain with opioids. The unimaginative approach of the 'prn' 4-hourly prescription, which is not regularly given, and which does not allow for the opportunity to titrate the dose and frequency against the needs of the patient, can lead to the emergence of extreme pain. The patient then becomes tense, sweaty and exhausted, and needs a large dose of opioid for adequate relief of pain.

The pain relief programme will depend on the severity, nature and cause of the pain. It may include a wide range of analgesics and, in addition, local anaesthetics and drugs that are specific for certain types of pain (e.g. colchicine for gout). It is impossible to specify regimens for all types of pain, but certain general rules should be followed:

1. The programmes must be flexible and aim at keeping the patient free of pain.

2. Many programmes have a continuous background of analgesia with facilities for a top-up (perhaps with a more powerful analgesic) if the pain breaks through.

3. A *combination* of drugs and treatments should always be considered. This can be very successful. Thus, paracetamol may be combined with an NSAID and an opioid—and a local anaesthetic technique may be used as well.

4. Patients vary considerably in their sensitivity to pain and response to analgesics so the programme should be individualized.

5. Anxiety markedly exacerbates the perception of pain. Explanation and reassurance are powerful tools with which to reduce anxiety and therefore the perception and distress of pain. Patients undergoing surgery must be given a full description of postoperative pain problems and the steps which will be taken for their relief.

6. In many hospitals there are specialized teams of doctors and nurses dedicated to the relief of acute pain.

Patient-controlled analgesia (PCA)
(Fig. 9.3)

Pain in postoperative and some terminally ill patients can be effectively controlled by the self-administration of analgesia via a syringe pump set up to deliver a pre-set dose of the drug when a delivery button is pressed by the patient. A number of PCA devices are commercially available, all designed so that dose, rate and frequency of administration can be controlled and pre-set. A number of drugs have been used successfully, including morphine and meperidine. Trials have demonstrated high levels of acceptance of PCA among patients in hospital and the community, where small, portable PCA machines have been used. Part of the success of PCA is related to the feeling of control it gives patients and the confidence that they will not have to wait for the nurse to give an injection to relieve pain. Nursing time is saved as, once the device is set up, it obviates the need to prepare and administer routine injections. However, nurses still have a responsibility for monitoring the adequacy of analgesia and the appearance of side-effects such as nausea or respiratory depression. This is best done by using written protocols which should define the monitoring and actions necessary to maintain adequate analgesia and to properly manage the side-effects of the drugs.

Patients must be taught how to use the device before they need it. For surgical patients this should be before their operation as a heavily

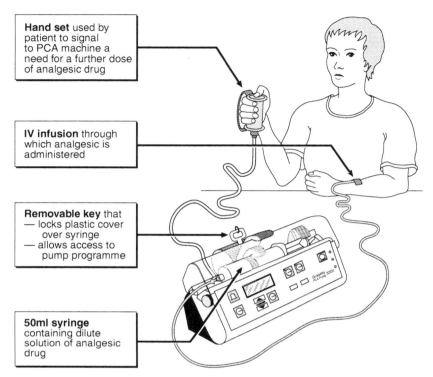

Hand set used by patient to signal to PCA machine a need for a further dose of analgesic drug

IV infusion through which analgesic is administered

Removable key that
— locks plastic cover over syringe
— allows access to pump programme

50ml syringe containing dilute solution of analgesic drug

Figure 9.3 An example of a machine/syringe pump used for PCA—patient-controlled analgesia. This machine, a specialized syringe pump, enables small bolus injections of analgesic to be given on demand. The minimum time between injections—the 'lock-out period'—is controlled. If required, a background, low-dose, continuous infusion is also possible.

These machines contain many safety features. The syringe is locked under a plastic cover and cannot, therefore, be interfered with by any unauthorized person. The *pump programme* used to control and alter the bolus size, the lock-out period, the continuous infusion rate and other functions, is only accessible using the same key that locks the plastic cover. This key should, therefore, be kept with ward keys or in some other secure place.

sedated postoperative patient will not be receptive to lengthy explanations. Patients going home with PCA machines should have the opportunity to become familiar with their use before they are discharged.

ANALGESICS IN PATIENTS WITH TERMINAL DISEASE

Pain is often a prominent feature of terminal disease, particularly cancer. Although the use of drugs is only part of the management of the dying, the correct use of analgesics can play a very important part in the care of these patients.

It must be realized that in this type of patient pain can arise in many ways and the cause should be determined as it may have a specific remedy. It may be related directly to the spread of the cancer; it may be the result of therapeutic measures such as surgery or wound procedures; it may be due to secondary deposits, particularly in bone; or it may even have some unrelated cause or be due to a combination of these factors.

Whatever the cause of the pain, unresolved fear or anxiety may make it worse. A vicious cycle of pain and distress is thus engendered, relieved only by resolution of the anxiety as well as the alleviation of physical pain. The concept

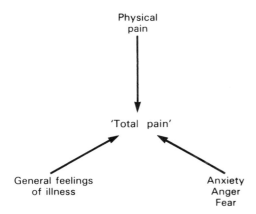

Figure 9.4   Factors which go to make up the concept of 'total pain' or anguish in the terminally ill patient.

of 'total pain' introduced by Cicely Saunders to incorporate physical, social and emotional factors is crucial if the patient's problems are to be fully addressed (Fig. 9.4).

In this situation the nurse has a fundamental role in the assessment of the patient's pain (Fig. 9.5). Nursing interventions may include regular administration of analgesia and also active listening to the patient's worries and anxieties. Evaluation of the response to such interventions is important in the ongoing care of that individual. Pain cannot be treated in isolation but must be regarded as one facet of the patient's physical and mental state.

For mild pain, weak analgesics may be adequate: paracetamol 500 mg–1.0 g every 4–6 hours to a maximum of 4.0 g in 24 hours; Co-proxamol (paracetamol + dextroproxyphene) 2 tablets every 6 hours or dihydrocodeine 30 mg every 4–6 hours (a bit constipating) are useful and, if given regularly, are a little better than paracetamol. For pain arising from secondary deposits in bone, anti-inflammatory analgesics (see p. 124) such as aspirin or naproxen are sometimes very effective alone or combined with opioids.

Moderate to severe pain should be treated by giving opioid analgesics regularly, titrated against the patient's pain.

The most effective drugs are morphine or diamorphine. As diamorphine is largely converted to morphine in the body their actions and efficacy are essentially the same. However, diamorphine is more soluble than morphine and is thus better for injection if a small volume is required.

The opioid should be *prescribed regularly* and *given regularly*. For the average patient morphine 10 mg orally as an elixir in chloroform water*, or as immediate-release tablets, may be satisfactory. Lower doses are required in elderly patients, very ill patients and sometimes in those with impaired liver or renal function. Higher doses will be necessary for those patients who

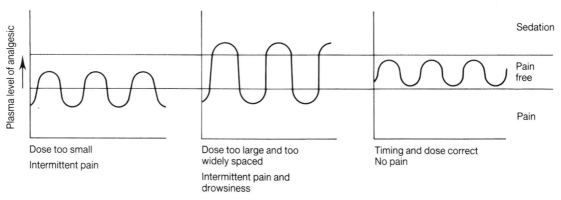

Figure 9.5   Adjusting the dose to keep the patient free from pain.

*The shelf-life of morphine in chloroform water is 3 months unopened, or 1 month if in use.

are already on, or have recently been on, opioids. The frequency of administration is commonly fixed at every 4 hours (2–6–10–14–18–22 hours), but this, like the dose, needs to be kept under regular review.

At first the patient may need additional doses 'p.r.n.' when the pain breaks through. This should be noted and incorporated in the regular 4-hourly schedule. *The object is to keep the patient pain-free.* It is easier to prevent pain with its attendant fear than to relieve a patient who is already distressed.

Once the correct dose of oral morphine has been established it may be convenient to change to Slow-Release (SR) morphine tablets which are only required twice daily and may be more effective in controlling the pain at night.

If possible the drug should be given orally. This saves repeated injections and also produces a smoother and more prolonged analgesic effect.

Dosage schedules should be reviewed every 24 hours and titrated against the patient's pain and well-being.

Side-effects may develop with the use of narcotic drugs (see Table 9.2). They should be anticipated and treated as necessary. Constipation may be a particular problem and a stool softener (docusate) combined with a bowel stimulant (Senokot) is very effective.

With this regimen, tolerance to the analgesic action of the drug does not usually develop. Need to increase the dose of the drug usually indicates advance of the disease.

The risk of dependence is not relevant in the terminally ill patient.

Other routes of administration. Sometimes it is necessary to give narcotics by injection intravenously or subcutaneously when the dose should be reduced. In very severe pain or when vomiting makes oral administration impossible opioids can be given by *subcutaneous infusion.* Diamorphine is used because of its solubility. The procedure is as follows:

1. A single 4-hour dose is given subcutaneously before the syringe pump is set up.
2. The 24-hour requirement of the analgesic is calculated and dissolved in water.

3. The syringe pump is started at a rate adjusted to give the correct dose over 24 hours. It should not be delivered at more than 1.4 ml/hour or absorption may be incomplete.
4. Anti-emetics can be included in the syringe. Cyclizine, prochlorperazine or droperidol are effective. Metoclopramide is not particularly effective and haloperidol is now rarely used.
5. Careful monitoring of the therapeutic effect and degree of sedation is necessary and adjustment of the dose as required.

Dextromoramide (p. 117) because of its short and rapid action can be given orally or sublingually before a painful procedure or for 'breakthrough' pain. The initial dose is 5.0 mg.

Oxycodone suppositories are useful in relieving pain at night, their action lasting for 8 hours, and are particularly useful for patients cared for at home.

Opioid-non-responsive pain

Certain types of pain respond poorly to opioid analgesics. These include pain due to pressure or infiltration affecting a nerve, or bone pain due to secondary deposits where movement may cause an acute exacerbation of pain which breaks through the opioid control. Nerve pain may respond to steroids which reduce surrounding oedema or to anticonvulsant drugs which stabilize the nerve and prevent its stimulation. Bone pain can be helped by radiotherapy (if this is possible), NSAIDs and by preventing movements which cause pain.

Entonox (50% oxygen + 50% nitrous oxide) by inhalation can be used to cover painful procedures.

Chlorpromazine is not only useful as an anti-emetic, but may increase the effectiveness of analgesics.

Amitriptyline (see p. 161) is a useful antidepressant to combat the psychotic depression which sometimes develops in these patients.

Other methods

The use of analgesics is not the only way to

relieve pain in terminal cancer. Radiotherapy is very effective, particularly in treating secondary deposits in bone. In recent years various types of nerve block either at the level of the peripheral nerve or in the spinal cord have been developed which can relieve pain without any systemic effects. These blocks may be temporary or permanent. Finally, much of the comfort and tranquillity of the patient will depend on the character and understanding of the nurse.

Analgesics in non-painful terminal disease

Many patients with malignant disease or dying from other diseases such as renal failure do not have pain, but they may experience considerable malaise and mental anguish. The use of opioids in these circumstances is more controversial. Some people consider that opioids should be used only for pain relief. Others, recognizing their undoubted euphoric action, would give them to reduce the anxieties and discomforts in the terminal stages if necessary, although, usually, relatively small doses are required. They are also useful in controlling cough and relieving the sensation of dyspnoea.

Analgesics and chronic non-terminal pain

In some types of chronic pain the cause is obvious (e.g. arthritis), in others it is obscure. Psychological factors play some part in most types of pain, but may play a major part in the more obscure varieties. This means that there are many types of treatment depending on the cause and severity of the pain and it is only possible here to make some general statements.

1. Before starting treatment it is very important to listen to patients and to assess their perception of the pain and how it affects their daily life.
2. Management with the appropriate drugs will be enhanced by considerable supportive therapy and various techniques for dealing with pain by psychotherapeutic methods are available.

3. Alternative methods of pain relief, i.e. nerve block, transcutaneous electrical nerve stimulation (TENS), which probably acts by closing the relay gate in the spinal cord, may prove helpful in some patients.
4. Do not forget that *depression* often presents as obscure chronic pain. In this case antidepressants are effective.
5. It is important to avoid drugs with a high risk of dependence. Even so-called 'low-risk' analgesics are not entirely safe, e.g. buprenorphine dependence does occur. In prescribing analgesics the patient should be assessed carefully and prescriptions should not be repeated endlessly.

The NSAIDs (see p. 124) are free from the risk of dependence, but not free from adverse effects.

TERMINAL CARE SERVICES AND THE PAIN CONTROL TEAM

The object of hospice care is to help maintain an acceptable quality of life whilst enabling a patient to die peacefully, with special reference to the person's values, preferences and outlook on life. This may be achieved through a team approach in various settings.

The hospice movement has expanded considerably over the last 25 years. There are about 500 units in the UK offering hospice facilities or home palliative care. Referral may be through the general practitioner or district nurse or arranged on hospital discharge.

A more recent development is the hospital support team, of which there are now about 370 in the UK. The team is usually multidisciplinary, sometimes working in conjunction with the radiotherapy or oncology departments. The hospital support team provides skills in symptom control and pain relief and can offer emotional support to patients and carers, while fulfilling an educational role within the hospital.

Pain control teams have been developed to cope with the problem of those in chronic pain. Although many of these patients have terminal cancer, there are other types of chronic pain such as post-herpetic neuralgia, various long-term pains following injury such as amputation, and pain for which there is no obvious cause but where psychological factors may play a part.

The team usually comprises one or two doctors who are interested in the subject (such as anaesthetists), nursing staff (often a sister who is specially trained) and a psychiatrist. They deal with patients referred to them in hospital; they may run an outpatient service and may also undertake home visiting.

Many types of chronic pain are made worse by depression, fear and anxiety and here the psychiatrist will be able to help by explanation, reassurance and the judicious use of drugs such as antidepressants. As in so many areas of treatment, the control of pain is becoming a team activity.

THE NONSTEROIDAL ANTI-INFLAMMATORY DRUGS (NSAIDs)

This is a large group of drugs. Their chief use is to treat minor pain, i.e. headaches, etc., and to control the pain and stiffness in rheumatic disorders and osteoarthritis. They are believed to act by suppressing the formation within the peripheral tissues of *prostaglandins*, which occur naturally and are released by cell damage and for various other reasons (see p. 206). One of the actions of prostaglandins is concerned with the production of painful stimuli, and they are also responsible for many of the features of inflammation (i.e. swelling and redness).

Two enzymes are concerned with the formation of prostaglandins: cyclo-oxygenase 1 (COX 1) and cyclo-oxygenase 2 (COX 2) (Fig. 9.6). Prostaglandins produced by COX 2 are responsible for pain and inflammation whereas those from COX 1 have a protective effect on the stomach lining (see p. 96). Most NSAIDs block both COX 1 and COX 2 and, although they relieve pain and inflammation, may cause peptic ulcers. NSAIDs are being introduced which inhibit only COX 2 and so should relieve pain without the risk of peptic ulceration.

The salicylates

Aspirin (acetylsalicylic acid). Aspirin is usually given by mouth and is rapidly absorbed from

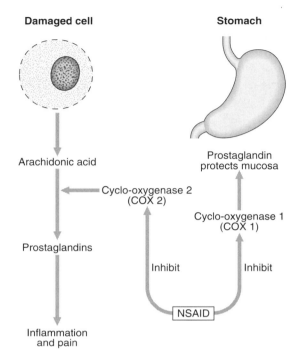

Figure 9.6 The action of NSAIDs. Most NSAIDs inhibit COX 1 and COX 2 thus reducing inflammation, but also the protective action of prostaglandin on the stomach lining. NSAIDs which inhibit only COX 2 may be available soon.

the intestinal tract and rapidly excreted by the kidney partly conjugated with glucuronic acid.

Aspirin is effective against pain of low intensity and particularly that of rheumatoid arthritis and acute rheumatic fever, when its anti-inflammatory properties are combined with its analgesic action. It is also useful in other minor pains such as headaches, sore throats and toothache.

Aspirin is also antipyretic—that is, it will lower a raised body temperature. The control of body temperature is regulated by a centre in the hypothalamus which balances heat production, resulting from metabolism, against heat loss. This is achieved either by increasing heat production by raising metabolism by such means as shivering, or by increasing heat loss by sweating or by dilating blood vessels in the skin. When a patient develops a fever the heat regulating mechanism is set at a higher level than normal. Aspirin acts on this centre and 'resets' it again at the normal level; this results in increased heat loss by sweating and by dilatation of blood vessels of the skin. These effects are only seen in patients with a raised temperature because aspirin does not lower the normal body temperature to any appreciable degree.

Therapeutics. To relieve pain the dose of aspirin is 300–600 mg given orally, and gastric irritation (see later) may be reduced if it is given with a meal. Aspirin is rapidly metabolized and excreted so that dosage every 4 hours is usually required to keep the patient free of pain. To suppress inflammation larger doses may be needed, up to 900 mg every 4 hours. Salicylates in high doses are particularly useful in the treatment of acute rheumatic fever. Within 2 or 3 days of starting the drug the patient's temperature should have dropped to normal levels and the swelling and pain in the joints will have disappeared.

In addition to these actions, aspirin decreases the tendency of platelets to form thrombi (see p. 87). For this purpose, 75 mg daily is usually adequate.

Soluble aspirin is a mixture of aspirin with calcium carbonate and citric acid. Its actions are similar to those of aspirin. It is more soluble, which aids absorption, and less irritant to the stomach, but it may still cause bleeding.

Adverse effects. In large doses aspirin produces effects on the eighth cranial nerve, i.e. dizziness, tinnitus, deafness and vomiting. This is associated with overbreathing due to stimulation of the respiratory centre and to acidosis.

In normal doses aspirin is a gastric irritant and in about 70% of people produces slight bleeding from the stomach. If it is taken continuously over a long period this may lead to anaemia. More rarely aspirin causes a severe haematemesis, usually from a superficial erosion of the stomach wall and is due to loss of the protective action of prostaglandins on the gastric mucosa and to local damage. This bleeding may occur with both aspirin and soluble aspirin. Although severe bleeding is rare when considered against the enormous amount of aspirin consumed, it should not be used in those with a history of peptic ulcer, haemophilia or liver disease or patients receiving anticoagulant drugs.

Occasionally aspirin causes bronchospasm and thus an asthma-like attack, due to reduced production of prostaglandins.

Aspirin should not be given to children under 12 years as it may rarely precipitate *Reye's syndrome* with coma and liver damage which can prove fatal.

Interactions. Aspirin increases the effects of anticoagulants and oral hypoglycaemic drugs.

Benorylate is a combination of paracetamol and aspirin which splits into its component drugs after absorption.

Paracetamol is a widely used minor analgesic and antipyretic. Although it has some cyclo-oxygenase inhibiting properties this action is very weak in the peripheral tissues and it has practically no anti-inflammatory action. Its analgesic effect must therefore be mediated by some action on the central nervous system which is not yet understood. Its main advantage is that unlike other drugs in this group it does not cause indigestion or gastric bleeding.

Therapeutics. The usual dose is 0.5–1.0 g every 4 or 6 hours and the total daily dose should not exceed 4.0 g. It is not very effective in rheumatoid arthritis because of its poor anti-inflammatory action.

Paracetamol is the preferred mild analgesic and antipyretic for children under 12 years old as it does not cause Reye's syndrome. In this age group it is frequently given as an oral suspension, the dose being:

3–12 months	—	60–120 mg
1–5 years	—	120–250 mg
6–12 years	—	250–500 mg

The child should be over 3 months old, except for postimmunization pyrexia, when 2 months is acceptable (dose 60 mg).

Adverse effects. These are uncommon at normal dosage but in overdose it causes dangerous liver damage (see p. 348). There is also some evidence that large doses taken over a long period may damage the kidneys (see later).

Mefenamic acid is a mild analgesic but is probably a little more powerful than aspirin. Its action may last longer than that of aspirin, but it may produce diarrhoea. It can also cause acute renal failure in the elderly. The dose is 250–500 mg every 8 hours.

Analgesic mixtures

There are many analgesic mixtures in which aspirin or paracetamol is combined with a small dose of weak opiate; thus the risk of dependence is minimal. These combinations are a little stronger than aspirin or paracetamol alone and are used for more severe pain. Whether in fact they are more effective than the single drugs is debated and certainly the risk of adverse effects and of danger in overdose is increased. Nevertheless, they are very popular and some are available over the counter.

Among those in common use are:

*Co-codaprin tablets:** codeine phosphate 8 mg + aspirin 400 mg per tablet. This is also available in a dispersible form.
*Co-codamol tablets:** codeine phosphate 8 mg + paracetamol 500 mg per tablet.
Co-dydramol tablets: dihyrocodeine tartrate 10 mg + paracetamol 500 mg per tablet.
Co-proxamol tablets: dextropropoxyphene 32.5 mg + paracetamol 325 mg per tablet.
Tylex: codeine phosphate 30 mg + paracetamol 500 mg per tablet.

Analgesic nephropathy

Some subjects take large quantities of minor analgesic drugs for recreational rather than therapeutic reasons. The favourite was phenacetin (no longer available) and this led to progressive kidney damage and, ultimately, renal failure. Paracetamol, which is related to phenacetin, probably carries the same risk but to a lesser extent. It appears that aspirin does not damage the kidneys in this way and the risk with other NSAIDs is very small (see NSAIDs and the kidney, page 128).

*Available without prescription.

Other nonsteroidal anti-inflammatory drugs

Indometacin. An NSAID which is used in various forms of arthritis and in acute gout. It is effective but minor adverse effects are fairly common.

Therapeutics. The incidence of side-effects is reduced by starting with a low dose (25 mg daily orally) and increasing the dose slowly. It is not usually helpful to give more than 75 mg daily. If morning stiffness is a problem, a 100 mg suppository at night is useful. In acute gout where a rapid effect is required, the initial dose should be 50 mg every 4 hours for the first 12 hours.

Phenylbutazone is a powerful NSAID. Unfortunately it has a number of serious adverse effects including agranulocytosis, gastric bleeding, salt and water retention and rashes. Its use is therefore restricted to the treatment of ankylosing spondylitis in hospital.

Newer NSAIDs

There is now a large number of NSAIDs available for use in rheumatoid arthritis and allied disorders. They are used to reduce the inflammatory element in osteoarthritis, though this use is more controversial as there is a suspicion that although they relieve pain they may hasten the degenerative changes in the joint. They are given to relieve pain in dentistry and that arising from soft-tissue and bony injuries and they can be used for the lesser pains of terminal illness. They provide useful analgesia, particularly after day surgery, when undue sedation has to be avoided. Some are listed in Table 9.4. They all act by reducing the production of prostaglandins (see p. 124) and thus reduce inflammation.

There are certain general principles which can be applied to this group:

1. There is no preferred drug—patients vary in their preference and if one drug is ineffective after 2 weeks of treatment a change should be made to another. It is, however, generally accepted that *ibuprofen* in doses usually recom-

Table 9.4 Newer NSAIDs

Drug	Trade name	Approximate dose	Side-effects and special features
Azapropazone	Rheumox	600 mg–1.2 g daily (600 mg daily in elderly patients)	High incidence of adverse effects. Use only if other NSAIDs are unsatisfactory
Diclofenac	Voltarol	25–50 mg t.d.s.	Indigestion, avoid in peptic ulceration. Rashes. Can be given by i.m. injection
Etodolac	Lodine	200–300 mg b.d.	
Fenbufen	Lederfen	600 mg night 300 mg morning	Indigestion, avoid in peptic ulceration. Produces a therapeutically active metabolite
Fenoprofen	Fenopron	300–600 mg t.d.s. or q.d.s.	Indigestion, avoid in peptic ulceration. Rashes
Flurbiprofen	Froben	50 mg t.d.s. or q.d.s.	Indigestion, avoid in peptic ulceration. Rashes
Ibuprofen	Brufen Ebufac	400 mg t.d.s. or q.d.s.	Indigestion, avoid in peptic ulceration. Rashes. Low incidence of side-effects but not so active as some of the group. Now available without prescription
Ketoprofen	Orudis	50 mg 2–4 times daily	Indigestion, avoid in peptic ulceration. Rashes
Meloxicam	Mobic	7.5–15 mg daily	
Nabumetone	Reliflex	1–2 g daily	Converted to active metabolite
Naproxen	Naprosyn	250–500 mg b.d.	Indigestion, avoid in peptic ulceration. Rashes. Twice daily dosage
Piroxicam	Feldene	20 mg once daily	Indigestion, avoid in peptic ulceration. Once daily dosage
Sulindac	Clinoral	100–200 mg twice daily with food	Rapidly converted to active metabolite in the body. Indigestion, avoid in peptic ulceration. Rashes. Dizziness

mended is rather less likely to produce side-effects, but is perhaps less effective. It is available over the counter without a prescription. *Azapropazone* has the highest incidence of adverse effects. The rest are all very similar.

2. It is useless to give two drugs of this type concurrently.

3. If a satisfactory response is obtained, use the lowest dose which is effective.

4. All these drugs may cause some gastric irritation and should be given with or after meals.

Several are available as suppositories (e.g. diclofenac, indomethacin, ketoprofen) or for injection (diclofenac).

Some NSAIDs, including ibuprofen, ketoprofen and piroxicam, are available without prescription as gels for topical application. Small amounts penetrate to deeper tissues and they appear to produce some improvement in soft-tissue injuries and arthritis. They should be rubbed in gently over the affected area and the hands washed after application. Occlusive dressings should not be used. Occasionally, excessive application can cause systemic adverse effects.

Adverse effects are similar for all these drugs. They are:

1. Indigestion.

2. Gastric bleeding and perforation. This is particularly common in elderly patients and is believed to be due to the inhibition of the gastric protective action of prostaglandins. They should not be given to patients with peptic ulcers or bleeding disorders but, if essential, they can be combined with omeprazole or possibly with misoprostol (see p. 97), an oral prostaglandin

preparation. They should also be avoided in the elderly, if possible.

3. Occasionally, salt and water retention.

4. Rarely, bronchospasm. They may make asthma worse.

Interactions. NSAIDs:

- antagonize the actions of diuretics and hypotensive drugs
- increase the effects of anticoagulants
- decrease the excretion and increase the effect of lithium (see p. 164).

NSAIDs and the kidney

NSAIDs very rarely damage the kidneys in normal subjects. However, in patients with heart failure, cirrhosis of the liver, renal disease or who are taking diuretics they can occasionally precipitate renal failure. This is believed to be due to an alteration of blood flow through the kidneys which follows inhibition of prostaglandin production. It usually recovers on stopping the drug but rarely NSAIDs cause irreversible renal damage. When this group of patients is given regular treatment with NSAIDs their renal function should be checked after a short period of treatment.

NSAIDs and the uterus

Prostaglandins can cause contraction of the uterus and are important in the initiation of labour. NSAIDs, by preventing prostaglandin formation, are useful in *reducing period pains* and have also been used to *prevent premature labour*.

RHEUMATOID ARTHRITIS

Rheumatoid arthritis is a common disorder affecting small and medium-sized joints and causing pain. In a proportion of patients it leads to considerable deformity and disability. Although the exact cause is not known, the inflammation in the joints is due to *prostaglandins*, which give rise to pain and swelling, and to *cytokines*, which are responsible for progressive damage to the joints leading to deformity.

Disease-modifying antirheumatic drugs (DMARDs)

This is a mixed group of drugs which inhibit the rheumatic process in various ways but, essentially, interfere with cytokine action and not only relieve pain but also reduce joint damage. Unlike the NSAIDs they may take up to 6 months to produce a full response.

Chloroquine appears to be of some benefit in rheumatoid arthritis and also in the skin lesions of lupus erythematosus. It is given in doses of 200 mg daily. Unfortunately, prolonged treatment may cause corneal opacities and, more serious, retinal damage. The former may be suggested by the patient reporting haloes round bright lights. Patients should have their eyes examined before starting treatment and be told to report any disturbance of vision. Thereafter, the eyes should be examined if it is considered necessary.

Gold in the form of *sodium aurothiomalate* suppresses the rheumatoid process, but its mode of action is unknown. It is usually given weekly by intramuscular injection, starting with 10 mg (test dose) and increasing gradually to 50 mg per week to a total of 1.0 g. It is then sometimes continued with monthly injections of 50 mg.

Adverse effects are common and can be serious and may require withdrawal of the treatment.

1. Itching followed by rashes which can progress to exfoliation requires treatment to be stopped.

2. Renal damage—urine must be tested for protein at each visit.

3. Bone marrow suppression requires weekly blood counts and the patient should report bleeding, bruising or sore throat.

4. Stomatitis.

An oral form of gold (*auranofin*) is available which is less toxic but less effective than the injection.

Penicillamine (see also p. 350) is used with some success in treating rheumatoid arthritis. Its mode of action is not clear, but in some way it suppresses the inflammation. The initial dose is 250 mg daily, which is increased. Its use is not without risk as it can cause nausea, depression of the blood count and, rarely, damage to the kidneys. It is therefore necessary to test the urine for protein and to perform a blood count at regular intervals.

Sulfasalazine (see also p. 99) also suppresses the rheumatoid process. It takes about 3 months to produce its full therapeutic effect, but is less toxic than gold or penicillamine. However, its use necessitates regular blood counts and liver function tests and the patient should be warned to report any sore throat, bleeding or bruising.

Methotrexate (see p. 279) is increasing in popularity as a second-line drug. It acts more rapidly than those discussed earlier and, if given in low doses of 5–20 mg orally *once weekly*, toxicity is acceptably low provided renal function is normal.

The main adverse effects are gastrointestinal upsets, liver cirrhosis and pulmonary fibrosis. It may be combined with folic acid to minimize these risks. Regular blood counts and liver function tests are necessary and a chest radiograph if a patient develops a persistent cough or dyspnoea.

Azathioprine and **Cyclophosphamide** can also be used when other treatments have failed.

Cyclosporin (see p. 252), which suppresses the rheumatoid process by interfering with T cell function, has also been used. It is particularly liable to cause renal damage.

Special points for patient education

Patients usually take these drugs long term and they must be aware of possible adverse effects and the importance of regular checks and of reporting warning symptoms.

TREATMENT OF RHEUMATOID ARTHRITIS

Treatment of patients with rheumatoid arthritis aims to control the symptoms of pain, stiffness and swelling of the joints and to prevent deformity. Until recently, therapy was usually started with an NSAID, the choice depending on the doctor's experience and preference. Some-

times it was necessary to add a simple analgesic, such as paracetamol to the NSAID, either on a regular basis to improve pain control or when pain became severe. Although this approach has been successful and symptoms are relieved, NSAIDs do not affect cytokines so damage to the joints continues.

Many doctors would now use a DMARD, either alone or in combination, early in treatment in an attempt to protect the joints from damage and minimize deformity. Opinions differ as to the best DMARD to use initially, but methotrexate and sulfasalazine are preferred at present. The long-term result of this approach has yet to be seen.

Steroids, although very effective, are rarely used over long periods because of the high incidence of adverse effects. However, they are sometimes given in low doses for a short time early in treatment, as they suppress both prostaglandins and cytokine activity.

Concurrent care includes various forms of physiotherapy and prevention of deformity, sometimes rest, occasionally surgery, the treatment of complications and advice and counselling.

Nursing point

Specialist rheumatology nurse practitioners are playing an increasingly important part in patient management.

GOUT

Gout is a metabolic disorder which tends to run in families. In gout there is an increase in the amount of uric acid in the body, probably due to increased production, and this precipitates around joints (particularly the big toe), producing an acute arthritis (Fig. 9.7). In longstanding cases uric acid may also accumulate in other parts of the body.

Drug treatment is used for two purposes:

1. To relieve the acute attack. NSAIDs may be used for this purpose. Indomethacin (see earlier) is very effective. It is used in large doses to produce a rapid effect, i.e. 50 mg every 4 hours

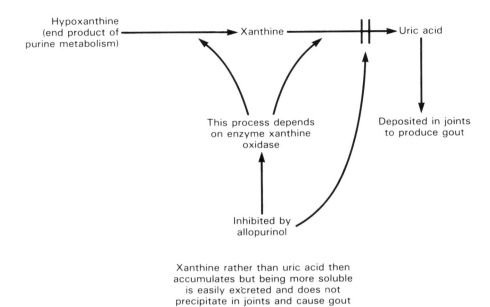

Figure 9.7 Mode of action of allopurinol.

until the pain subsides (usually about 12–24 hours) and then at a reduced dose for a week. An older remedy is colchicine.

2. To decrease the amount of uric acid in the body and thus prevent further attacks. This can be achieved by increasing its excretion in the urine by uricosuric drugs or by preventing the production of uric acid by giving allopurinol.

Colchicine. An alkaloid obtained from the autumn crocus or meadow saffron.

It is not an analgesic in the strict sense of the word because it relieves only one type of pain— that associated with an acute attack of gout. Its mode of action in gout is complicated, but it probably inhibits some actions of inflammatory cells in gouty tissue.

Therapeutics. The pure alkaloid colchicine is used in the treatment of gout. The dose for the acute attack is 500 micrograms two or three times daily to a maximum of 10 mg for the course. Do not repeat for 3 days. Sometimes toxic effects (vomiting and diarrhoea) may cause premature cessation of treatment.

Uricosuric drugs

These drugs increase the excretion of uric acid by the kidney.

Probenecid increases the excretion of uric acid by the kidney, probably by an action on the renal tubular cells. It can be given over long periods. Side-effects are rare but gastrointestinal upsets and rashes may occur.

Sulphinpyrazone is a very powerful uricosuric agent. Its effects are blocked by simultaneous administration of citrates or salicylates.

Drugs preventing the production of uric acid

Allopurinol slows the production of uric acid by inhibiting an enzyme (xanthine oxidase) which is concerned with the synthesis of uric acid within the body (Fig. 9.7). It is given orally, the usual dose being 300 mg daily. It is excreted via the kidneys and care is necessary if it is used in renal failure. Skin rashes are particularly common if retention of the drug occurs. It must not be combined with the anticancer agent *6-mercaptopurine* as it prevents the breakdown of this drug and greatly increases its effect. It has proved particularly useful in the long-term management of gout, particularly if the attacks are frequent, and will usually need to be continued for the rest of the patient's life.

Nursing points

1. Uricosuric drugs and allopurinol may cause an acute attack of gout in the first 2 months of treatment, probably because deposits of uric acid are mobilized, and should therefore be combined with an NSAID during this period.
2. If uricosuric agents are used the patient should be advised to maintain a high fluid intake to prevent the formation of uric acid crystals in the renal tract.
3. Remember that diuretics and pyrazinamide can cause attacks of gout.

FURTHER READING

Akil M, Amos RS 1995 Rheumatoid arthritis—treatment. British Medical Journal 310: 652

Alison M C et al 1992 Gastrointestinal damage associated with the use of NSAI drugs. New England Journal of Medicine 327: 7949

Arthur V, Clifford C 1998 Evaluation of information given to rheumatology patients using NSAIDs. Journal of Clinical Nursing 7: 175

Courtney M 1998 Oral analgesics: aspirin and paracetamol. Nursing Times 94(5): 59

Current Problems in Pharmacovigilance 1994 Relative safety of oral non-aspirin NSAIDs 20: 9

Editorial 1991 Post-operative relief of pain and non-opioid analgesics. Lancet 337: 524

Editorial 1994 Drug-induced end-stage renal disease. New England Journal of Medicine 331: 1711

Editorial 1995 Methotrexate in rheumatoid arthritis. Drugs and Therapeutics Bulletin 33: 17

Editorial 1994 Pain control, TENS machines. Nursing Times 91: 51

Editorial 1997 Disease modifying drugs in rheumatoid arthritis. British Medical Journal 314: 766

Editorial 1998 Modifying disease in rheumatoid arthritis. Drug and Therapeutics Bulletin 36(1): 3

Edwards S 1992 Evaluating syringe drivers. Nursing Times 88 (3): 46

Hodges C 1998 Easing pain in children. Nursing Times 94(10): 55

Jordan S 1992 Drugs update—drugs for severe pain. Nursing Times 88 (2): 24

Levy M H 1996 Pharmacological treatment of cancer pain. New England Journal of Medicine 335: 1124

Macleod G A, Davies M T O, Colvin J B 1995 Shaping attitudes to post-operative pain relief—the role of the acute pain team. Journal of Pain and Symptom Management 10: 30

McLintock T et al 1990 Analgesic requirements in patients previously exposed to positive intra-operative suggestion. British Medical Journal 301: 788

Melzack R, Wall P D 1991 The challenge of pain. Penguin Books

O'Neill W M 1993 Pain in malignant disease. Prescribers Journal 33: 250

Reynolds F, Crowhurst J A 1997 Opioids in labour—no analgesic effect. Lancet 349: 4

Richmond C E, Bromley L M, Woolf C J 1993 Pre-operative morphine preempts post-operative pain. Lancet 342: 73

Shady P 1992 Patient-controlled analgesia: can education increase outcomes. Journal of Advanced Nursing 17: 408

Wolfe M M, Lichtenstein D R, Gurkipal Singh 1999 Gastrointestinal toxicity of NSAIDs. New England Journal of Medicine 340: 1888

10

Hypnotic drugs

INSOMNIA

Approximately 20% of the adult population consider they do not get enough sleep. This is a subjective opinion and in only a few does their health suffer. However, insomnia can cause feelings of anxiety, inability to concentrate and general debility.

Sleep requirements vary with age. Teenagers need about 10 hours sleep, adults about 8 hours and the elderly about 6 hours, but there is also considerable interperson variation.

Hypnotics are drugs which produce sleep that is comparable with normal sleep (Fig. 10.1). They

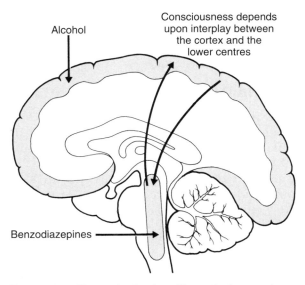

Figure 10.1   The mode of action of hypnotic drugs and tranquillizers.

do not relieve pain. Before prescribing hypnotics it is important to ascertain whether the patient is not getting enough sleep, as some people exaggerate their insomnia, and to find out if there is some reason for failing to sleep. Among these reasons may be:

- Anxiety and stress
- Depression
- Physical illness e.g. heart failure, chronic lung disease and sleep disordered breathing
- Pain
- Caffeine, alcohol and steroids taken before retiring.

If these are remedied, sleep should occur naturally. Various simple measures can be tried—a walk, a bath, a rather unexciting book before retiring or a glass of milk at bedtime may be sufficient. More comprehensive programmes are detailed by Espre (1993).

Although hypnotic drugs may be required in some circumstances, for example during periods of stress or for certain chronic insomniacs, their use should be discouraged. Tolerance to their action often develops in 2–3 weeks with some degree of dependence. Withdrawal at this stage can lead to increasing wakefulness at night for a few days or longer. This is particularly important in hospitals where they are often prescribed much too freely and where a lifetime of habituation to these drugs may start. Patients should not as a general rule be sent home from hospital receiving hypnotic drugs.

THE NATURE OF SLEEP

Sleep is not just a state into which one lapses on going to bed and from which one emerges on waking. It is a series of cycles each lasting about 90 minutes. After falling asleep the subject becomes progressively more relaxed with slow pulse and respiration rate; this phase lasts about 80 minutes and ultimately the state of 'deep sleep' is reached. Then follows a phase lasting about 10 minutes with dreaming, increased muscle tone, rapid eye movements and increased heart rate, known as *rapid eye movement* (REM) sleep. The whole cycle is then repeated about six times per night.

It has been shown that if a subject is deprived of REM sleep he or she will show psychological changes during waking hours. Many centrally acting drugs and alcohol do in fact suppress REM sleep and thus do not really produce completely natural sleep.

HYPNOTIC DRUGS

Chloral hydrate and its derivatives have been used as hypnotics for many years and have established a reputation for being especially useful for children. Chloral hydrate is rapidly absorbed and produces sleep in about 30 minutes, by causing interference in functioning of the brain cells. The drug is conjugated in the liver and excreted via the kidneys. Its hypnotic action lasts about 4 hours.

Therapeutics. Chloral has an unpleasant taste, is a gastric irritant and can cause rashes. Although an effective hypnotic, its popularity has declined and it is no longer the hypnotic of choice, even for children. If required, its derivative, **triclofos**, is preferred, being less of a gastric irritant.

Adverse effects and interactions. Chloral is relatively safe but may cause gastric upset. It should be used with caution in liver or renal failure. It enhances the effect of warfarin.

Promethazine is an antihistamine which is sometimes used as a hypnotic drug, especially in children. By blocking the action of histamine in the brain it produces sleep. It is not a particularly good hypnotic drug, having rather a long action with sedation next morning, and because it has an anticholinergic action it can cause a dry mouth and interfere with bladder function. It is available without prescription.

The dose for an adult is 25 mg orally and for children from 2–5 years 15 mg and 5–10 years 20 mg.

Chlormethiazole. This drug, which is related to vitamin B_1, is now rarely used as a hypnotic because of the risk of dependence. It can be given orally or intravenously. Its action is short-lived.

Therapeutics. Chlormethiazole is used particularly in elderly subjects, for patients who are agitated and confused and for controlling withdrawal symptoms in alcoholics, although *dependence* on chlormethiazole may develop. As a hypnotic drug the usual dose is one capsule (containing 192 mg base). To control alcohol withdrawal symptoms the dose is three capsules three times daily and reduced as necessary. Chlormethiazole can also be given intravenously to terminate status epilepticus or control delirium tremens. It is given as a 0.8% solution and usually, an initial loading dose may be continued at a lower dose if necessary. When given in this way there is a danger of respiratory depression and hypotension and the patient requires careful observation and direct medical supervision. *The infusion should not usually be continued for more than 18 hours.*

Adverse effects are rare but some patients complain of stuffiness in the nose shortly after taking the drug.

The benzodiazepines (see also p. 158)

Several members of this group of drugs can be given as a hypnotic. They bind to a specific receptor and enhance the effect of GABA, a naturally occurring inhibitor substance in the brain. There is very little to choose between them in efficacy, their main difference being in their duration of action. This is shown in Table 10.1. Those with a prolonged action may produce a hangover effect the next day if given in a dose sufficient to produce sleep. They are easy to use and pleasant to take and are the most commonly prescribed hypnotic drugs.

Nitrazepam. This was the first benzodiazepine to be recommended as a hypnotic drug. Although it has been claimed that this drug is unlikely to confuse elderly patients, this is not true. In addition, some sedative effect may persist well into the following day.

Diazepam. Although more usually used as a minor tranquillizer, diazepam is a fairly good hypnotic drug if there is some background anxiety and sedation lasting into the next day is needed.

Temazepam. This drug has a shorter half-life and length of action than most other benzodiazepines and it does not produce metabolites which

Table 10.1 Benzodiazepines used as hypnotic drugs

Drug	Dose*	Half-life	Duration of action
Nitrazepam	5–10 mg	20 hours	Fairly long-acting
Diazepam	2–10 mg	30 hours	Long-acting, also active breakdown product
Temazepam	10–20 mg	5–6 hours	Short-acting
Flurazepam	15–30 mg	60 hours	Residual effects
Flunitrazepam	Fairly long-acting		
Loprazolam	Short-acting		
Lormetazepam	Short-acting		

*The lower doses should be used in the elderly.

are also hypnotics. It is, therefore, less liable to cause drowsiness into the next day.

Flunitrazepam has a fairly prolonged action. Because it is tasteless, it can be added to drinks, etc., and has gained a reputation for being used when rape is intended. It is subject to prescribing constraints.

Adverse effects. The benzodiazepines are remarkably free from serious adverse effects, although continued use can cause fatigue, memory problems and, rarely, behavioural disturbances. The main problem is the *development of dependence.* This may occur after 2 weeks or less when they are used as hypnotics. Withdrawal then results in considerable difficulty in sleeping for several days or even weeks, and the temptation is to resume taking them.

When stopping treatment with benzodiazepines, particularly if they have been taken for a long time, the dosage should be reduced stepwise, reducing it about every 14 days, depending on symptoms, and finally withdrawing it altogether.

Zopiclone and Zolpidem

These short-acting hypnotics, although differing in structure from the benzodiazepines, also bind to the benzodiazepine receptors and increase the sedating activity of gamma aminobutyric acid (GABA) in the brain.

Zopiclone is rapidly absorbed and produces sleep lasting 6–8 hours. There may be some drowsiness the next morning. The available evidence suggests that tolerance may develop and dependence occur. In general it is very similar to the short-acting benzodiazepines. The usual dose is 7.5 mg at bedtime; for the elderly patients this is reduced to 3.75 mg.

Adverse effects. A bitter metallic taste in the mouth is fairly common. Sometimes nausea and hallucinations and other psychological phenomena have been reported. It should not be used during pregnancy or given to children.

Interactions. Increased drowsiness if used with other central depressants (alcohol, benzodiazepines).

Zolpidem in doses of 10 mg is similar, sleep lasting about 6 hours, and there are few after effects the next morning. Dependence potential is low but can occur.

Adverse effects include drowsiness, headache and nausea.

Neither of these hypnotics is ideal and whether they are preferable to the short-acting benzodiazepines (e.g. temazepam) is not clear but they are more expensive. As with the benzodiazepines, they should only be used after careful consideration and should not be taken for more than 2–4 weeks.

Ethyl alcohol. Alcohol is occasionally used as a sedative at night, particularly in the elderly. It is not a good hypnotic and though it may help patients to get to sleep, they often waken during the night due to rebound insomnia. It is important to remember that patients who take alcohol regularly may become restless and have difficulty in sleeping if it is stopped suddenly.

The use and choice of hypnotics

The first essential is to make certain that a hypnotic drug is necessary to relieve the patient's insomnia. Insomnia may be considered in three categories.

1. *Transient insomnia* occurs in people who usually have no sleep problem and is due to altered circumstances, i.e. admission to hospital or travel. In these cases a short-acting benzodiazepine such as temazepam is appropriate.

2. *Short-term insomnia* may be due to anxiety, illness, etc. Here a short-acting benzodiazepine can be used, but if anxiety is prominent, a drug such as diazepam may be more useful as its effect will last into the next day. It is important that the drug is not given for more than 2 weeks and that intermittent dosing is introduced as early as possible as there is a *definite risk of dependence developing*. The nurse has an important part to play by listening to the patient's worries and by relieving any physical discomfort if possible.

3. *Chronic insomnia.* Careful analysis is necessary in these patients. Some will be suffering from psychiatric illness, particularly depression. In other cases an excess of coffee or alcohol may be the cause. If these can be excluded, a change in lifestyle with regular exercise and reduction of stress (if possible) can be tried.

Diazepam is the most suitable hypnotic drug, preferably on an intermittent basis, for a month. If this fails, trial of an antidepressant is appropriate. The long-term management of this type of patient is often difficult.

There is little indication for the use of hypnotic drugs other than the benzodiazepines, but if an alternative is required zopiclone is probably the most satisfactory substitute.

Hypnotic drugs in special circumstances

In renal failure. Some hypnotic drugs are excreted via the kidney so that accumulation occurs in patients with renal failure. Nitrazepam does not fall into this group and is satisfactory, but small doses should be used initially.

In liver failure. Temazepam is satisfactory, but should be used with care.

In respiratory disease. All hypnotic drugs produce some depression of respiration so they must be used with great care in patients with

---

Nursing points

Dependence can occur with long-term use of all hypnotics. Use the minimum dose for the minimum time.

Do not forget that depression causes insomnia.

respiratory failure and during attacks of asthma. Temazepam is as good as any.

In the elderly hypnotics should be avoided if possible. If nocturnal confusion is a problem thioridazine (see p. 154) is preferred.

Sedatives prior to minor procedures

Patients often require some sedation before such manoeuvres as gastroscopy, etc. Benzodiazepines are useful because they are both sedative and also produce amnesia for the event. **Diazepam** is often used intravenously. It is, however, irritant to the vein. A specially prepared non-irritant solution of diazepam, Diazemuls, is preferable. Alternatively, **midazolam**, which has an action lasting about 2 hours, can be given.

Following injections of this type the patient should be warned not to drive until the next day and to avoid alcohol or other depressants.

Adverse effects and interactions. There have been a number of reports of respiratory depression and cardiac arrest after midazolam, especially in elderly patients who do not eliminate the drug as rapidly as younger subjects. This is usually due to excessive dosage and care should be taken.

The action of midazolam is increased by erythromycin.

JET LAG

Rapid long flights, crossing several time zones, give rise to fatigue and loss of concentration and appetite on arrival. Flights to the West lead to early wakening and to the East, difficulty getting to sleep. This is due to the body clock becoming out of phase with the local time and it may take 2 or 3 days to adjust.

Melatonin which is secreted by the brain, helps this adjustment and there is some evidence that, if given orally in the evening, it helps sleep and reduces jet lag. It is not licensed as a medicine in the UK but is available in the USA and elsewhere. Until its use is regulated it is probably best avoided.

FURTHER READING

Burton E 1992 Drugs update: something to help you sleep? Nursing Times 88(8): 52

Editorial 1995 Management of anxiety and insomnia. MeReC Bulletin 6(10): 37

Editorial 1995 Zopiclone and zolpidem. MeReC Bulletin 6(11): 41

Editorial 1998 Melatonin for jet lag? Drug and Therapeutics Bulletin 36(2): 15

Espre C A 1993 Practical management of insomnia. British Medical Journal 306: 509

Gillin J C, Byerley W F 1990 The diagnosis and management of insomnia. New England Journal of Medicine 322: 239

Hodgson L A 1991 Why do we need sleep? Relating theory to nursing practice. Journal of Advanced Nursing 16: 1503

Kupfer D J, Reynolds C F 1997 Management of insomnia. New England Journal of Medicine 336: 341

Lader M 1988 A practical guide to prescribing hypnotic benzodiazepines. British Medical Journal 293: 1048

Reid E 1997 Intravenous sedation for short procedures and investigations. Nursing Standard 12(5): 35

Swift C G, Shapiro C M 1993 Sleep and sleep problems in elderly people. British Medical Journal 306: 1468

Tyrer P 1993 Withdrawal from hypnotic drugs. British Medical Journal 306: 706

11

Anaesthetics. Muscle relaxants. Cardiac arrest and resuscitation. Local anaesthetics

GENERAL ANAESTHESIA

General anaesthesia for surgery was first used in 1842 by William E. Clark, of Rochester, New York, for a dental extraction. He used **ether**, a drug that is still in use in parts of the world where more recent and expensive drugs are unavailable. Horace Wells, a dentist in Hartford, Connecticut, introduced **nitrous oxide** in 1844, also for dental extractions (he first persuaded a travelling lecturer in chemistry to give him nitrous oxide whilst a fellow dentist took out one of his teeth before he then used it successfully on his own patients). Nitrous oxide is still widely used as part of almost every general anaesthetic. **Chloroform** was introduced, in 1847, by James Y. Simpson, of Edinburgh, for use in general surgery and obstetrics. It was administered to Queen Victoria, in 1853, at the birth of Prince Leopold. Chloroform remained popular for over 100 years but is no longer used as a general anaesthetic.

PREMEDICATION

Premedication before general anaesthesia may be given to allay anxiety and, sometimes, to reduce oral secretions. However, this is not essential and it is now common practice not to administer any premedication.

The best treatment for anxiety is to listen to the patient, to allow sufficient time for them to fully express their concerns and worries, and to give clear and simple explanations and reassurance whenever possible. The nurse looking after the patient probably plays a more important part in this respect than anyone else.

Most patients are anxious before anaesthesia and surgery. Some feel a general sense of nervousness or apprehension, but have no particular concern or worry. Others may have one or more specific fears which may be of injections, of dying, of waking up in the middle of the operation, of waking up in pain, of talking during the anaesthetic (and perhaps giving away personal secrets), of the embarrassment of nakedness, or of the loss of control over themselves and their environment brought on by the sedative effects of drugs.

Drugs used to reduce anxiety or its effects include the *benzodiazepines, chlorpromazine derivatives,* and *opioids.* Oral and tracheal secretions are reduced using anticholinergic drugs. See Table 11.1 for a list of the commonly used drugs.

Premedication, if used, is given 1–2 hours before anaesthesia. Temazepam given orally is the usual choice; intramuscular injections are rarely used.

Nursing point

Always try to give patients the opportunity and time to ask any questions they wish and to fully express their anxieties before anaesthesia and surgery.

Table 11.1 Drugs used for premedication

Drug	Trade name	Dose	Usual route	Comments
Benzodiazepines				
Diazepam	Valium Diazemuls	10–20 mg	Oral, i.m. or i.v.	Potent anxiolytic but has no analgesic action. Good amnesic effect in larger doses. i.v preparation is Diazemuls
Lorazepam	Ativan	1–3 mg	Oral	Similar to diazepam but longer action
Temazepam		10–20 mg	Oral	Similar to diazepam but shorter action. A popular drug for premedication
Chlopromazine derivatives				
Promethazine	Phenergan	25–50 mg	Oral or i.m.	
Trimeprazine	Vallergan	2 mg per kg	Oral	Used for children only. Can cause marked pallor
Opioids				
Morphine		10–15 mg	i.m.	Good euphoric effect. Potent analgesic which may provide useful initial postoperative pain relief. Commonly causes nausea and sometimes vomiting after surgery. May cause respiratory depression in large doses or in combination with other drugs or in sick patients
Papaveretum		7.7–15.4 mg	i.m.	Similar to morphine (it is a mixture of alkaloids originally obtained from the poppy and of which the major component is morphine)
Meperidine		50–100 mg	i.m.	Less sedative and shorter action than morphine
Anticholinergic drugs				
Atropine		0.3–0.6 mg	Oral or i.m.	Dries mouth by reducing secretion of saliva. Causes marked tachycardia if given i.v. No sedative action
Glycopyrronium (Glycopyrrolate USP)	Robinul	0.2–0.4 mg	i.m. or i.v	Similar to atropine but causes less tachycardia when given i.v.
Hyoscine	Scopolamine	0.2–0.4 mg	i.m.	Similar to atropine but also has a potent sedative action

INTRAVENOUS INDUCTION AGENTS

Intravenous drugs, or induction agents, are usually used to start general anaesthesia, although a 'gas' induction using any of the inhalational anaesthetic agents is sometimes used, particularly for children. Intravenous induction agents only act for a few minutes and anaesthesia is then continued using inhalational anaesthetics and other intravenous drugs.

Thiopentone was first used in 1934 and is still in widespread use. It is a barbiturate. *Unconsciousness* occurs about 20 seconds after injection and continues for several (5–10) minutes. The termination of its action occurs as the drug is redistributed away from the brain into other tissues, particularly muscle and fat.

It is *metabolized very slowly* (several hours) and thus cannot be used as a continuous intravenous infusion as it would accumulate and lead to prolonged sleepiness or unconsciousness when discontinued (compare with propofol).

Loss of muscle tone and therefore of normal airway control occurs immediately after injection, as does a short period of *hypoventilation* (respiratory depression) and sometimes *apnoea*. It is therefore important to have facilities for lung ventilation and the delivery of oxygen immediately at hand.

It causes a small *drop in blood pressure*, mainly due to a reduction in peripheral resistance; a marked fall in blood pressure may occur if the injection is too rapid, the dose is too large or the patient is sick.

Accidental *intra-arterial injection* results in immediate and severe pain in the arm distal to the site of injection and, if concentrations greater than 2.5% are used, this may be followed by arterial spasm, loss of peripheral pulses and permanent ischaemic damage to parts of the arm. The risk of this occurrence is reduced by injecting the drug into a vein on the dorsum of the hand where arteries are rarely found, although extravascular injection can also result in tissue damage.

Methohexitone was first described in 1957. It is also a barbiturate and is similar to thiopentone, although it has a slightly shorter duration of action and is metabolized more quickly, but not fast enough to be used as a continuous infusion.

It is frequently *painful on injection* but the pain is along the line of the vein and does not reflect any damage to tissues. *Involuntary muscle movements, twitching and hiccups* are common minor side-effects of the drug. Intra-arterial or extravascular injection does not lead to tissue damage. It is rarely used except for ECT (electroconvulsive therapy—a treatment for depression).

Etomidate was first used in 1973. It is not a barbiturate. It is metabolized more quickly than either of the barbiturates and recovery is probably faster than from methohexitone. It also causes pain on injection and involuntary muscle movements.

It has *minimal or no effect on blood pressure* and for this reason is sometimes chosen for use in patients with cardiac problems. It is otherwise not commonly used.

Propofol, a commonly used agent, was first used in 1977, although it was not released for general use until 1986. It is dissolved in the oil phase of an emulsion of soybean oil and purified egg phosphatide and is white and looks like milk (like Diazemuls).

It is *very rapidly metabolized* (in a few minutes) and can therefore be used as a continuous low-dose intravenous infusion to provide prolonged periods of anaesthesia or to sedate patients for hours or days in intensive care wards.

Recovery from its effects is more rapid and complete than from any of the other induction agents; it is therefore commonly used for short procedures and in outpatients.

Like methohexitone and etomidate, propofol causes pain on injection, which can be considerably reduced by mixing it with lidocaine. It possibly causes more hypoventilation, apnoea and hypotension than the other agents (apart from ketamine), particularly if injected rapidly.

Ketamine is unique among the induction agents. Some of the differences between ketamine and other induction agents are:

1. It can be given *intramuscularly* as well as intravenously.
2. It has *potent analgesic activity* and produces a state known as dissociative analgesia in which the patient looks dreamily half awake and may move around a little but is, in fact, unaware of his or her surroundings and is free of any pain.

3. *Muscle tone is maintained* and therefore the patient retains the ability to maintain his or her own airway despite being unconscious. It is thus of particular use when adequate access to the head and neck is not possible as occurs in children receiving radiotherapy, some civilian transport disasters and casualties in the field of battle.

4. It causes a *rise in blood pressure* and is therefore popular for use in children with severe congenital heart disease.

5. During recovery *nightmares and hallucinations*, referred to as emergence phenomena, are common, except, apparently, in children. These effects are so unpleasant in adults that the drug is rarely used for adults except in the unusual circumstances mentioned in paragraph 3 above.

Nursing point

After ketamine has been used let the patient wake up peacefully, preferably in a quiet room with subdued lighting, and don't prod and shout at the patient to wake him or her up more quickly. This will reduce the incidence and severity of emergence phenomena—nightmares and unpleasant hallucinations.

MAINTENANCE OF ANAESTHESIA

There are three important groups of drugs used to maintain anaesthesia after the effects of the induction agents have worn off:

1. Inhalational anaesthetics
2. Short-acting opioids
3. Muscle relaxants.

INHALATIONAL ANAESTHETICS

Nitrous oxide is the original 'gas' or 'laughing gas', so called because it causes some patients to laugh during the induction of anaesthesia if used on its own. It is a faintly smelling gas that is compressed and stored as a liquid in cylinders (coloured blue in the UK). Even in concentrations up to 80% it is only a weak anaesthetic and it needs to be combined with other inhalational agents or intravenous drugs. Unlike the other inhalational anaesthetics, it has a powerful analgesic effect in concentrations less than those required to produce unconsciousness.

Entonox takes advantage of its analgesic properties. It is a 50 : 50 mixture of nitrous oxide and oxygen, stored as a compressed gas in cylinders (coloured blue and white in the UK). It is used for pain relief in labour, and by ambulance crews and others for pain relief outside hospital.

Halothane, enflurane, isoflurane and sevoflurane are potent halogenated hydrocarbons and have very similar structures and effects. Some of the differences between them are listed in Table 11.2. They are volatile liquids that require a carrier gas, usually oxygen and nitrous oxide, to deliver them, and vaporizers capable of delivering accurate concentrations in the range of 0.25–8%. Unlike nitrous oxide, they have no analgesic properties in sub-anaesthetic concentrations. Halothane is the oldest, but is now little used as it causes cardiac arrhythmias and, very rarely, severe hepatitis; isoflurane, the most commonly used, has little effect on cardiac output and is associated with a rapid recovery from anaesthesia. Sevoflurane is the most expensive but is particularly useful for inducing anaesthesia in children as it has a weak and not unpleasant smell and, in a high concentration of 8%, induces anaesthesia extremely rapidly—within a few breaths.

Desflurane, another recently introduced halogenated hydrocarbon, is not widely used; its place in general anaesthetic practice has yet to be established.

Ether is, of course, an historically important drug, but is no longer used except in a few parts of the developing world where resources and skills are limited. It is cheap, potent, fairly safe and can be used with simple and portable equipment using room air instead of cylinder oxygen. Induction of, and recovery from, anaesthesia are, however, very slow, and it has a pungent and unpleasant smell and is explosive.

SHORT-ACTING OPIOIDS

Long-acting opioids, such as morphine, are described elsewhere. In patients whose lungs

Table 11.2 Some inhalational anaesthetics

	Halothane	Enflurane	Isoflurane	Sevoflurane
Trade name	Fluothane	Ethrane	Forane	
First use in humans	1956	1966	1971	
Equipotent concentrations	0.8%	1.6%	1.2%	2.0%
Boiling point	50°C	56.5°C	48.5°C	58.5°C
Cardiac arrhythmias	+++	+	0	0
Hypotension	+	+	++	+
Cost	+	++	+++	+++++
Amount of absorbed drug metabolized	20%	2%	0.2%	5%
Potential for organ damage	Very rarely causes severe hepatitis	Causes mild, reversible renal tubular damage in large doses	None	None

are ventilated by machine during anaesthesia, potent and short-acting opioids are commonly used and safe. They have three very useful actions contributing to general anaesthesia:

1. Profound analgesia
2. Sedation and, in large doses, hypnosis
3. Intense respiratory depression (in this situation, a useful effect!).

They have almost no effect on blood pressure and, in large doses, they reduce the need for inhalational anaesthetic agents to a minimum. Of the three commonly available, **fentanyl** is the most popular. The only significant differences between them are the doses required and their duration of action (see Table 11.3).

If necessary, as with the longer-acting opioids, their action may be easily reversed at the end of an anaesthetic using **naloxone**. This may be necessary to correct any respiratory depression but, of course, it will also reverse any analgesia and may leave the patient in pain.

Remifentanil is a new and different class of opioid. Unlike any other opioid it is rapidly metabolized by non-specific tissue esterases and thus its elimination is unaffected by renal or hepatic function. The action of remifentanil is so short—a few minutes—that it is generally given

Table 11.3 Short-acting opioids

	Approximate equipotent doses	Approximate duration
Alfentanil	500 micrograms	10 min
Fentanyl	100 micrograms	30 min
Phenoperidine	1 mg	60 min
Morphine	10 mg	4 hours

as a continuous infusion. Because of its potency, short action and lack of cardiovascular side-effects it is likely to find a useful place in the management of general anaesthesia for major operations on patients with heart disease whom it is planned to wake up quickly at the end of surgery. It does not have a place in the management of postoperative pain.

MUSCLE RELAXANTS (NEUROMUSCULAR BLOCKING AGENTS)

The introduction of muscle relaxants into anaesthetic practice in the 1940s has been claimed as the greatest single advance in anaesthesia made this century.

Curare was the first such drug to be used and is an alkaloid extracted from the bark, leaves

Table 11.4 Muscle relaxants

Drug	Type of blocker	Duration of action	Reversal of action	Other points
Atracurium Vecuronium	Competitive	20–30 minutes	Neostigmine (with atropine or glycopyrronium)	The most commonly used
Cisatracurium	Competitive	20–30 minutes	Neostigmine (with atropine or glycopyrronium)	Causes less histamine release than atracurium
Rocuronium	Competitive	20–30 minutes	Neostigmine (with atropine or glycopyrronium)	Fastest onset of action of all competitive blockers
Mivacurium	Competitive	10–15 minutes	Neostigmine (with atropine or glycopyrronium)	Often causes marked histamine release leading to cutaneous flushing and tachycardia
Gallamine Pancuronium	Competitive	45–60 minutes	Neostigmine (with atropine or glycopyrronium)	Older, rarely used drugs. Should not be used in renal failure as renal secretion is significant
Suxamethonium	Depolarizing	2–5 minutes	Cannot be reversed with drugs	Causes postoperative muscle pains and tenderness. Prolonged action in 1 in 2800 patients

and vines of the tropical plant, *Chondrodendron tomentosum*, found around the upper reaches of the Amazon. Crude preparations of this plant have long been used by South American Indians to poison the tips of their arrows. Since the 1940s many new relaxants have been produced and those in current use, and some of the differences between them, are listed in Table 11.4.

Clinical use

Most anaesthetics involve the use of muscle relaxants for which there are three main indications:

1. To facilitate intubation of the trachea with an endotracheal tube at the start of an anaesthetic.
2. To relax muscles sufficiently to make surgery possible. This applies particularly to abdominal surgery for which relaxed abdominal musculature is necessary for easy access to, and closure of, the abdomen.
3. To enable easy ventilation of the lungs by machine or hand. There are many situations in anaesthesia when it is better to ventilate lungs mechanically than let patients breathe spon-

taneously. These include lengthy surgery, chest surgery and severe cardiorespiratory disease.

Mechanism of action

These drugs act at the neuromuscular junction (or motor end plate) by blocking the transmission of nerve impulses from nerve to muscle (see Fig. 11.1). When a nerve supplying a voluntary muscle is stimulated, *acetylcholine* is liberated from vesicles in the nerve ending and acts on special receptor sites on the muscle to produce a change known as depolarization. This is followed by contraction of the muscle fibre. The *acetylcholine* is then rapidly broken down by the enzyme cholinesterase and repolarization occurs. The muscle is now ready to be stimulated again. Should depolarization persist (see Depolarizing muscle relaxants) then the muscle would remain unresponsive to further stimulation.

Competitive or non-depolarizing muscle relaxants

Two types of block are produced by muscle relaxants. Most are competitive blockers—that

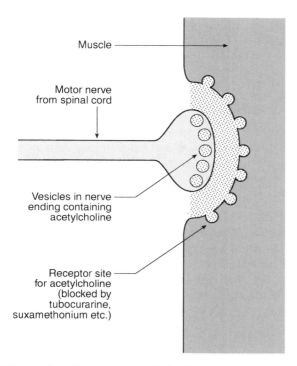

Figure 11.1 The neuromuscular junction.

is, they occupy receptor sites for acetylcholine and so render ineffective the acetylcholine that is released following nerve stimulation.

Atracurium and vecuronium have a medium duration of action of 20–30 minutes and are the most commonly used competitive blockers. **Neostigmine** reverses their effects more quickly than the longer-acting drugs. Only minimal vecuronium, and no atracurium, is excreted by the kidney.

Cisatracurium is a single isomer of atracurium and leads to less histamine release than atracurium, and therefore less cutaneous flushing and drop in blood pressure.

Rocuronium has the most rapid onset of action of all the non-depolarizing muscle relaxants, particularly if given in a high dose.

Mivacurium has a short duration of action of 10–15 minutes, which is so short that it is rarely necessary to reverse its action with **neostigmine**. It causes marked histamine release with consequent cutaneous flushing, tachycardia and sometimes hypotension.

Gallamine and pancuronium are much older drugs with a long duration of action of 45–60 minutes; they are rarely used. Their effects may be reversed by the anticholinesterase drug **neostigmine**. They are predominantly excreted by the kidney.

Depolarizing muscle relaxants

These drugs also occupy receptor sites for acetylcholine. However, they initially stimulate the muscle to contract (visible as the 'twitching' that occurs almost immediately after they are injected) and then produce a state of persistent depolarization during which no further stimulation is possible.

Suxamethonium is the only representative of this group in current use. It has a short duration of action of 2–5 minutes and is mainly used for endotracheal intubation at the beginning of anaesthesia and for very short procedures requiring relaxation.

A total of 1 in 2800 of the population will have a prolonged period of paralysis of up to 2 or 3 hours (suxamethonium apnoea) due to a genetically determined and familial abnormality of the enzyme cholinesterase that is normally responsible for the rapid breakdown of this drug.

A common side-effect is muscle pain and tenderness, particularly in the chest and abdomen, often severe, and occurring about 24 hours after it has been given.

> **Nursing point**
>
> 'Suxamethonium pains'. Look out for patients, mostly young adults, who complain, about 24 hours after surgery, of pain and tenderness in their muscles, usually of the abdomen and chest. These symptoms may follow the use of suxamethonium and can sometimes be very severe.

Anticholinesterases

These drugs have two main uses:

1. Reversal of muscle relaxants
2. Treatment of myasthenia gravis.

Reversal of muscle relaxants

The effects of the competitive, non-depolarizing, muscle relaxants may be allowed to wear off spontaneously. However, the effects can be reversed more quickly by using one of the anticholinesterase drugs. (Compare the depolarizing muscle relaxant, suxamethonium, whose effects cannot be reversed with drugs.) Anticholinesterases act at the neuromuscular junction where they temporarily inhibit the enzyme *cholinesterase*, which normally breaks down acetylcholine, and so allow *acetylcholine* to rise in concentration and therefore increase its duration of action. This helps the return of normal neuromuscular transmission and muscle strength.

Neostigmine is the drug of this group most commonly used to reverse muscle relaxants.

Edrophonium is also effective in reversing muscle relaxants, although, possibly, less so than neostigmine when used to reverse the effects of the long-acting muscle relaxants.

Myasthenia gravis

This disease is due to progressive destruction of the neuromuscular junction of voluntary muscles by antibodies and is characterized by muscle weakness and fatigue. *Acetylcholine* is no longer as effective as normal as a transmitter at the neuromuscular junction and therefore the symptoms of weakness and fatigue may be completely or partially relieved with anticholinesterases which, by inhibiting the enzyme *cholinesterase*, increase the amount of *acetylcholine* available.

Pyridostigmine is the longest-acting anticholinesterase and probably has the least side-effects. It can only be given orally.

Neostigmine, given orally, acts for up to 4 hours. It can be given intravenously for the emergency management of myasthenia gravis, but side-effects are common by this route and it must be given with atropine.

Edrophonium is the shortest acting, can only be given intravenously and is mostly used to establish the diagnosis of myasthenia gravis.

Corticosteroids, because of their immuno-suppressive action, improve the majority of patients. It is important to start with a low dose, which is slowly increased until optimal results are obtained. Occasionally patients become temporarily worse after starting steroids.

Side-effects of anticholinesterases

Unfortunately, anticholinesterases also have cholinergic effects at sites other than the neuromuscular junction: namely, at peripheral parasympathetic nerve endings. The most important effects of this are:

1. A bradycardia—this can be very marked and therefore dangerous
2. An increase in salivation and tracheo-bronchial secretions
3. An increase in peristaltic activity in the gut, causing colic and diarrhoea.

Fortunately, these effects can be prevented by giving one of the anticholinergic drugs (atropine or glycopyrronium—see below) at the same time as the anticholinesterase.

Anticholinergic drugs

These drugs temporarily block the effects of acetylcholine, particularly at postganglionic parasympathetic nerve endings, and have three uses during anaesthesia:

1. To reduce tracheobronchial and salivary secretions. They may be included as part of premedication for this purpose.
2. To increase the pulse rate.
3. To prevent the unwanted effects of the anticholinesterases.

Atropine (see p. 49), glycopyrronium and hyoscine are the drugs used for these purposes. Glycopyrronium has a longer duration of action than atropine and causes less temporary tachycardia when given with neostigmine. Hyoscine also causes marked sedation and can therefore *only* be used as part of premedication.

Malignant hyperpyrexia

Susceptibility to this extremely rare disorder is

familial and genetically determined. Malignant hyperpyrexia may be triggered by exposure to *suxamethonium* (but not to any of the non-depolarizing muscle relaxants) and to any of the halogenated hydrocarbon inhalational anaesthetics—*halothane, enflurane, isoflurane, sevoflurane* or *desflurane*—but not to nitrous oxide or, curiously, almost any other drug. It starts with excessive metabolic activity in muscle cells which leads to muscular rigidity, a high temperature and widespread severe metabolic disturbances. It used to have a high mortality.

Dantrolene, if given promptly and combined with aggressive treatment of the metabolic problems, markedly reduces mortality from this disorder. It acts at an intracellular level and reduces the excessive metabolic activity in the muscle cells. Every operating department should stock sufficient amounts of this drug to treat one patient although, of course, it will very rarely be required. It is very expensive.

MISCELLANEOUS RELAXANTS

Patients with disorders of the musculoskeletal system and of the central nervous system may suffer from muscle spasm. This spasm can produce pain and deformity, and, if the spasm could be relieved without altering normal muscle function, patients could be helped considerably.

There are now several drugs which claim to relax such spasm, probably by damping down reflexes in the spinal cord.

Diazepam acts on the spinal cord and has some antispasmodic effects. Fairly large doses, i.e. 10 mg t.d.s., are usually required and sedation can be a problem.

Baclofen is similar to diazepam but is less sedating. The dose is 5–20 mg t.d.s. but this may cause nausea, particularly with the larger doses.

Dantrolene has a direct inhibiting effect on skeletal muscle and reduces spasm in this way. However, muscle power is reduced in parallel with the decrease in spasticity and this limits dosage. The initial dose of 25 mg daily is slowly increased.

LOCAL ANAESTHETICS

Local anaesthesia for surgery was first used in 1884 when **cocaine** was used for ophthalmic surgery by Carl Koller, in Vienna. The use of cocaine for nerve blocks was first described by William S. Halstead in 1885; unfortunately, Halstead soon became addicted to cocaine after he had experimented on himself with too many nerve blocks.

Local anaesthetics produce a reversible inhibition of conduction along nerves and, in sufficient concentration, produce a complete sensory and motor blockade.

However, the fine, unmyelinated, nerve fibres that conduct pain sensation are more easily blocked by local anaesthetics than the thicker, heavily myelinated, motor fibres to muscle, and so, if an appropriate low dose or concentration of local anaesthetic is used, it is possible to provide good analgesia without the loss of too much motor function. This is best illustrated by observing the effects of an epidural during labour in which there is good pain relief and yet the patient is still able to move her legs.

There are several ways of giving local anaesthetics:

1. Direct application to mucous membranes
2. Direct application to the skin
3. Intradermal injection
4. Local infiltration of subcutaneous tissues, or deeper to involve muscles, other soft tissues or periosteum
5. Local nerve blocks
6. Extradural injection (an 'extradural', 'epidural' or 'caudal')
7. Subarachnoid injection (a 'spinal')
8. Intravenous injection (a 'Bier's block').

A **Bier's block**, otherwise called intravenous analgesia, is established as follows. The arm is elevated for a few minutes to encourage the drainage of as much blood as possible. Further exsanguination may be achieved by applying an Esmarch bandage. A previously applied blood pressure cuff is inflated to above arterial blood pressure. 40 ml of 0.5% prilocaine is then injected into a previously inserted cannula in a vein in the dorsum of the hand. The prilocaine now spreads through all the vessels in the arm below the blood pressure cuff and after a few minutes this will produce complete analgesia of the arm below the cuff. A similar procedure can be undertaken in the leg, but requires 100 ml of 0.5% prilocaine.

Nursing point

Do not forget that the patient will be conscious during procedures carried out under local anaesthesia. Conversation between staff should be at a minimum, but the patient should be reassured throughout.

Vasoconstrictors and local anaesthetics

Some local anaesthetics are vasodilators which, by increasing local blood flow, hasten the removal of the drug from the site of action. If **epinephrine** is mixed with the drug, then the vasoconstriction it produces will delay the removal of the drug and so prolong the duration of its action.

Felypressin (Octapressin), is a safer alternative to epinephrine. It is an analogue of vasopressin and is a powerful vasoconstrictor, but has none of the potentially serious effects that epinephrine has on the heart.

Epinephrine must never be used with local anaesthetics given intravenously, as in a Bier's block, because of its obvious dangerous effects on the heart. Neither should vasoconstrictors be used for blocks around the base of the penis or for 'ring' blocks of the fingers or toes; they may severely interrupt the blood supply and cause permanent ischaemic damage to the penis or digit.

Toxicity of local anaesthetics

All local anaesthetics have dangerous side-effects at doses only a little above those used for the more extensive blocks. Care must therefore be taken to calculate the total dose used when establishing any block. See Table 11.5 for maximum doses.

Nursing point

A 1% solution equals 1 g in 100 ml
or 10 mg in 1 ml

Only by knowing this can the amount of drug given be calculated.

Table 11.5 Summary of important local anaesthetics

Drug	Trade name	Maximum dose		Main uses
		plain	with adrenaline	
Lidocaine	Xylocaine Xylocard Xylotox	200 mg	500 mg	ALL local anaesthetic techniques Cardiac arrhythmias
Bupivacaine	Marcaine	150 mg	150 mg	All infiltration techniques Epidurals, caudals and spinals (NEVER for intravenous analgesia—Bier's blocks)
Ropivacaine	Naropin	200 mg	—	As for bupivacaine
Prilocaine	Citanest	400 mg	600 mg	Intravenous analgesia (Bier's blocks) Dental blocks (often mixed with felypressin) Constituent (with lidocaine) of EMLA cream
Amethocaine				Surface analgesia in the eye
Oxybuprocaine				Surface analgesia in the eye
Cocaine		100 mg	—	Surface analgesia for intranasal surgery Surface analgesia in the eye

Signs of toxicity start with tinnitus, tremor and restlessness and progress to convulsions and cardiac and respiratory depression.

Lidocaine (Lignocaine) is the most commonly used local anaesthetic. It has a rapid onset of action and a duration of action of approximately 1–2 hours. It is a mild vasodilator and so has a much longer duration of action if mixed with epinephrine.

It is available in various concentrations and preparations, including an aerosol spray for use on mucous membranes, most commonly in the mouth, pharynx or trachea.

Lidocaine also depresses myocardial excitability and so is used to suppress ventricular arrhythmias such as may follow myocardial infarction or cardiac arrest. For this purpose it is given as a bolus injection or as a continuous, low-dose, intravenous infusion. (It will, of course, like all local anaesthetics, cause myocardial depression in overdose.)

Prilocaine is similar to lidocaine, although it has a slightly longer duration of action, is less potent and less toxic. Because it is less toxic than lidocaine, it is the preferred drug for intravenous analgesia, a 'Bier's block'. It is commonly used, with felypressin, for dental blocks. In doses greater than twice the recommended maximum, it causes cyanosis due to the formation of *methaemoglobin*.

Bupivacaine has a slower onset of action than lidocaine, but about twice the duration of action. It is particularly popular and suitable for continuous epidural analgesia in labour and for postoperative pain relief. It is probably markedly more toxic on the heart than other local anaesthetics and must therefore never be used for intravenous analgesia, a 'Bier's block'.

Ropivacaine is a new local anaesthetic whose duration of action is similar to that of bupivacaine but it is less cardiotoxic and, more interestingly, is associated with less motor blockade for the same degree of sensory blockade. This means that epidural and spinal analgesia produced by using ropivacaine leaves patients with greater power in, and better use of, their legs than they would have if bupivacaine had been used to provide the analgesia.

Amethocaine (Tetracaine) has a slow onset and a long duration of action. It is a vasodilator. It is, however, very toxic and can therefore never be given by injection. It provides excellent surface analgesia and is mostly used for conjunctival analgesia in the eye. It may also be used to provide skin analgesia for venepuncture (see below).

Oxybuprocaine is only used as a local anaesthetic in the eye. It causes less initial stinging sensation and has a shorter duration of action than amethocaine.

Cocaine (see page 309), the first of the local anaesthetics, is a very different drug.

It is an alkaloid obtained from the leaves of a tree, *Erythroxylon coca*, found in Bolivia, Brazil, Peru and other South American countries. For centuries it has been chewed by the peoples of these countries to produce euphoria and to increase their capacity for physical work.

It is absorbed well by mucous membranes and is used to provide surface analgesia in eye surgery and nose and throat surgery, where its intense local vasoconstrictor action is also a useful feature. It is available as a paste, and as solutions of various concentrations, for these purposes. It is too toxic for use by injection.

It has widespread sympathomimetic actions causing mydriasis (dilatation of the pupil), marked vasoconstriction, hypertension, tachycardia and ventricular arrhythmias; in overdose, sudden death due to ventricular fibrillation occurs. Headache, nausea, vomiting and abdominal pain are common. It causes excitement, restlessness, euphoria and confusion, and with increasing dosage, central nervous system depression, coma and convulsions.

It is a drug of addiction, which occurs after only a few doses. Not surprisingly, it is a controlled drug.

EMLA cream (Eutetic mixture of local anaesthetics) is a unique preparation. If powders of lidocaine and prilocaine are mixed together, a eutectic mixture is formed—that is, the consistency changes from a powder to a paste. Substances are then added to this paste to make a cream, containing 2.5% lidocaine and 2.5% prilocaine, suitable for application to the skin.

Absorption through the skin is slow, but application for at least 45 minutes produces adequate analgesia and EMLA cream is now used extensively to allow pain-free venepuncture, particularly in children.

Amethocaine gel (Ametop) is another preparation designed to allow pain-free venepuncture. It may have a quicker onset of action than EMLA cream and it may cause more vasodilation and so make venepuncture easier. It should be removed after 60 minutes as it may cause marked skin irritation if left on too long.

There are many other local anaesthetics, old and new, amongst which are **procaine**, **mepivacaine** and **benzocaine**, all of which are still available, although they are rarely used. They are sometimes used as constituents of proprietary drug mixtures.

DRUGS USED FOR CARDIOPULMONARY RESUSCITATION

Useful guidelines to basic life support and advanced life support are given by the Resuscitation Council (UK) in *Resuscitation* (1997) 24: 104.

Basic life support

Once it is established that a patient is unconscious and unresponsive, then basic life support may be needed and consists of three parts:

1. *Airway*. The patient's airway should be cleared and kept open.
2. *Breathing*. If the patient is not breathing, then the lungs should be ventilated using mouth to mouth, or other, techniques as appropriate.
3. *Circulation*. If there is no pulse then cardiac massage should be started.

Advanced life support

If the appropriate drugs, equipment and skills are available, as they are in any hospital, then advanced life support is now started. Initially three things are done:

1. *Oxygen*, instead of the resuscitator's expired gas, is used to ventilate the lungs and, often, *tracheal intubation* is undertaken to facilitate efficient lung ventilation.
2. An *intravenous infusion* is established, preferably into a central vein, i.e. a large vein in the neck or groin, from where drugs will reach the heart quickly in an arrested circulation.
3. An *ECG machine is connected* so that the exact rhythm disturbance and the effects of treatment can be seen.

Treatment is now aimed at reversing the life-threatening arrhythmia using drugs and defibrillation as indicated in the algorithm in Figure 11.2.

Epinephrine (adrenaline) is used to convert asystole to ventricular fibrillation, which may then be converted to sinus rhythm by defibrillation. Epinephrine does not, of course, convert ventricular fibrillation to sinus rhythm. Epinephrine is also important because it raises peripheral resistance and, therefore, blood pressure and so improves coronary and cerebral circulation. It also increases myocardial contractility. It should be given every 2–3 minutes during resuscitation in a dose of 1 mg (1 ml of 1 in 1000 or 10 ml of 1 in 10 000).

Large doses of epinephrine cause dilatation of the pupils and this effect may be misinterpreted as evidence of persistent and severe brain damage during and shortly after resuscitation.

Atropine is given to increase cardiac rate. Bradycardia is common during recovery from

---

Nursing point

1 mg of epinephrine = 1 ml of '1 in 1000'
or 10 ml of '1 in 10 000'

This information is important during cardiopulmonary resuscitation. (It is unfortunate that the concentration of epinephrine is still given in such a curious manner—1 in 1000 means 1 g in 1000 ml. The concentration of NO other drug is indicated in this way.)

ADULT ADVANCED LIFE SUPPORT

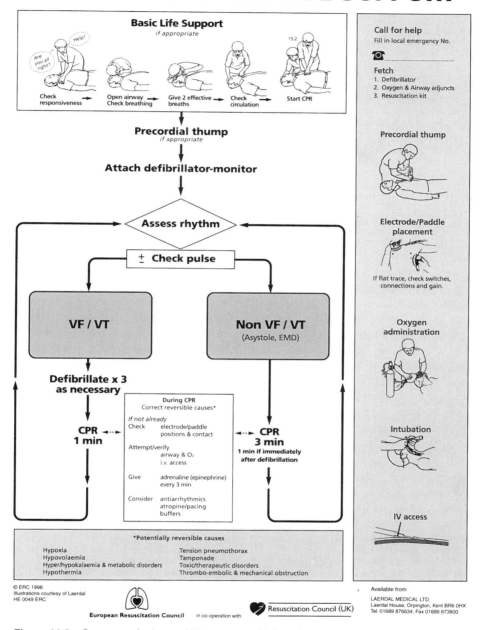

Figure 11.2 Summary of advanced life support guidelines for use in the UK, 1998.
(Reproduced by permission of the Resuscitation Council (UK) and Laerdal Medical Ltd.)

cardiac arrest. Atropine, like epinephrine, causes dilatation of the pupils.

Lidocaine reduces the excitability of myocardial cell membranes and so reduces the incidence of abnormal rhythms that appear during resuscitation. It also reduces the incidence of reversion of sinus rhythm back to ventricular fibrillation that sometimes occurs after successful defibrillation. Dosage must, however, be limited as it is also a potent myocardial depressant.

Calcium chloride, once popular, is no longer recommended for routine use during resuscitation except when there is a specific indication, e.g. hypocalcaemia, hyperkalaemia or calcium antagonist toxicity. Nevertheless, it is still sometimes used, and is effective, during electromechanical dissociation in an otherwise normal heart.

Sodium bicarbonate is used to correct the metabolic acidosis that occurs following prolonged inadequate tissue perfusion. Overenthusiastic use can cause serious hypernatraemia and, paradoxically, intracellular acidosis. It should therefore be withheld for the first 30 minutes of resuscitation and then be given in small amounts (e.g. 50 mmol) or in response to the measurement of blood acid–base status.

Adenosine, amiodarone, digoxin, esmolol, isoprenaline, magnesium, potassium and verapamil may all be used occasionally for the treatment of peri-arrest arrythmias.

Route of administration of drugs during CPR

The ideal route for the administration of drugs is via a *central vein*, i.e. a vein in the neck or the groin, from where drugs can easily reach the coronary circulation where they are required. If a *peripheral vein* is used then the drug should be flushed generously through the vein with saline or 5% glucose as the peripheral circulation will be sluggish.

Lidocaine and atropine are also absorbed fairly reliably through the *lungs*, if given in twice the normal dose down the endotracheal tube. This route may thus be worthwhile using if intravenous access has not been established. However, it is doubtful if sufficient epinephrine can be absorbed via this route.

Intra-osseous administration is effective and is gaining popularity in children. Finally, the use of the long *intracardiac needle* to administer drugs is dangerous and should rarely, if ever, be used: there is a danger of intramyocardial injection, intrapericardial haemorrhage and pneumothorax.

FURTHER READING

Adams A P, Cashman J N 1991 Anaesthesia, analgesia and intensive care. Edward Arnold, London
Drachman D B 1994 Myasthenia gravis. New England Journal of Medicine 330: 1797
Guidelines for Resuscitation 1997 European Resuscitation Council, Antwerp, Belgium
Nieman J T 1992 Cardiopulmonary resuscitation. New England Journal of Medicine 327: 1075
Wicker P 1994 Local anaesthesia in the operating theatre. Nursing Times 90: 34

12

Drugs used in psychiatry

INTRODUCTION

Mental illness is one of the major causes of ill health. During the last 40 years many drugs have been produced with the hope that they would have some therapeutic effect. Certain mental illnesses, particularly depression and schizophrenia, are linked with chemical abnormalities in the brain. The nature of some of these abnormalities is known, but there are considerable gaps in our knowledge.

Most drugs used in psychiatry interfere with the action of transmitter substances on receptors. The important known transmitters are acetylcholine, epinephrine and norepinephrine, dopamine, and 5-hydroxytryptamine (5-HT), GABA (gamma aminobutyric acid) and neuropeptides. Most of these substances have, in addition, well-defined actions outside the brain (see p. 35). Acetylcholine probably acts as a transmitting agent between nerve cells in the brain. Epinephrine and norepinephrine may act in a similar fashion. If the amounts of epinephrine and norepinephrine are increased in the brain by giving drugs (amine oxidase inhibitors) which retard their breakdown or interfere with their reabsorption (tricyclic antidepressants), an awakening and stimulating effect is produced. If the amount of these substances in the brain is reduced, a tranquillizing or depressing effect is produced. 5-HT also seems to be concerned with mood. GABA exerts a sedating inhibiting effect. Dopamine stimulates more than one class of receptor. It causes nausea and vomiting but also appears to be concerned with the schizoid state.

One further point is worth remembering. Formerly it was considered that the cerebral cortex was the part of the brain largely concerned with consciousness. It is now realized that the reticular formation, a band of tissue running through the brain stem, is also important, and it is the interaction between this formation and the cerebral cortex which maintains the state of wakefulness. It seems that some drugs which are used in psychotherapy act on this area of the brain. In addition, the limbic system is concerned with various emotions entering consciousness.

During the last 40 years many drugs which might be useful in mental disease have been produced, but testing them is difficult. At the animal level it is impossible to reproduce exactly in the laboratory psychological disorders which are seen in humans and therefore the drugs are put through a battery of tests which it is hoped will pick out those which are potentially useful as therapeutic agents. Trials of these drugs in humans are also fraught with difficulty and not all of their alleged usefulness will stand up to scientific examination. The nurse, therefore, must be on guard against extravagant claims for new drugs in this field and should temper enthusiastic claims with careful and impartial observations.

Special points in the administration of drugs to psychiatric patients

1. In hospital many psychiatric patients are not confined to bed and drugs may be given out at a central point rather than having a 'drug round'.

2. Two nurses should always be concerned with drug administration.

3. In psychiatric patients compliance may be a problem and it is necessary to ensure that medication is actually taken.

4. In some patients, especially schizophrenics, drugs may be given by injection as depot preparations to get round the problem of non-compliance.

5. Occasionally a patient's paranoia may extend to drugs they are given.

6. Drug education for when the patient returns home is very important and relatives may have to be involved. Non-compliance is an important hazard as the patient's illness may relapse if treatment is stopped. It should also be possible for patients or relatives to ring up for information if problems arise.

7. The nurse should observe the effects of drug treatment.

8. On discharge, care should be taken not to prescribe excessive quantities of drugs, particularly if there is a suicide risk.

NEUROLEPTICS

These drugs are particularly useful in controlling the states of agitation found in acute schizophrenia, mania and some other forms of delirium and in paranoia. Their exact mode of action in these conditions is not known but most of them block the action of dopamine on D_2 receptors in the mesolimbic system of the brain and this seems important in their sedative and antipsychotic action (Fig. 12.1). They also block the action of dopamine on the CTZ and are thus anti-emetic (see p. 105), and in the extrapyramidal system which may cause various disorders of movement and posture (see later).

The phenothiazines

1. They have an antipsychotic effect. Restlessness, agitation and hallucinations are reduced and this has made them especially useful in treating schizophrenia.

2. They produce some sedation with a feeling of detachment from external worries and troubles.

3. Many of them have some anti-emetic action.

4. Chlorpromazine is sometimes used to control persistent hiccup.

In addition, peripheral effects include anticholinergic blockade and some blockade of α-adrenergic receptors.

Most of the phenothiazines are well absorbed after oral dosage. They are largely metabolized in the liver to numerous breakdown substances.

A number of phenothiazines are now used in treatment: some are preferred for one type of

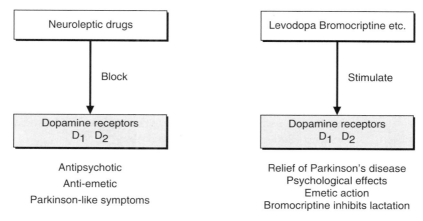

Figure 12.1 Effect of drugs on dopamine receptors in the brain. The exact part played by D_1 and D_2 receptors and other subgroups is not known.

disorder, some for another. Table 12.1 gives some of the most commonly used drugs in the group.

The doses of these drugs are very variable and depend on the disorder being treated and the response and age of the patient. In long-term administration, it is not worth altering the dose more than once a week *because of their variable and prolonged action.*

Adverse effects are not uncommon and the incidence varies from drug to drug. They include:

1. Jaundice. This occurs with chlorpromazine and is due to blocking of the bile canaliculi in

Table 12.1 Classification of phenothiazines

Name	Trade name	Salient feature	Dose* (24 hour)
Group I—sedative			
Chlorpromazine	Largactil	Widely used as a sedative in confused patients. Occasionally as an anti-emetic or in the anxious	50–300 mg orally. Can be given by injection.
Promazine	Sparine	Weaker than chlorpromazine, otherwise similar	50–400 mg orally
Group II—moderately sedative, less extrapyramidal effect			
Thioridazine	Melleril	Useful in agitated elderly patients. Can cause retinal damage	150–600 mg orally
Group III—less sedative, marked extrapyramidal effects			
Prochlorperazine	Stemetil	Used for vomiting and vertigo	15–75 mg orally. Can be given by injection
Trifluoperazine	Stelazine		5–15 mg orally.
Fluphenazine	Modecate	Used for depot injection in schizophrenia	12.5–100 mg as a single dose deep intramuscular every 14–35 days
Zuclopenthixol acetate	Clopixol	Used by injection for short-term management	50–150 mg i.m.

*These doses are only an approximate range. Low doses should be used in the elderly.

the liver. It is presumed to be an allergic effect, and recovery occurs when the drug is stopped.

2. Various disorders of movement due directly or indirectly to a dopamine blocking action in the brain. *These may occur with all neuroleptics.*

a. Parkinson-like syndrome.

b. Akathisia, which is a feeling of restlessness with an inability to stand still.

c. Dystonia, which is uncontrolled movements.

All these may commence soon after starting treatment and require a reduction of the dose if possible. Akathisia may be helped by a benzodiazepine and dystonic reaction and Parkinsonism by anticholinergic drugs such as benztropine.

d. *Tardive dyskinesia*, consisting of abnormal movements of the mouth and tongue and sometimes the upper limbs. It develops in about 20% of patients on longer-term neuroleptics. Its onset is usually delayed for a while. Control is difficult and it may not stop even if the drug is withdrawn.

3. Depression of white cells in the blood.

4. Skin rashes including light sensitivity and contact dermatitis when the drug is handled. A sunscreen is advised with chloropromazine.

5. An α-blocking effect on the sympathetic nervous system leading to a fall in blood pressure and faintness.

6. In elderly patients hypothermia may be precipitated.

7. There may be considerable weight gain and the development of gynaecomastia and impotence with these drugs.

8. Dry mouth can be troublesome.

9. Sedation, greatest with chlorpromazine.

10. Rarely, the *neuroleptic malignant syndrome* with hyperpyrexia, coma and muscular rigidity may develop; this requires urgent treatment.

In treating psychotic patients large doses of phenothiazines are often used and may have to be continued for many months or even longer. This means that a careful watch must be kept for side-effects, especially those involving the nervous system.

Therapeutics. The phenothiazines are used in psychiatry to reduce restlessness, anxiety and agitation in psychotic patients and to reduce the severity of hallucinations. They are thus useful in controlling schizophrenics who show these symptoms. They are sometimes used in low doses in psychoneurosis with anxiety.

They are, in addition, used as anti-emetics, in severe pruritus and in association with anaesthetic agents.

In the present state of knowledge it is impossible to say which is the best drug of this group. Patients seem to vary in their response to individual drugs and trial and error seems to be the only way to decide which is the best for any particular patient.

Nursing point

Staff should avoid contact with chlorpromazine (i.e. crushing tablets, etc.) because of the risk of contact sensitization.

The thioxanthenes

These are rather similar to the phenothiazines. They are antipsychotic and anti-emetic and are largely used in the treatment of schizophrenia. They are less sedative than the phenothiazines, but akathisia is rather common. Among them are:

Flupentixol used as an injected depot preparation every 2 weeks or as tablets daily.

The butyrophenones

This group of drugs has actions rather similar to those of the phenothiazines, they are less sedative, but are liable to produce extrapyramidal side-effects.

Haloperidol is widely used in doses of 0.5–2 mg three times daily orally and may be increased. It is particularly useful in the management of manic or confused patients when 2–10 mg 6 hourly by intramuscular injection may be used. In doses above 5 mg daily symptoms of Parkinsonism may develop.

Droperidol is similar but acts more rapidly. It can be given orally or by injection.

Other neuroleptics

Pimozide is an antipsychotic drug used in the treatment of schizophrenia and manic states. It is long-acting, less sedative than chlorpromazine.

Adverse effects. Pimozide can cause dangerous cardiac arrhythmias and should not be given to those who suffer from them. An ECG should be taken before starting treatment and repeated at 6-monthly intervals for those receiving high doses.

Sulpiride has a more specific dopamine-blocking action than the other neuroleptics but with less adverse effects. However, it can still cause the various disorders of movement.

Atypical antipsychotic drugs

This group of drugs differ from older neuroleptics in that they not only have overall less D_2 blocking action but the blockade may be confined to those areas of the brain believed to be concerned with schizophrenia (the mesolimbic system); in addition, they also block serotonin (5-HT) and adrenoreceptors. The result is that they seldom cause disorders of posture and movement and may be effective when older neuroleptics fail.

Clozapine is used for patients who have proved resistant to neuroleptic treatment. Because of its adverse effects profile, treatment should be started in hospital under careful supervision.

Adverse effects. These can be serious. About 3% of patients taking this drug for 1 year develop neutropenia, so monitoring of the blood count is mandatory. Other adverse effects include fits, hypotension, excessive salivation and sedation. It is also very expensive. Because of these problems clozapine is at present reserved for specially selected cases.

Risperidone blocks several receptors in the brain, including dopamine receptors. It appears to be useful in the negative symptoms of schizophrenia and extrapyramidal side-effects seem to be uncommon.

Olanzapine is similar to the above but, unlike clozapine, it does not depress the white count. It does, however, cause drowsiness and weight gain.

At present, it is impossible to say which is the preferred drug in this group, but they appear to offer advantages over the older neuroleptics. They are considerably more expensive and their use will probably be confined to patients who run into difficulties with standard neuroleptics. Other drugs in this group are becoming available.

Depot injections

Several antipsychotic drugs are given as depot injections including fluphenazine and flupentixol, because patients with severe mental disease often fail to take their pills regularly. Depot preparations given by deep intramuscular injection into the upper and outer part of the buttock or the lateral aspect of the thigh, using the Z technique, get round this problem. However, this dosage scheme is inflexible and there is difficulty if a patient develops some adverse effect. These injections may be very painful and seepage of fluid can result in inaccurate dosage unless the injection technique is well executed. Currently, newer and more effective ways of delivering depot injections are being tested.

Nursing point

Do not forget the adverse effects of this group of drugs, particularly those affecting the nervous system. With long-term use careful surveillance is also required on withdrawal of treatment as the re-emergence of symptoms may be delayed for several weeks.

Nursing point

Special care is needed if neuroleptics are given to:

1. Patients with Parkinson's disease as symptoms may be increased.
2. Epileptics or patients with alcohol withdrawal symptoms as fits may be precipitated.
3. Elderly patients who may get postural hypotension.
4. Pregnant and lactating mothers.

THE DRUG TREATMENT OF SCHIZOPHRENIA

Schizophrenia is a mysterious disease. It may take many forms but the essential feature is a change of personality with disordered thought processes which may be associated with hallucinations, delusions and withdrawal. Once it has developed complete recovery is unusual, although considerable improvement is possible. It usually starts in young people.

There are several theories as to its cause. It seems most likely that it is a complex biochemical disorder in the brain. The fact that symptoms can be relieved in many patients by dopamine blocking drugs supports the view that it is due to overactivity of the dopamine system, probably involving D_2 receptors in the mesolimbic system of the brain. However, not all patients respond to D_2 receptor antagonists and other receptors are probably involved. Although few would now support the idea that it is a disorder of personality development due to faulty interaction with the family in early life, it is probably made worse, or even precipitated, in susceptible individuals by periods of stress and difficulty.

The total management of the schizophrenic patient has many facets but the introduction and use of neuroleptic drugs have greatly improved treatment (Table 12.2). They have enabled many patients who, without treatment, would be confined to a mental hospital, to take their place in the community and lead a reasonable life. This requires very efficient social services to ensure that patients are properly supported. The dosage requires individual titration for each patient and drug treatment must be combined with support and management, especially the avoidance of stressful situations.

Drug treatment is started as soon as the diagnosis is confirmed. Haloperidol, up to 15 mg daily, or one of the other standard neuroleptics is used and symptoms should remit in 2 or 3 weeks. If a patient does not respond, a change can be made to an atypical antipsychotic drug. When the disorder is controlled, long-term maintenance treatment is required, either oral or by depot injection, and usually for life. Compliance may be poor and supervision is essential, otherwise relapses will occur.

Table 12.2 Some drugs used in treating schizophrenia

Drug	Sedation	Extrapyramidal effects	Usage
Chlorpromazine	++	++	Acute and long-term
Promazine	+	++	Acute and long-term
Haloperidol	+	+++	Acute, sometimes long-term
Pimozide	+	(+)	Long-term only
Flupentixol	+	+++	Depot injection
Clozapine	(+)	(+)	Subjects who do not respond to older drugs
Risperidone	+	(+)	
Olanzapine	++	(+)	

Nursing point

A schizophrenic patient receiving appropriate drugs may well behave normally, but, if treatment is stopped suddenly, there may be a catastrophic relapse.

MINOR TRANQUILLIZERS

The benzodiazepines

In addition to their use as hypnotics, this group of drugs is widely used as minor tranquillizers in anxious patients. It is believed that they act on the reticular formation and limbic system in the brain. There are specific receptors for benzodiazepines and they appear to enhance the action of a substance called GABA which is produced by the brain and which depresses brain function (Fig. 12.2).

All the benzodiazepines have much the same effect, being tranquillizing and sedative, but vary in their duration of action. The variation is due to different rates of breakdown in the body and some of them produce breakdown products which are themselves sedative and which thus prolong the action.

Although the benzodiazepines are effective in relieving anxiety they have two disadvantages:

1. They become less effective with prolonged use.

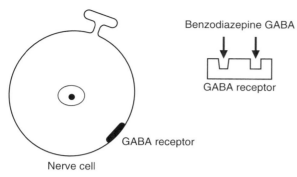

Figure 12.2 GABA and benzodiazepine receptors are closely related. Benzodiazepines enhance the inhibitory action of GABA.

Table 12.3 Benzodiazepines used as tranquillizers

Drug	Dose/day	Duration of action (approx.)	Special features
Diazepam	4–30 mg	24 hours	Can be used i.v. in status epilepticus
Chlordiazepoxide	30–60 mg	24 hours	
Oxazepam	45–120 mg	12 hours	
Lorazepam	1–4 mg	12 hours	May be more liable to cause dependence
Clonazepam	4–8mg	24 hours	Largely used in epilepsy
Clorazepate	15 mg	30 hours	

2. If the drug is stopped suddenly, even after a relatively short period of use (e.g. 2–3 weeks), about a third of patients will develop some withdrawal symptoms. These are anxiety and sleeplessness for a few days, but after prolonged and heavy dosage may include fits, psychotic symptoms, muscle pains and twitching. They usually occur within a week of stopping the drug and earlier if it is short-acting. This suggests that dependence has developed and in severe cases patients may take some months to recover. Patients, therefore, require slow and stepwise withdrawal of the drug over several weeks.

They should only be used for acute agitation, panic attacks and for anxiety if it is severe and disabling, and the treatment should be the lowest effective dose for no more than 2 weeks and combined with other treatment.

Previously, they have been used in acute emotional crises, but by preventing the patient responding to the painful situation they may delay psychological adjustment.

Diazepam and clonazepam are also given intravenously in treating status epilepticus (see p. 170) and diazepam and midazolam as sedatives before various investigations.

Diazepam also has some muscle relaxing properties and is used in combination with an analgesic to relieve pain and spasm in lumbago and related disorders.

The benzodiazepines are metabolized in the liver and often produce further active com-

pounds. For example, diazepam is partially converted to desmethyldiazepam which also has a prolonged sedative action.

Table 12.3 gives some of the benzodiazepines used as tranquillizers (see also table of hypnotics, p. 135).

Duration of action is also dependent on the dose and to some degree on the individual. Although the actions of these drugs are very similar the price varies considerably—diazepam is cheap and usually adequate.

Adverse effects and interactions. The group is very safe generally. Overdose can cause marked sedation, incoordination, memory difficulties and occasionally respiratory depression, but this is rarely serious in healthy individuals though fatalities have been reported. Interactions with other CNS depressants (e.g. alcohol) increase sedation and can be dangerous. Diazepam is irritant when given intravenously and should be given as an emulsion (Diazemuls).

The problem of dependence has been considered.

Flumazenil is a benzodiazepine antagonist. It is given intravenously and reverses benzodiazepine-induced sedation in a few minutes. It has been used in overdose and to speed recovery in patients who have been anaesthetized with midazolam (see p. 137). However, its effect only lasts about 1 hour so repeated doses may be required with long-acting benzodiazepines.

Buspirone is an attempt to produce an anxiolytic drug without adverse effects. It reacts with a group of 5-HT receptors. Buspirone appears to have no sedative action or risk of dependence; its only adverse effects are occasional nausea and headache. However, its onset of action is delayed for about 2 weeks and it seems to be ineffective in treating the symptoms of benzodiazepine withdrawal.

THE TREATMENT OF ANXIETY

Anxiety is a universal phenomenon and a certain amount is useful to the individual, acting as a stimulant and increasing efficiency. However, when it becomes disproportionate to the stimulus an anxiety state develops and this degree of anxiety may interfere seriously with the patient's life.

There are three main types of anxiety:

1. *General anxiety disorder (GAD)* in which the patient feels apprehensive and tense for no particular reason or as a result of some minor problem. In addition, there may be muscle aches, nausea, sleep problems and various other symptoms.
2. *Panic attacks* are unexpected attacks of anxiety, often with marked physical symptoms such as tremor, palpitation and dry mouth due to overactivity of the sympathetic nervous system.
3. *Phobic states* in which the patient fears certain situations. The commonest is agoraphobia in which the subject is frightened to go out and acute anxiety is precipitated by supermarkets or travelling on trains and buses, etc.—the syndrome of the homebound housewife.

Various methods of treatment may be used, including simple counselling, relaxation techniques and cognitive and analytical therapy.

Drugs may be given as part of the management plan, but they do not reveal or relieve the underlying cause. Benzodiazepines are the most commonly prescribed drugs and they are useful in controlling panic attacks. Prolonged use carries the risk of dependence and generally they should be avoided or used intermittently or for 1–2 weeks only.

β blockers such as propranolol 20 mg three times daily suppress the physical concomitants of anxiety (tremor and palpitations).

Buspirone can be useful, but there is a delay of several weeks before it becomes effective.

Antidepressants, both tricyclic and 5-HT, re-uptake inhibitors, in small doses are also helpful.

Phobic states are treated largely by behavioural methods and drugs play a minor part, though monoamine oxidase inhibitors are sometimes used.

THE MANAGEMENT OF ACUTE CONFUSIONAL STATES

Acute confusional states have many causes. They may be part of a psychiatric illness but often develop as a result of a serious 'organic' illness or may be due to drug dependence, e.g. alcohol withdrawal.

1. It is important that such patients are nursed in quiet surroundings. The nurses' approach must be calm and as much explanation given as is feasible.
2. If possible drugs should be given orally. The choice lies between a benzodiazepine such as diazepam, or a neuroleptic such as haloperidol. Chlorpromazine should not be given intramuscularly as it forms deposits in the muscle and may also cause hypotension. More seriously disturbed patients can be given lorazepam i.m. or droperidol i.m. *Patients confused as a result of alcohol withdrawal should not be given neuroleptics owing to the risk of fits.*

ANTIDEPRESSANT DRUGS
Depression

Depression is a common and normal emotion and people naturally become depressed as a result of unfortunate domestic and social conditions. Sometimes, however, the depression is disproportionate to the precipitating factors or there may be no obvious cause at all. This is an illness called *endogenous* or *psychotic* depression and is commoner in older people. Some psychiatrists recognize a further type of depressive illness in which environmental factors play a more promi-nent part and this is sometimes called reactive depression or *depressive neurosis*. Sometimes depression may alternate with attacks of mania. This is known as *bipolar depression* or *manic-depressive psychosis*.

In depression the mood is at its lowest in the morning and improves throughout the day. The patient is disinterested and may be irritable and anxious. The appetite is poor and vague symp-toms including headache and odd pains are common. *Suicide is a special risk in depressed patients*.

The cause of depression is not known but there is evidence that a major factor is a reduction in the amount of amines such as 5-HT or norepinephrine at the junctions between nerve cells in the brain. Many of the drugs used to treat depression increase the amount of these substances in the brain, thus providing some evidence that amines are connected with changes of mood.

The following groups of drugs are used to relieve depression:

- Tricyclic antidepressants
- Tricyclic anxiolytics
- 5-HT re-uptake inhibitors
- Other antidepressants
- Monoamine oxidase (MAO) inhibitors
- Lithium.

Tricyclic antidepressants

There are several tricyclic antidepressants in use and there is not a great deal of difference bet-ween them. They are well absorbed after oral administration and undergo considerable break-down in the liver; some of these metabolic pro-ducts are therapeutically active (Table 12.4). It is believed that they produce their therapeutic effect by preventing the re-uptake of amines at nerve endings in the brain which thus increases the concentration of these substances available for receptor uptake (Fig. 12.3).

Some members of the group (i.e. nortriptyline and desipramine) have a greater effect on norepinephrine concentration and others

Table 12.4   Other tricyclic antidepressants

Drug	Dose*/24 hours	Special features
Nortriptyline	20–50 mg	
Protriptyline	15–60 mg	Least sedative
Clomipramine	10–100 mg	Particularly useful in obsessional features
Lofepramine	140–210 mg	Least side-effects, sedation minimal

*Low doses should be used initially and in the elderly.

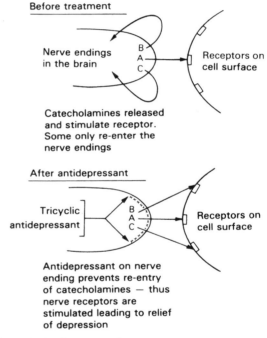

Figure 12.3   The mode of action of the tricyclic antidepressant drugs.

(imipramine and amitriptyline) on 5-HT con-centration.

Imipramine. The first of these drugs to be used. The usual dose is 25–150 mg daily.

Amitriptyline is very similar to imipramine but is rather more sedating. The usual dose range is 25–150 mg daily.

Both these drugs have a long action and need only be given once a day. If amitriptyline is given in the evening its sedative action will help sleep, which is often disturbed in depression.

Therapeutic use. After starting treatment the sleep disorders associated with depression usually respond fairly quickly, but it is important to remember that *it may take several weeks before the depression itself is relieved.*

The drug should therefore be continued for 6 weeks before deciding that treatment has failed. About 80% of depressed patients will ultimately respond.

Tricyclic antidepressants are also used in the treatment of pains of obscure origin such as atypical facial pain.

Blood concentration. Owing to the considerable intersubject variation in the breakdown of these drugs blood levels may vary widely. Extensive investigation has been carried out on the measurement of blood levels to control treatment but it is doubtful whether this is helpful in controlling dosage.

Adverse effects:

1. Anticholinergic effects. Dry mouth can be troublesome and may be mitigated by lemon juice. Elderly male patients may experience difficulty with micturition, and constipation can be a problem, particularly in depressed patients already preoccupied with their bowels. Owing to a dilating effect on the pupil of the eye, they should not be given to patients with glaucoma.

2. Postural fall in blood pressure with occasional faintness, especially in elderly patients.

3. Increased appetite and weight gain.

4. In patients with epilepsy, the tendency to fits is increased and the dose of anti-epileptic drugs may require alteration if tricyclic antidepressants are used.

5. They depress conduction in the heart, and a number of sudden deaths have been reported in patients with heart disease taking tricyclics. They are therefore best avoided in this group of patients.

6. Tricyclic antidepressants are dangerous in overdose, producing cardiovascular disturbance, fits and coma.

7. Withdrawal symptoms develop if the drug is stopped suddenly (see p. 165).

Interactions with other drugs occur, including antiepileptics, sympathomimetic drugs (but not local anaesthetics) and with other antidepressants and MAO inhibitors. They may reverse the effect of some hypotensive agents and their action is enhanced by alcohol, so care should be taken when combining tricyclics with other drugs.

Imipramine is used for *nocturnal enuresis* (bed wetting) in children. The dose is:

8–11 years	25–50 mg	2 hours before
12–16 years	50–75 mg	bedtime.

It is important to explain to the child's parents that:

1. The effect may be delayed for 2–3 weeks.
2. The tablets must be stored in a childproof place.
3. Treatment should not usually be given for more than 3 months.

Anxiolytic tricyclic antidepressants

Doxepin/Dosulepin. These drugs are similar to the tricyclic antidepressants, but have a weaker antidepressant action and are particularly useful when anxiety complicates mild depression. They are also more rapidly effective than the standard tricyclics.

Dose:

- Doxepin—50–100 mg at night
- Dosulepin—75–100 mg daily.

Adverse effects. Similar to the tricyclics but generally less marked. They are still dangerous in overdose.

Maprotiline is not a tricyclic drug, but is a re-uptake inhibitor. Its action and adverse effects profile is very similar to the tricyclics. It is also cardiotoxic.

Selective serotonin/5-HT re-uptake inhibitors (SSRI)

5-HT is concerned with mood and behaviour and a deficiency in the brain is believed to be a factor in depression. Several drugs have been introduced which specifically inhibit 5-HT re-uptake at nerve junctions and thus raise its concentration in the brain. Those available at present are:

Drug	Special points
Fluvoxamine	Dangerous interaction with methylxanthines
Fluoxetine	Long half-life (48 hours) and active metabolite. Rarely, serious hypersensitivity reaction.
Sertraline	
Paroxetine	Rarely, dystonic reaction
Citalopram	

In relieving depression these drugs are about as effective as the tricyclics and they have also been used in anxiety states. Their advantage lies in the lack of many of the adverse effects of the former group.

- They are not cardiotoxic and therefore less dangerous in overdose.
- They do not cause hypotension.
- There are no anticholinergic effects.
- They do not cause weight gain.
- They do, however, have other adverse effects.

Adverse effects. Nausea, diarrhoea, weight loss, headaches and insomnia are fairly common. Various hypersensitivity reactions can occur with fluoxetine and may herald a serious vasculitis. Blood dyscrasias are rare. Fluoxetine has been claimed to cause suicidal ideas and to produce personality changes beyond its antidepressive action, but this is dubious.

Interactions are important. Combination with lithium or MAO inhibitors can cause hyperthermia, coma and fits (serotonin-like syndrome) and an adequate gap must be left between stopping MAO inhibitors and starting these drugs. They may increase the blood level of tricyclic antidepressants.

It seems likely that ultimately they may replace tricyclic antidepressants on grounds of safety, but at present they are much more expensive (Table 12.5).

Other antidepressants

There are several other antidepressants which act by modifying the amount of amines in the brain but do not fit the above categories.

Table 12.5   Comparison of tricyclic and 5-HT re-uptake inhibitor antidepressants

	Tricyclics	5HT re-uptake inhibitors
Cardiotoxicity	++	−
Anticholinergic effects	+++	−
Sedation	+++ or +	−
Weight gain	++	−
Nausea	−	++
Price	Low	High

Trazodone has a mixed action on 5-HT receptors.

Therapeutic use. It is an antidepressant and also an anxiolytic. It is not cardiotoxic and may therefore be useful for patients with cardiac disease. It is fairly sedative and, at present, much more expensive than the standard tricyclics.

Venlafaxine is a combined 5-HT and norepinephrine re-uptake inhibitor. Its main advantage is that it relieves depression more rapidly than most antidepressants. Anticholinergic side-effects are rare but nausea and rashes can be a problem.

Nefazodone appears to be rather similar to trazodone.

Mirtazepine increases the concentration of norepinephrine and 5-HT in the brain and, by blocking some types of 5-HT receptors, has a more specific action on depression. It appears to be about as effective as the older antidepressants with a low incidence of side-effects. Rarely, it can produce depression of the white count.

Although these drugs are effective, they are rather expensive and rarely offer any special advantage.

Monoamine oxidase (MAO) inhibitors

These drugs irreversibly inhibit monoamine oxidase and thus interfere with the breakdown of epinephrine, norepinephrine and 5-HT in the brain and this leads to an accumulation of these substances. It is tempting to link this action with the antidepressive action of these drugs, but this has not been finally proved.

They produce a mood change with increase in cheerfulness, energy and well-being in about half of patients with depression. The main use for the MAO inhibitors is in atypical depression and phobic anxiety states. The long list of possible adverse effects limits their usefulness and they should only be prescribed by those who are familiar with the problems which may arise. The most important members of the group are:

Phenelzine which is given three times daily by mouth.

Isocarboxacid is similar.

Moclobemide is a *reversible* inhibitor of monoamine oxidase and has less risk of interactions with items of diet or with other drugs. However, the precautions outlined in the following are still necessary. The initial dose is 100 mg three times daily after food.

Adverse effects and interactions. Monoamine oxidase inhibitors can cause postural hypotension, insomnia and nervousness, difficulties with micturition and, rarely, jaundice.

Interactions are important and can be dangerous. They may exaggerate the effects of such centrally acting drugs as the barbiturates, alcohol, cocaine, morphine and particularly meperidine.

They also lead to over-action by vasopressors such as epinephrine and amfetamine and a number of vasoconstrictor drugs which are included in widely used 'cold-cures' may cause headaches, hypertension, restlessness and even coma and death. Similar effects may also occur if these MAO inhibitors are taken with various articles of food including cheese, meat, yeast extracts, some wines and beers, game, broad bean pods and pickled herrings. Hospitals often have their own cards listing restrictions. This is because these foods contain vasopressor substances which are normally broken down by MAO. If this breakdown is inhibited, the vasopressors accumulate and produce toxic effects. Therefore, the utmost care must be taken in administering these drugs and all those concerned with patients should be informed. If a surgical operation is to be undertaken, when it may be necessary to give such drugs as morphine or meperidine, the MAO inhibitors should be stopped 2 weeks previously. *It is dangerous to combine MAO inhibitors with tricyclic antidepressants or 5-HT re-uptake inhibitors.* There

---

> **Nursing point**
>
> A persistent headache is often a warning of rising blood pressure in a patient on MAO inhibitors.

should be a gap of 5 weeks between treatment with fluoxetine and MAO inhibitors.

Lithium

Lithium is treated by the body in a similar way to sodium. It is believed to modify neurotransmission in the brain. Lithium is used in treating patients with *bipolar depression (manic-depressive psychosis)*. It is given regularly to prevent mood swings in these patients. It will control acute mania, but is slow to produce a therapeutic effect and haloperidol is usually preferred in this situation. Before starting treatment with lithium, renal function must be checked as retention of the drug may occur if it is impaired. The dose usually lies between 0.4 and 1.2 g daily, and is adjusted to produce a blood level of 0.4–0.9 mmol/litre in a blood sample taken 12 hours after dosing. If the slow-release preparation (Priadel) is used, the tablet must be swallowed whole. Because lithium is excreted slowly it takes some days of treatment before a steady blood level is reached and it is usual to start measuring blood levels 1 week after starting treatment. Blood should be taken 12 hours after dosing and it is important not to collect it in tubes which use lithium heparin as the anticoagulant. Once a satisfactory dose is established monitoring is only required monthly.

Adverse effects can be divided into two groups—those due to overdosage and those which do not appear to be dose-related.

Overdose	Not dose-related
Weakness	Thyroid deficiency
Drowsiness	Increased urine secretion
Confusion	Weight gain
Coma	

Anything which depletes the body of sodium increases the toxicity of lithium. This includes not only diuretics (see later), but prolonged vomiting or diarrhoea.

Interactions. If a thiazide or loop diuretic is combined with lithium the excretion of lithium by the kidney is reduced and toxicity may develop. Under these circumstances the dose of lithium must be reduced and the blood level carefully monitored. Interaction can also occur with NSAIDs, ACE inhibitors and other antidepressants.

Special point for patient education

Different preparations of lithium vary in their bioavailability and patients should receive only one preparation. They should also maintain a reasonable fluid intake.
  Record cards are available for patients taking lithium.

Special points for patient education

Patients must understand that the response to treatment may be delayed for up to 6 weeks with tricyclics.
  They must be told of possible adverse effects and how to make the best of them.
  They must be informed of the important interactions and how to avoid them.
  They must realize that most of the drugs are dangerous in overdose.

Nursing point

Non-compliance is an important cause of treatment failure.

THE MANAGEMENT OF DEPRESSION

Most patients with mild to moderate depression are managed at home. Indications for hospital admission are severe depression, risk of suicide and those who cannot care for themselves. All patients need support and encouragement.

The main physical methods of treatment are drugs and electroconvulsive therapy (ECT). There is considerable debate as to whether the tricyclic or the 5-HT re-uptake antidepressants should be the drug group of choice. They are equally effective and both have adverse effects, but those of the tricyclics are rather more unpleasant than those of the 5-HT re-uptake group. The tricyclics are certainly more dangerous in overdose. However, the 5-HT re-uptake drugs are much more expensive. If tricyclics are used *amitriptyline* is preferred in patients with sleep problems as it is fairly sedative, otherwise *imipramine* is satisfactory. The other members of this group are used in special circumstances. Because of their long half-life, once daily dosage, usually before retiring, is sufficient. Sleep problems respond promptly, but it may take several weeks for the depression to lift. The initial dose of both drugs would be 50–75 mg as a single dose at night for an outpatient, but larger doses may be used for in-patients. In elderly patients 25 mg is a safer starting dose and twice daily dosing may be

necessary if postural hypotension is a problem. Patients who are at special risk from tricyclics such as elderly patients with bladder or eye problems or those with heart disease should be given a 5-HT re-uptake inhibitor. Some authorities think that the use of 5-HT re-uptake inhibitors should largely replace tricyclics. In severe depression, especially if there is a serious risk of suicide or antidepressants have failed, ECT is often used.

In depressive neurosis when environmental factors are playing a part MAO inhibitors are sometimes used and can be combined with a benzodiazepine. Tricyclic antidepressants must not be combined with MAO inhibitors as this may cause excitement and pyrexia. Normally there should be a 2-week gap when changing from one type of antidepressant to another (five weeks following fluoxetine).

Treatment for depression is usually continued for at least 4 months after recovery. Shorter periods of treatment increase the risk of relapse. The drug should then be phased out over about 6 months otherwise withdrawal symptoms may ensue. These consist of anxiety, diarrhoea, insomnia and restlessness or relapse may occur.

In *bipolar depression* (manic-depressive illness) the manic phase can be controlled by a neuroleptic (usually haloperidol, see p. 156) and the depressive phase by a tricyclic antidepressant. The long-term use of lithium to prevent the mood changes has revolutionized the treatment of this condition. Sometimes it is more effective if *carbamazepine* is combined with lithium (see p. 168).

DRUGS IN DEMENTIA

Dementia is a clinical state with various underlying causes, some of which are amenable to drug treatment. Myxoedema-associated dementia responds to replacement with thyroxine and dementias related to chronic alcoholism are often improved by vitamins of the B group.

Alzheimer's disease, which affects about one-quarter of those over 85 years, presents a more difficult problem. Its causes are not yet fully understood and, as yet, there is no specific remedy.

Donepezil inhibits cholinesterase (p. 48) in the brain and thus facilitates the function of nerve cells. It is given orally and produces a moderate improvement in about 40% of patients with mild Alzheimer's disease.

Nursing point

Drugs used either therapeutically or for recreation can cause a variety of organic mental states.

FURTHER READING

Ballinger B R 1990 Hypnotics and anxiolytics. British Medical Journal 300: 456

Behavioural emergencies 1991 Drug and Therapeutics Bulletin 29: 62

Buckley N A et al 1995 Relative toxicity of benzodiazepines in overdose. British Medical Journal 310: 219

Culshaw F 1994 Composition and effects of commonly used neuroleptics. Nursing Times 90: 38

Editorial 1988 Benzodiazepines and dependence. Bulletin of the Royal College of Psychiatrists 12: 107

Editorial 1988 Tardive dyskinesia. British Medical Journal 296: 150

Editorial 1994 Risperidone for schizophrenia. British Medical Journal 308: 1311

Editorial 1995 The drug treatment of patients with schizophrenia. Drug and Therapeutics Bulletin 33: 81

Editorial 1996 Three new antidepressants. Drug and Therapeutics Bulletin 34(9): 65

Editorial 1997 Donepezil for Alzheimer's disease. Drug and Therapeutics Bulletin 35(10): 75

Editorial 1999 Acetylcholinesterase inhibitors for Alzheimer's disease. British Medical Journal 318: 615

Edwards J G 1994 Selective serotonin re-uptake inhibitors in the treatment of depression. Prescribers Journal 34: 197

Gram L F 1994 Fluoxetine. New England Journal of Medicine 331: 1354

Henry J A, Alexander C A, Sener E K 1995 Relative mortality from overdose of antidepressants. British Medical Journal 310: 221

Jefferson J W 1998 Lithium. British Medical Journal 316: 1330

Lader M 1994 Treatment of anxiety. British Medical Journal 309: 321

Macgabhann L 1998 A comparison of two depot injection techniques. Nursing Standard 12(39): 41

Pathare S R, Paton C 1997 Psychotropic drug treatment. British Medical Journal 315: 661

Quartermaine S 1995 A comparative study of depot injection techniques. Nursing Times 91(30): 36

Smith L 1995 Clozapine: indications and implications for treatment. Nursing Times 91(30): 40

Song F et al 1993 Selective serotonin reuptake inhibitors: meta-analysis of efficacy and acceptability. British Medical Journal 306: 683

Tyrer P 1988 The Nottingham study of neurotic disorder. Lancet ii: 235

13

Antiepileptics and drugs used in Parkinson's disease

ANTIEPILEPTICS

Antiepileptic drugs are used in the treatment of epilepsy. There are several varieties of epilepsy and they vary in their response to drugs. In focal epilepsy the attack arises from a focal electrical discharge in the brain. This may produce a brief *aura* which is a feeling or movement. If the discharge becomes generalized the patient falls unconscious and passes through the typical tonic and clonic phases, regaining consciousness after a varying interval. This is known as a *tonic–clonic (grand mal) seizure*. Sometimes the spread of the discharge is limited (*partial seizure*) producing psychological disturbances (*psychomotor seizure*) or various involuntary movements. Alternatively, the electrical discharge is widespread from the start, and causes *absence (petit mal) seizure*, which is a brief interference with consciousness. These attacks are common in childhood. The object in treating epilepsy is to completely abolish the attacks by means of drugs. Although there are now a number of drugs which are useful in controlling epilepsy, it is usually best to start treatment with one drug and only use multiple drug regimens in resistant cases. The initial dose should be low and it should be increased until control of the fits is achieved or adverse effects develop.

Patients with epilepsy should be warned against driving vehicles, swimming and working under conditions where a fit could produce disaster.

DRUGS USED IN TONIC–CLONIC AND PARTIAL SEIZURES

Phenytoin. Phenytoin sodium is well absorbed by mouth and does not produce drowsiness or sleep. It probably acts by reducing the excitability of nerve cells and by preventing the abnormal discharge from spreading in the brain.

Therapeutics. Its effectiveness as an anticonvulsant and the incidence of side-effects depend largely on the blood level of the drug, which should be 10–20 mg/litre. Finding the correct dose may be difficult for several reasons:

1. Patients vary considerably in the rate at which they break down phenytoin so there is a wide variation of dose requirements between patients.
2. The relationship between dose and blood level is not linear: this means that a small increase in the dose may cause a considerable rise in the blood level (Fig. 13.1).
3. Because phenytoin is slowly broken down, once daily dosage is adequate. It takes about a week for the blood level to become steady; this means that the dose should not be altered at less than fortnightly intervals.

The initial dose is usually 150 mg once daily after food and is increased by 50 mg fortnightly until the correct dose is found as judged by the control of fits, the absence of toxicity and the blood level.

Adverse effects. These are fairly common with phenytoin and include:

1. If dosage is too high the patient is sedated, ataxic and may show nystagmus.

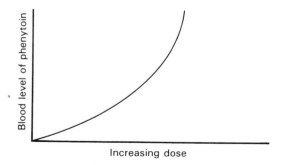

Figure 13.1 Relationship between dosage and blood level of phenytoin.

2. Greasy skin and hirsutism may cause problems in women.
3. Macrocytic anaemia due to folic acid deficiency.
4. Gum hypertrophy—dental care is important.
5. Lymph node enlargement.
6. A variety of rashes.

Interactions. These are common and indicate the need for regular measurement of plasma levels of phenytoin.

Phenytoin levels are altered by chlorpromazine, carbamazepine, diazepam, ethanol, isoniazid and sodium valproate.

Phenytoin alters the levels of hydrocortisone, oral contraceptives, theophylline, tricyclic antidepressants and thyroxine among others.

Carbamazepine is widely used in the control of tonic–clonic and partial seizures. It is also used to relieve the pain of trigeminal neuralgia (see p. 174) and in the treatment of bipolar depression (see p. 165). Carbamazepine is given orally and is fairly slowly absorbed from the intestine. It is interesting that its rate of breakdown in the body increases with prolonged use. The usual initial dose is 100 mg twice daily and this is increased until the fits are controlled. Estimation of blood levels may help to determine the correct dose.

Children may break down the drug rapidly so they may require three or four doses daily.

Adverse effects include rashes, dizziness and drowsiness, blurring of vision, depression of the white cells of the blood and occasionally jaundice and excessive salivary secretion.

Interactions occur with warfarin and erythromycin.

Phenobarbital is one of the barbiturate group of drugs. It is slowly absorbed, the major portion is broken down in the body and the rest slowly excreted by the kidneys. Its action is therefore prolonged over about 12 hours.

Therapeutics. Phenobarbital is particularly effective in the treatment of tonic–clonic seizures, but may also be used in other types of epilepsy.

Adverse effects are not uncommon. Drowsiness and ataxia may be troublesome and occasionally a rash resembling measles is seen. Phenobarbital is a powerful inducer of enzymes in the liver, particularly those which break down other drugs. For example, phenobarbital increases the rate of breakdown of anticoagulants and estrogens whose effects are therefore reduced.

Primidone is in many ways similar to phenobarbital and is effective against tonic-clonic attacks. It is important to start treatment with low dosage and gradually increase the dose, otherwise *adverse effects* such as drowsiness, vertigo and vomiting may occur. It should not be combined with phenobarbital.

Sodium valproate. This drug increases the amount of gamma-aminobutyric acid (GABA) in the brain. GABA is a naturally occurring inhibitory substance and sodium valproate is effective in both tonic–clonic and absence seizures. The initial dose is 600 mg daily after food and may be increased.

Adverse effects. Sodium valproate fairly commonly causes a modest fall in the platelet count. Occasionally this is severe and the patient should be warned to report any bruising or bleeding. It is advisable to carry out a platelet count before major surgery. Very rarely it causes serious liver damage, particularly in those with pre-existing liver disease or in mentally retarded children. Drowsiness, thinning of the hair and weight gain are not uncommon.

Vigabatrin inhibits the breakdown in the brain of GABA, which accumulates and suppresses fits. It is particularly effective in partial seizures and is also used in tonic–clonic seizures. It is taken orally and, although fairly rapidly excreted, its action lasts for 24 hours, so once daily dosage is possible.

Therapeutic use. Vigabatrin is used when the older antiepileptic drugs have proved unsuccessful. The initial dose is 1 g daily.

Adverse effects. Sedation may occur and occasionally, gastric upsets and headaches. Behavioural problems such as irritation, aggression, hallucination and memory faults occur in about 15% of patients. Occasionally, visual field defects develop and may require withdrawal of the drug.

Lamotrigine inhibits the release in the brain of the exciting substance *glutamate* and thus prevents fits. It is effective in partial and tonic–clonic fits and has been shown to be as effective as carbamazepine and better tolerated. It is a useful addition to the range of antiepileptic drugs and may also be effective when other antiepileptics have failed.

Therapeutic use. If combined with other antiepileptic drugs, dose adjustment is necessary. Higher doses may be required with phenytoin or carbamazepine and lower doses with sodium valproate.

Adverse effects. Ataxia, headaches, nausea and rashes which may be dangerous and occur particularly in children. It should not be used in patients with hepatic or renal impairment.

Clonazepam is related to the benzodiazepine drugs and may act by enhancing the inhibiting effect of GABA (see earlier). It is effective in all forms of epilepsy. It is also useful in treating status epilepticus (see later).

Gabapentin binds to specific receptors in the brain. It is used to control partial and general seizures, but is no more effective than the older drugs in use. It is also excreted fairly rapidly by the kidney so thrice daily dosage may be necessary.

Adverse effects. Sleepiness, ataxia and fatigue. There is no known serious interaction.

Outcome of treatment

About 80% of patients with tonic–clonic seizures are controlled by a single drug. When the patient has been free of fits for 5 years, the treatment can be slowly withdrawn. Many subjects will have no further fits, but about 40% (rather less in children) will relapse.

It is important that anticonvulsants are not discontinued too suddenly as this may precipitate fits.

DRUGS USED IN ABSENCE SEIZURES

Ethosuximide is the drug of choice. It may aggravate tonic–clonic seizures and may, if necessary, be combined with a drug which controls this type of attack.

Adverse effects include sleepiness, gastric upsets and headaches.

Dose: Ethosuximide 0.5–2.0 g daily.

Children—10–20 mg/kg once daily.

Sodium valproate (see earlier) is also effective.

DRIVING

A patient may be allowed to drive a car after being free from fits for 1 year, but not a heavy goods or public service vehicle.

DRUG COMBINATIONS

In most patients with epilepsy, complete control can be obtained with a single drug. This is desirable as it minimizes the adverse effects and there is no problem with interactions between the drugs. Sometimes, however, a combination of drugs is required to achieve better control.

STATUS EPILEPTICUS

In status epilepticus the patient has a series of fits, rapidly following each other. These patients require careful nursing so that they do not injure themselves. They should be nursed in the lateral semi-prone position, dentures removed and the airway established; oxygen should be given by mask. *The patient should not be left unattended until the fits have ceased.* The most effective drugs are *diazepam* (as *Diazemuls*) in a dose of 10 mg intravenously or lorazepam 4.0 mg slowly intravenously. In young children rectal diazepam using rectal tubes (*Stesolid*) in a dose of 5 mg for those aged 1–3 years and 10 mg for older children is rapidly effective and useful particularly if intravenous injection is difficult. Diazepam should control fits within 10 minutes and if the fits persist the dose may be repeated. Although diazepam will usually stop the fits, relapse quite commonly occurs within the next hour. To prevent this *phenytoin* 15 mg/kg is injected intravenously, no faster than 50 mg/minute. Phenytoin has some action on the heart so should not be given via a central line and should be monitored by ECG and blood pressure measurements. If the fits persist *chlormethiazole*

should be given intravenously and the dose adjusted to produce a satisfactory therapeutic effect. Finally, if all else fails, *thiopentone* (see p. 141) can be given by intravenous injection. When this drug is used *it is essential to have an anaesthetist* to help as intubation may be necessary and the procedure is not without risk.

Nursing point
The use of chlormethiazole and thiopentone requires considerable expertise and should, if possible, be carried out in an intensive care unit with expert guidance.

Paraldehyde has been used for many years. It is an oily liquid with a pungent smell. It is a central nervous system depressant which controls status epilepticus. It is given rectally, diluted in saline, or by deep intramuscular injection but, being an irritant, care must be taken to avoid the sciatic nerve. The dose is 5–10 ml (not more than 5 ml at one site). It is not the first line treatment for status epilepticus but, because it is a relatively safe drug, it can be used when facilities for close monitoring and respiratory support (if needed) are not available.

Nursing point
The renewal of seizures or the emergence of toxicity after a period of good control may be due to poor compliance or to an interaction with a newly prescribed drug.

FEBRILE CONVULSIONS

About 3% of infants and young children have a fit when feverish. Of these only some 1% will ultimately develop true epilepsy.

The *immediate treatment* is to lie the child semi-prone and most convulsions stop within a few minutes. If the fit persists, rectal diazepam as for status epilepticus (see earlier) is the safest and easiest treatment. Hospital admission may be necessary to exclude serious infection.

Prevention. The parents should be taught to reduce fever by removing excess clothing, keeping the environment cool, supplying cool drinks and giving paracetamol paediatric elixir. If attacks recur with fever the alternatives are:

1. To give rectal diazepam when the child develops a fever.
2. To give continuous medication. Phenobarbital is effective in most children, but side-effects may limit its use and it is rarely required.

Finally, parents will require reassurance as the majority of convulsions of this type are short-lived and cause no long-term problems.

Answers to parents' questions

1. There is a 30% chance it will happen again if the child has a fever, but, becomes rare after 4 years of age.
2. Only 1 in 100 children become epileptics.
3. Brain damage is very rare.

Nursing point

Although febrile convulsions are nearly always benign, nurses must remember that they may signify a serious illness (e.g. meningitis). Any unusual features call for a rapid assessment by an expert.

ANTIEPILEPTICS AND PREGNANCY

There is evidence that antiepileptic drugs given during pregnancy are associated with an increased incidence of fetal malformation. If possible a single antiepileptic should be used and the dosage controlled by repeated measurement of blood levels. Fetal abnormalities occur early in pregnancy and women who are taking antiepileptic drugs should be advised of the risk before becoming pregnant.

Carbamazepine and sodium valproate may cause neural tube defects and phenytoin may cause a variety of abnormalities. At present, there does not appear to be an entirely safe drug. To minimize the risk, women should receive supplementary folic acid before (if possible) and throughout pregnancy.

Many antiepileptic drugs induce liver enzymes and thus increase the rate of breakdown of oral contraceptives, so the *patient's method of contraception* may need to be reviewed.

Eclampsia

The control of seizures is important in the treatment of eclampsia. In the UK this has usually been attempted by using phenytoin or diazepam. It has been shown that intravenous **magnesium sulphate** is probably more effective. Its mode of action in these circumstances is not clear, but it may relieve cerebral ischaemia by vasodilation or minimize brain damage. It is given by intravenous infusion, initially as a bolus of 4.0 g over 20 minutes, followed by 1 g/hour.

DRUGS USED IN PARKINSON'S DISEASE

Parkinson's disease is characterized by rigidity of muscle, by tremor and by slowness of movement. It is due to degenerative changes in nerve cells in the basal nuclei of the brain.

The essential feature of these changes appears to be a considerable decrease in the concentration of *dopamine* in the basal ganglia and thus the balance between *acetylcholine* and *dopamine* in this region of the brain is upset (Fig. 13.2). It can be seen, therefore, that relief of symptoms can be achieved by reducing cholinergic activity or by increasing the amount of dopamine.

Nursing point

The nurse should remember that the symptoms of Parkinson's disease can be caused by treatment with neuroleptic drugs. In the majority of patients these symptoms will disappear when the drug is stopped.

DRUGS WHICH DECREASE CHOLINERGIC ACTIVITY

Originally drugs of the belladonna group were used for this purpose but they have now been replaced by synthetic substitutes. These drugs reduce tremor, but have less effect on rigidity.

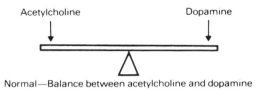

Normal—Balance between acetylcholine and dopamine

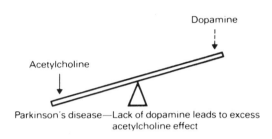

Parkinson's disease—Lack of dopamine leads to excess acetylcholine effect

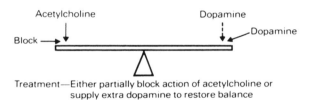

Treatment—Either partially block action of acetylcholine or supply extra dopamine to restore balance

Figure 13.2   The use of drugs in Parkinson's disease.

They may be used in mild cases, but they have troublesome adverse effects and have also been largely replaced.

Trihexyphenidyl (Benzhexol) is given orally and the dose is gradually increased until a satisfactory response is obtained or the limit of tolerance is reached.

Orphenadrine has the advantage of having a general stimulating effect as well as relieving the symptoms of Parkinsonism. This is useful as these patients are often depressed.

Benztropine is in many ways similar to benzhexol. It is particularly useful in the excessive salivation often found in Parkinsonism and in muscular rigidity.

It is liable to cause drowsiness and is best given as a single dose at bedtime.

Adverse effects of these drugs include nausea, constipation, giddiness, dry mouth, urinary retention and glaucoma; in overdose, confusion and hallucinations may also occur.

DRUGS WHICH INCREASE DOPAMINE (Fig. 13.3)

Levodopa. It is not possible to restore the deficiency in the brain by giving dopamine, as this substance will not enter the brain. Therefore levodopa is used. This is a precursor of dopamine which passes freely into the brain where it is converted to dopamine. It is particularly useful in reducing rigidity, but has less effect on tremor.

Levodopa and a decarboxylase inhibitor. Levodopa is broken down by an enzyme called *dopa decarboxylase* which is found particularly in the gut wall and liver. If this enzyme is inhibited by a drug which can be administered in combination with levodopa, the effects of levodopa are enhanced and prolonged and a much smaller dose of levodopa is required. This reduces the incidence of some side-effects. Two preparations which are widely used are:

- Levodopa + carbidopa (Sinemet, Co-careldopa)
- Levodopa + benserazide (Madopar, Co-beneldopa).

Therapeutics. Adverse effects are very troublesome when levodopa is used alone, so treatment is usually started with a small dose—either half a tablet of Sinemet Plus (levodopa 50 mg) or Madopar 125 (levodopa 50 mg) three times daily after food. This is gradually increased until a satisfactory control of symptoms is obtained, usually 3–8 Sinemet Plus tablets (levodopa 300–800 mg) daily. A controlled-release preparation is available and contains 100 or 200 mg of levodopa together with a decarboxylase inhibitor.

Adverse effects. Nausea and vomiting are very common but can be minimized by giving the drug in divided doses with meals. **Domperidone** (see p. 107) is a useful anti-emetic because it blocks the effect of dopamine on the CTZ in the brain stem, but does not interfere with the therapeutic action of dopamine at the basal ganglia.

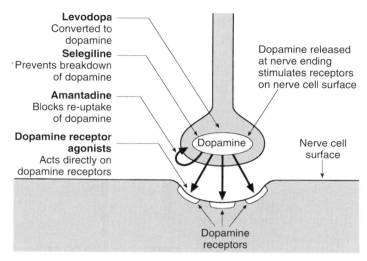

Figure 13.3   Sites of action of drugs used in Parkinson's disease.

Some postural fall in blood pressure is common, but rarely causes symptoms. Blood pressure should be measured before and during treatment.

A few patients become restless, and at higher dose levels involuntary movements, usually affecting the face, may occur.

Constipation will require a good fluid and fibre intake.

Interactions. Levodopa/decarboxylase inhibitor combinations should not be combined with MAO inhibitors. Concomitant use of halothane, cyclopropane or trichlorethylene carries an increased risk of cardiac arrhythmias and the drug should be stopped 8 hours before an operation.

Selegiline inhibits the breakdown of levodopa in the brain. It is often used in combination with levodopa with or without a decarboxylase inhibitor and this allows a smaller dose of levodopa to be used and prolongs its action. It is usually given as a single dose in the morning.

Adverse effects are confusion and nausea.

Amantadine increases the concentration of dopamine in the basal ganglia and thus relieves the symptoms of Parkinson's disease. It is not as effective as levodopa and is useless in some patients, but can be used when that drug is contraindicated. The initial dose may be increased after 1 week if necessary.

Adverse effects include nausea, central effects and swelling of the ankles.

Dopamine receptor agonists

This group of drugs stimulate dopamine receptors in the remaining cells of the basal ganglia. They are prescribed when treatment with levodopa is ineffective or requires supplementation, and sometimes in early cases, but adverse effects can limit their use.

Bromocriptine and **cabergoline** are almost identical. Both drugs can cause nausea and postural hypotension and dosage requires careful adjustment.

Lisuride, Pergolide and Ropinirol have similar actions, pergolide being effective for about 5 hours and lisuride for 3 hours.

Adverse effects. A few patients develop postural hypotension, but the most common problem is nausea which can be controlled by domperidone (see p. 107)

Apomorphine is a powerful dopamine receptor stimulant in the CTZ (see p. 106) and has been used as an emetic. Treatment is difficult and requires close supervision and considerable patient education. It should be initiated in hospital and domperidone is started three days before apomorphine to control vomiting. Apomorphine is given by multiple subcutaneous injections or by continuous subcutaneous infusion.

THE TREATMENT OF PARKINSON'S DISEASE

As can be seen from the preceding discussion there are a number of drugs which are useful in relieving the symptoms of this disease, but they do not prevent its progression. There is no unanimous opinion as to the order in which they should be given. In mild cases a start may be made with an anticholinergic drug such as benzhexol, especially if tremor is a problem. If this is ineffective or tolerance develops it can be changed to amantadine or levodopa. There is no evidence that selegilene should be used early in treatment for its supposed neuroprotective action. It may indeed increase mortality. For most patients, particularly those with more severe symptoms, it is usual to start with levodopa combined with a decarboxylase inhibitor. If a very high dosage of levodopa is required to control symptoms (e.g. more than 600 mg daily), a dopamine receptor agonist may be added to the regime.

About three-quarters of patients with Parkinson's disease respond to drugs. Rigidity is usually most amenable to treatment and tremor less so.

Unfortunately, in more than half the patients being treated by levodopa its efficacy decreases after about 5 years, so that increasingly frequent dosage is required to maintain its effect and prevent the 'on-off' phenomenon during which there are periods of weakness and loss of movement. These fluctuations can be reduced by frequent dosage or by using a controlled-release preparation. If this fails, selegiline can be added to the regime. Finally, if levodopa becomes ineffective an oral agonist or injections of apomorphine can be used.

TRIGEMINAL NEURALGIA

This is an unpleasant disorder of unknown aetiology which produces attacks of severe pain in the face (i.e. in the distribution of the trigeminal nerve).

Treatment has been considerably improved by the use of **carbamazepine**. The initial dose is 100 mg twice daily and is subsequently modified according to the response of the patient. About 70% of patients are relieved. If drug treatment fails, it may be necessary to resort to surgery.

FURTHER READING

Brodie M J, Dichter M A 1996 Antiepileptic drugs. New England Journal of Medicine 334: 168
Calne D B 1993 The treatment of Parkinson's disease. New England Journal of Medicine 329: 1021
Chadwick D 1994 Gabapentin. Lancet 343: 89
Dichter M A, Brodie M J 1996 New antiepileptic drugs. New England Journal of Medicine 334: 1583
Eclampsia Trial Collaboration Group 1995 Which anticonvulsant for women with eclampsia? Lancet 345: 1455
Editorial 1989 Withdrawing anti-epileptic drugs. Drug and Therapeutics Bulletin 27: 29
Editorial 1999 Developments in the treatment of Parkinson's disease. Drug and Therapeutics Bulletin 37: 5: 36
Editorial 1994 Epilepsy and pregnancy. Drug and Therapeutics Bulletin 32(7): 49
Editorial 1995 Selegiline in Parkinson's disease. British Medical Journal 311: 1583
Editorial 1996 Stopping status epilepticus. Drug and

Therapeutics Bulletin 34(10): 73
Editorial 2000 The treatment of early Parkinson's disease. British Medical Journal 321: 1
Freely M 1999 Drug treatment of epilepsy. British Medical Journal 318: 106
Marson A G, Kadir Z A, Chadwick D W 1996 New antiepileptic drugs. British Medical Journal 313: 1169
Neville B G R 1997 Epilepsy in childhood. British Medical Journal 315: 924
Quinn N 1995 Drug treatment of Parkinson's disease. British Medical Journal 310: 575
Rosman N P et al 1993 A controlled trial of diazepam to prevent the recurrence of febrile seizures. New England Journal of Medicine 329: 79
Valman H B 1993 Febrile convulsions. British Medical Journal 306: 1743

Guidance for group protocols for variation of prescriptions by Parkinson's disease nurse specialists are available from the RCN.

14

The endocrine system

The endocrine or ductless glands are small islands of tissue in various parts of the body (Fig. 14.1). Each gland secretes a substance, and in some cases, several substances, called *hormones*. These are released into the bloodstream and circulate through the body. Their speed of action is variable; the effects of some hormones are seen immediately after release, whereas others may take hours or even days to show their effect. After release, these hormones act upon a receptor mechanism in the organ or organs which they influence, thus producing their specific actions. The actions of the various hormones differ widely, one group being concerned with metabolic processes, another with secondary sexual characteristics and so on. Sometimes a hormone will act on another endocrine gland and stimulate it to produce a further hormone. This two-stage, or even three-stage series of events is particularly likely to involve the anterior lobe of the pituitary gland (see later).

Most of these hormones have been isolated and their structure determined. This has made it possible to prepare synthetically either the hormones or analogues which are sometimes more active than the hormones themselves.

The endocrine glands can be divided roughly into three groups:

1. The pituitary, which secretes hormones that exercise a controlling influence over the rest of the endocrine system
2. Those affecting metabolism
3. Those affecting the reproductive system.

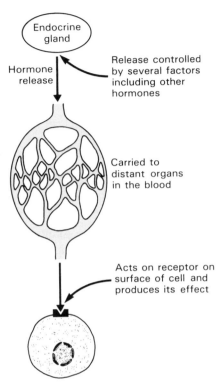

Figure 14.1 Endocrine glands and hormone action.

SECTION I: THE PITUITARY

The pituitary is a small endocrine gland attached to the brain by a stalk and lying, almost surrounded by bone, in the base of the skull. It consists of anterior and posterior lobes (Fig. 14.2). In spite of its small size, it is of great importance. It secretes a number of hormones which not only affect various processes in the body, but also the activity of nearly all the other endocrine glands. It is of interest that the activity of the pituitary itself may be influenced by other hormones, so that a balance is maintained between the pituitary and other endocrine glands.

The release of pituitary hormones is a complex function and it appears that for many of them there is a specific *releasing hormone* which is probably produced in the brain. Thus thyrotrophic hormone is released into the circulation after the pituitary has been stimulated by thyrotrophic releasing hormones. Releasing hormones are only just becoming available on a commercial scale for general use.

POSTERIOR LOBE

Two hormones can be extracted from the posterior lobe of the pituitary (Fig. 14.3).

Oxytocin. This hormone causes contraction of the uterus and is considered on page 207.

Vasopressin, Argipressin (synthetic vasopressin). Vasopressin has two actions. In large doses it causes vasoconstriction with a concomitant rise in blood pressure, but its more important effect from the therapeutic aspect is concerned with water balance as it is the *antidiuretic hormone*.

If the intake of water is limited, the blood becomes slightly more concentrated. This affects special receptors in the base of the brain, which in turn stimulate the posterior pituitary to secrete more vasopressin. The vasopressin increases the reabsorption of water by the renal tubules and thus decreases the amount of urine and conserves the body water. If the intake of water is increased the production of vasopressin drops and the output of urine by the kidneys is increased—thus balancing the intake and output of water by the body.

Therapeutics. Occasionally damage to the posterior pituitary or closely related structures produces a disease called *diabetes insipidus*, in which little or no vasopressin is produced. There is thus a continuous high output of urine, which in turn requires the drinking of vast quantities of water if dehydration is to be avoided.

The disorder can be controlled by the administration of vasopressin, which is given as an injection of 5–20 units 4 hourly. It was previously used as a snuff, but has now been replaced by desmopressin (see below).

Desmopressin is a synthetic drug allied to vasopressin. It can be given nasally or intramuscularly. It has a very long action so that one or two doses daily suffice to control diabetes insipidus and it is now the preferred preparation. Unlike vasopressin it does not cause vasoconstriction. Treatment should aim at reducing

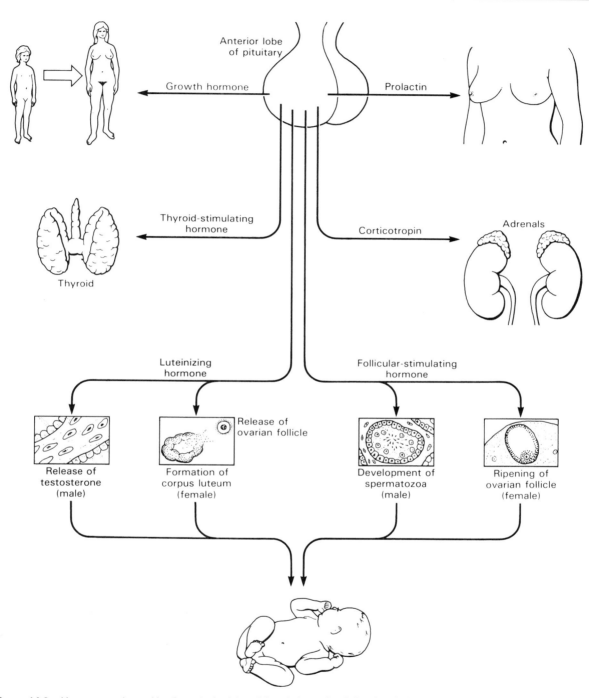

Figure 14.2   Hormones released by the anterior lobe of the pituitary gland showing their main sites of action.

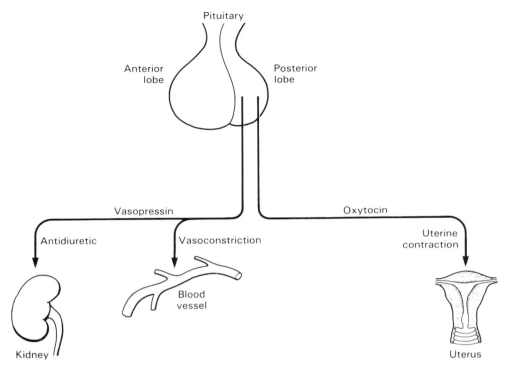

Figure 14.3 Hormones released by the posterior pituitary and their sites of action.

the patient's urine output to about 2 litres a day. Desmopressin can also be used to treat *nocturnal enuresis*, in patients with normal pituitary function, by reducing the night-time urine volume. Care must be taken to prevent fluid overload.

The vasoconstrictive properties of vasopressin can be used in the treatment of bleeding from oesophageal varices. The vasoconstriction lowers pressure in the portal vein and allows the bleeding vein to clot. Twenty units are given very slowly intravenously (over 15 minutes); the patient may complain of abdominal colic.

Lypressin is similar to the above and is given by nasal spray.

The dose and route of administration depend on the condition being treated. To control diabetes insipidus, desmopressin is given orally, intranasally or by injection. To treat oesophageal varices, terlipressin or vasopressin are given intravenously. To prevent nocturnal enuresis, desmopressin is given orally or intranasally at bedtime.

ANTERIOR LOBE

Several hormones are produced by the anterior lobe of the pituitary. They may be divided into:

1. Those which stimulate the release of other hormones
2. Those which inhibit hormone release
3. Those which act directly on their target organs. These include luteinizing hormone and follicular stimulating hormone (see p. 200).

Those releasing other hormones

Corticotropin (ACTH) stimulates the release of cortisol by the adrenal cortex. Its rate of release is partly controlled by the circulating level of cortisol—high levels of cortisol suppress corticotropin production and vice versa, thus providing a self-regulatory mechanism between the adrenal and pituitary glands (see Fig. 14.5). Large doses of cortisol or similar hormones decrease the production of corticotropin and in time will cause the adrenal gland to atrophy. It is therefore important not to cease steroid treatment suddenly, but to reduce it gradually to stimulate a return to normal adrenal production.

Corticotropin is no longer available, but a synthetic analogue, tetracosactide, is used mainly for testing adrenal function.

Tetracosactide is available as a rapidly acting preparation for intramuscular or intravenous use.

The rapidly acting preparation is used to test adrenal function. A dose of 250 micrograms is injected intramuscularly. Blood levels of cortisol are measured before and 30 minutes after injection. If the adrenals are working properly the injection is followed by a release of cortisol and a rise in the blood level.

Gonadotrophins. The pituitary secretes two hormones which affect the gonads. They are concerned with reproduction and are considered on page 199.

Thyroid stimulating hormone (thyrotrophic hormone, TSH). The stimulation of the thyroid gland by this hormone indirectly increases the metabolism of the body.

If the thyroid function is depressed by drugs or other means the pituitary secretes large amounts of TSH. It is used in various tests of thyroid function.

The release of TSH is itself stimulated by a further hormone **thyrotrophin-releasing hormone (protirelin)**, which is produced in the hypothalamus. It is used in doses of 200 micrograms intravenously for tests of thyroid function.

Those which act directly on target organs

Somatotrophin (growth hormone). This hormone stimulates growth both in soft tissue and in bone. Its release from the pituitary is complicated as there are at least two substances from the brain which control its secretion. Unfortunately, most animal somatotrophin is ineffective in humans so human growth hormone must be used. This has now been synthesized by using biological technology and the product is called **somatropin**. In patients with dwarfism due to

hormone deficiency, treatment must be started before epiphyseal fusion has occurred and continued until growth is complete. Somatropin is given subcutaneously weekly and the dose adjusted as necessary. It is expensive.

Overproduction of somatotrophin by the pituitary gland will produce *gigantism* in children and *acromegaly* in adults.

Somatostatin is a naturally occurring hormone which inhibits the release of somatotrophin from the pituitary; a synthetic analogue **octreotide**, with a similar action, is being used increasingly in various conditions.

Therapeutics. By suppressing the release of somatotrophin in acromegaly, octreotide can control the symptoms when surgery is impossible or incomplete. The main problem in its use is the need for dosage up to three times daily by injection and it is expensive. Octreotide suppresses the release of several hormones in the stomach and intestine and reduces the blood flow to the gut. As a result of these actions it can be given to control certain types of diarrhoea, including that due to AIDS, and it is also used to reduce the bleeding from oesophageal varices and in the treatment of certain tumours of the intestine.

Adverse effects. Gastritis and gallstone formation.

Lactogenic hormone. Prolactin, the lactogenic hormone, produces its maximum effect on the breast which has already been prepared throughout pregnancy by estrogens and progesterone. Its production by the pituitary can be suppressed by bromocriptine (see below) which is used when it is necessary to suppress lactation.

Prolactin also has a powerful inhibitory effect on ovarian function and high blood levels during the period of lactation are probably responsible for the delayed return of menstruation after pregnancy.

Bromocriptine. This interesting drug is related to ergot. It acts on the pituitary in the same way as the naturally occurring substance dopamine and inhibits the release of various hormones, particularly prolactin and growth hormone. It also stimulates dopamine receptors in the basal ganglia and thus relieves the symptoms of Parkinson's disease (see p. 173).

Therapeutics. Increased production of pro-lactin by the pituitary can cause impotence in men and amenorrhoea in women. By suppressing the production of prolactin, bromocriptine is successful in reversing these symptoms, though treatment may have to be continued for some time. The initial dose is 1.0 mg at night with food to decrease nausea and *slowly* increased.

By inhibiting growth hormone release, it is of some value in the management of acromegaly. It has also been used in the treatment of Parkinson's disease.

Bromocriptine is not now recommended to suppress lactation.

It is important to start with a small dose which can be increased gradually, otherwise the side-effects, nausea, vomiting, low blood pressure and drowsiness, are troublesome.

Cabergoline and **Quinagolide** are similar to the above and have the same indications. They can be used for patients who are intolerant of bromocriptine.

FURTHER READING

Editorial 1992 Cyclical breast pain – what works and what doesn't. Drug and Therapeutics Bulletin 30: 1
Editorial 1995 New drugs for hyperprolactinaemia. Drug and Therapeutics Bulletin 33: 65
Lambert S W J et al 1996 Octreotide. New England Journal of Medicine 334: 246
Smail P 1991 The GP, specialist and HGH. Prescriber Issue 38: 28

SECTION II: HORMONES AFFECTING METABOLISM

THE THYROID

The thyroid consists of two lobes connected by an isthmus and is situated in the neck, in front of the trachea. Circulating iodine is picked up by the cells of the thyroid gland and incorporated to form two hormones, thyroxine (T_4) and tri-iodothyronine (T_3). These are stored in the thyroid as thyroglobulin. With appropriate stimu-

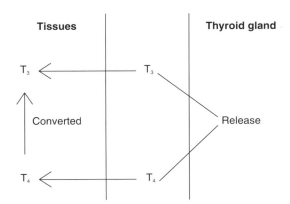

Figure 14.4 Production, storage and release of thyroid hormones.

lation both thyroxine (T_4) and triiodothyronine are released into the bloodstream. On reaching certain tissues thyroxine is converted to tri-iodothyronine (T_3), which is the more active hormone (Fig. 14.4).

The effect of these thyroid hormones is to increase tissue metabolism and thus to raise the basal metabolic rate. They are also important in promoting growth. The release of thyroid hormone is controlled by the thyroid stimulating hormone (TSH) from the pituitary which, in turn, is controlled by thyroid releasing hormone (TRH). In normal people the release of thyroid hormone is nicely adjusted to maintain the metabolic rate at a satisfactory level. Under certain conditions, a considerable excess of thyroid hormone is produced and metabolism is greatly increased which, together with over-activity of the sympathetic nervous system, give rise to the clinical condition known as *thyrotoxicosis* or *Graves' disease.* Exophthalmos, which is a characteristic sign of thyrotoxicosis, is not due to thyroid hormone or to TSH, but is partially due to sympathetic overactivity and also to a rather mysterious hormone called 'long-acting thyroid stimulator' (LATS). Suppression of the thyroid by drugs or by surgery (see later) will not therefore relieve exophthalmos.

Conversely, the thyroid may produce little or no hormone, with a resulting fall in metabolic rate and the appearance of the state known as *cretinism* in infants or *myxoedema* in adults. Both these disorders may be treated by replacement with thyroxine.

THYROID DEFICIENCY

There are two preparations which are effective in treating thyroid deficiency. They are *levothyroxine*, which is the pure hormone synthetically prepared and is used for long-term treatment, and *liothyronine*.

Levothyroxine sodium (Thyroxine sodium) tablets given orally are absorbed from the intestinal tract, but their full effects are not seen for about 10 days. If they are given to patients with cretinism or myxoedema they will cause them to return to normal. Large doses will cause an excessive rise in metabolic rate and the symptoms of thyrotoxicosis, with loss of weight, tachycardia, nervousness and tremors.

Therapeutics. It is important to start treating cretins as soon as possible because if they are left in a hypothyroid state too long, the change may be irreversible. The initial dosage of levothyroxine for infants with cretinism is 5.0 micrograms/kg daily, which is subsequently modified according to the response of the patient.

In myxoedema it is very important to start with a small dose or the undue stimulating effect on the heart may cause untoward effects, including anginal pain. Treatment should be started with 50 micrograms of thyroxine (25 micrograms in elderly patients or those with heart disease) and this is cautiously increased until the desired effect is produced, the usual maintenance dose being 100–400 micrograms once daily.

Early in treatment the patient should be kept warm, hypnotics should be avoided and constipation, which is common, should be relieved.

In both cretinism and myxoedema it is usually necessary to continue treatment for the rest of the patient's life.

Although the dose can be monitored by the clinical response of the patient, it is preferable to measure the plasma T_4 and TSH occasionally to ensure that the correct amount of hormone is being given.

Thyroxine is sometimes used to stimulate the metabolism of obese patients and thereby cause a loss of weight. It should not be used for this purpose as dangerous amounts of the drug are required to cause much weight loss.

Liothyronine is the official name of triiodothyronine. Its actions are similar to those of thyroxine, but are much more rapid in onset, the maximum effect being seen after 3 days.

Therapeutics. Liothyronine is not so useful as thyroxine in treating myxoedema as the control of the disease is apt to be uneven, but it is useful if a rapid effect is required.

In treating myxoedema coma the dose is 5–20 micrograms i.v. repeated at 12-hourly intervals as required. The initial oral dose is 10–20 micrograms daily, increasing to 20–60 micrograms daily.

EXCESS THYROID HORMONE (THYROTOXICOSIS)

Overproduction of hormone by the thyroid gland may be treated by surgical excision of most of the thyroid gland or by drugs. There are several drugs which decrease thyroid hormone production. Some of the most important are discussed.

Iodine. Iodine will temporarily depress thyroid function and relieve the symptoms of thyrotoxicosis.

It is usually given orally as *aqueous iodine solution (Lugol's iodine)*. The maximum effect is seen after about 2 weeks and is not maintained. It is therefore not used for the long-term treatment of thyrotoxicosis, but is valuable in preparing thyrotoxic patients for operation. The dose of aqueous iodine solution is 0.3–1.0 ml daily and it may be given in milk to improve the taste. Rarely it can cause sensitivity reactions.

Radioactive iodine (^{131}I) is used therapeutically. It is given by mouth and rapidly absorbed from the stomach and intestines. In the treatment of thyrotoxicosis large doses are given to stop production of thyroid hormone permanently. This takes several weeks and after about 1 month replacement treatment with thyroxine is begun to prevent the development of myxoedema and continued indefinitely. Radioactive iodine should not be used to treat thyrotoxicosis during pregnancy or if the mother is breast feeding and there is doubt about its use in children and young women. It will also destroy malignant cells in certain patients with carcinoma of the thyroid.

Special care will be required in the handling of and disposal of urine, etc., from these patients.

Carbimazole. Carbimazole suppresses the overproduction of thyroid hormones and is most commonly used in the treatment of thyrotoxicosis. After absorption it is converted in the blood to *methimazole*, which is the active agent.

Therapeutics. The initial dose is 20–60 mg daily by mouth and it usually takes 1–2 months to return the thyroid function to normal, although the thyroid gland itself often enlarges. The dose is then reduced to 5–15 mg daily and continued for about 18 months, after which treatment may be further reduced and eventually stopped. About 60% of patients will remain well, but 40% will relapse and either require further drug treatment or surgery.

Adverse effects include rashes, joint pains, enlarged lymph nodes and fever. Transient depression of the white cell count develops in around 10% of patients and, rarely, dangerous agranulocytosis; therefore *severe sore throats or other infections should be reported immediately.*

Carbimazole should be given with care to pregnant women as excessive dosage may suppress the fetal thyroid, causing goitre and hypothyroidism. It is also excreted in maternal milk and may have similar effects on the newborn.

Propylthiouracil may be used in a similar way.

β blockers (see p. 47). These drugs reduce those symptoms of thyrotoxicosis due to sympathetic overactivity, including tachycardia, tremor, sweating and anxiety. In addition to their actions on the sympathetic system, they reduce the conversion of T_4 to T_3 in the tissues. They are useful for the rapid control of these symptoms, particularly in the preparation for operation and may be continued with digitalis if atrial fibrillation develops. It must be remembered, however, that they do not cure thyrotoxicosis, so that if they are stopped the symptoms will return.

The treatment of thyrotoxicosis

For otherwise healthy patients with thyrotoxicosis either surgery or drug treatment with carbimazole or ^{131}I produces satisfactory results, and the complications and failure rates are about equal for both methods of treatment. Surgery has the advantage of getting a quick result, but some patients prefer to avoid an operation and treatment with radioactive iodine is being increasingly used. For nodular goitres surgery is indicated. Prior to operation it is usual to make the patient euthyroid with carbimazole and to follow this with a short course of aqueous iodine solution which, in addition to keeping the patient euthyroid, makes the thyroid less vascular and easier for the surgeon to handle. β blockers can also be used to prepare patients for operations.

If β blockers are used alone the drug must be continued for 10 days after operation to prevent a thyroid crisis.

In elderly patients or those with some other complicating disease ^{131}I is very satisfactory.

Patient education in the recognition of the symptoms of thyroid disorders and the adverse effects of drugs used in treatment is important.

THE ADRENAL GLANDS

The two adrenal glands are situated at the upper pole of the kidneys. They consist of an outer layer or cortex and a central portion or medulla. These two parts of the adrenal glands produce hormones of very different composition and function and they will therefore be considered separately.

THE CORTEX

There are a number of hormones produced by the adrenal cortex. They also belong to the class of chemical substances known as steroids and three main groups may be defined.

1. Mineralocorticoid hormones

These are concerned with salt (sodium) and water control; the most important is aldosterone.

Aldosterone increases reabsorption of sodium by the kidney, thus raising the amount of sodium in the body, which in turn causes water retention. The main trigger to the release of aldosterone is the renin mechanism (see p. 67) and its main function is to ensure that the volume of fluid in the circulation and tissue spaces is kept constant.

Excess of aldosterone gives rise to hypertension and sometimes oedema. It is not available for clinical use as a drug, but very rarely aldosterone-producing tumours arise in the adrenal gland causing *Conn's syndrome*, which is characterized by hypertension and low plasma potassium with muscle weakness.

2. Sex corticoid hormones

Normally these are only secreted in small amounts and are of little importance. Excessive secretion leads to virilism.

Disorders may occur as a result of deficiency of these hormones following disease of the adrenal gland or from overproduction of one or more of their hormones by hyperplasia or tumour of the adrenals.

Although these conditions may affect only one group of hormones, it is common for a mixed picture to be produced.

3. Glucocorticoid hormones, corticosteroids, steroids

The glucocorticoids are concerned with metabolism of carbohydrate, fat and protein and will also modify the response of the body to injury.

The chief glucocorticoid released from the adrenal is *cortisol*. Its release is controlled by corticotropin, which is in turn produced by the pituitary. The mechanism is such that when the amount of cortisol in the blood increases it 'switches off' the release of corticotropin by the pituitary (negative feedback) and this prevents

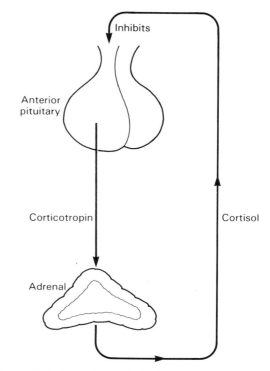

Figure 14.5 Control of cortisol release.

large changes in the blood cortisol concentration (see Fig. 14.5). In addition to cortisol, there are a number of synthetic hormones with similar actions and the whole group is sometimes called the *corticosteroid* or *steroid hormones* (Fig. 14.5).

Cortisone and cortisol (hydrocortisone). The actions of these two hormones are essentially the same and they will be considered together. Cortisol is the naturally occurring hormone and cortisone is a synthetic substitute. They are carried in the blood to their various sites of action; they penetrate the plasma membrane and act on intracellular structures. Their main actions are:

Carbohydrate metabolism. They stimulate the production of glucose from protein and decrease sensitivity to insulin. Prolonged treatment may rarely give rise to diabetes mellitus. *Deficiency* of glucocorticoids leads to weight loss.

Effect on electrolytes. They cause retention of sodium and water and loss of potassium via the kidneys, though they are not so powerful as aldosterone. The retention of sodium and water may lead to oedema and hypertension in some patients. Potassium loss may be replaced by potassium supplements (see p. 216) in patients who are receiving large doses over long periods. *Deficiency* leads to sodium loss through the kidneys and low blood pressure.

Effect on inflammation. They suppress all inflammatory processes and also the generalized reactions of inflammation such as pyrexia and malaise. This action may be very dangerous, for inflammation is the body's method of dealing with infections. If no inflammatory reaction occurs the bacteria can spread widely without the seriousness of the position being apparent to the doctor or the patient. Such patients require urgent treatment with antibiotics and an *increase* in steroid dosage.

Effect on the stomach. They may increase gastric acidity and at times appear to exacerbate ulcers which are already present. It is doubtful if enteric-coated tablets have any advantage. If perforation of the ulcer occurs, their effect on inflammation may mask the symptoms of the perforation, with disastrous results. *Deficiency* leads to loss of appetite.

Effects on immunity. The immune reaction is suppressed and patients become more vulnerable to infections. This is partly due to damping down the antigen–antibody response and possibly also to the reduced production of antibodies. For the same reasons allergic reactions of various types are inhibited.

Effects on bone. They reduce bone production and prolonged treatment can cause osteoporosis.

Psychological effects. They usually produce a feeling of well-being; however, occasionally serious mental disease may follow their administration; it usually occurs in those with a background of mental ill health.

Effect and response to stress. Stress causes an increased secretion of cortisol. Failure of this response leads to a shock-like state.

Miscellaneous effects. In large doses they will produce a picture similar to that of Cushing's disease, with a round 'moon-like' face, hair on the face and body, a tendency to acne and purple striae on the trunk. Occasionally, muscle weakness and wasting occur and the skin becomes thin and very susceptible to bruising.

It should be noted that many of these effects are only seen if glucocorticoids are given in large doses and not at the physiological levels normally found in the blood.

Prednisolone; prednisone; dexamethasone; betamethasone; triamcinolone; beclomethasone; budesonide. These synthetic substances have powerful anti-inflammatory actions, but less sodium-retaining properties than cortisone. They are therefore used when an anti-inflammatory action is required. Side-effects are similar to those produced by cortisone. In addition, marked muscle wasting has been reported with triamcinolone. Beclomethasone and budesonide are given by inhalation in the treatment of asthma.

Fludrocortisone has very powerful sodium-retaining properties with minimal anti-inflammatory action.

Therapeutics. The therapeutic uses of corticosteroids may be considered under two headings:

1. Suppression of some disease process when relatively large doses are required.
2. Replacement of steroid hormones which, for some reason, are deficient. In this situation small (physiological) doses are needed.

Suppression of disease processes

Anti-inflammatory actions. This effect is used in treating certain patients with systemic lupus, polyarteritis nodosa, temporal arteritis and, rarely, rheumatoid arthritis. In these disorders, much higher concentrations of the drugs are required than those which occur naturally to suppress the inflammation and thus relieve the patients of their symptoms. It must again be stressed that these drugs are only useful in certain types of inflammation; in inflammation due to bacterial infection they may actually favour spread of infections and are thus dangerous.

The best drugs to use when anti-inflammatory effects are required are those with little sodium-retaining action such as prednisolone.

Anti-allergic actions. By suppressing allergic reaction these drugs are useful in such disorders as asthma, hay fever and eczema.

In asthma they are reserved for those patients who do not respond to more usual measures, particularly status asthmaticus when 200 mg of cortisol (hydrocortisone) intravenously and repeated every 6 hours may be life saving. In the long-term treatment of asthma, steroids (beclomethasone) can be given by inhalation to produce a maximum local action with minimum systemic effect. In hay fever and eczema cortisol (hydrocortisone) may be applied locally and it is also used as eye drops.

They are also used to suppress immunity and thus prevent rejection after organ transplant.

Antitumour actions. Steroids have some anti-lymphocyte action and are used in combination with cytotoxic drugs to treat lymphomas and some leukaemias. Large doses (i.e. prednisolone 30–60 mg daily) are given over 1 or 2 weeks. Dexamethasone in doses of 16 mg daily is given in the palliative treatment of either primary or secondary cerebral tumours. It probably acts by reducing oedema.

Miscellaneous uses. Steroids produce an improvement in idiopathic thrombocytopenic purpura, in certain acute haemolytic anaemias and in certain types of the nephrotic syndrome. In these disorders large doses are usually required.

Dose. The dose required in treating the above disorder is the smallest amount which produces a satisfactory therapeutic effect. This varies considerably. Common practice is to start treatment with a fairly large dose of steroid (e.g. prednisolone 20–60 mg daily) and, when a suitable result is obtained, to reduce the dose stepwise until a low maintenance dose is achieved (Table 14.1). The incidence of adverse effects depends on the dosage and duration of treatment and, if possible, the maintenance dose should be below 7.5 mg of prednisolone daily.

If *rapid action* is required hydrocortisone hemisuccinate can be given intravenously.

Ideally, steroids should be given with food at breakfast. At this time natural steroid production is at a maximum so least suppression of adrenal function results. In children, long-term treatment with steroids retards growth. This may be minimized by giving the hormone on

Table 14.1 Potencies of various steroids

Drug	Anti-inflammatory effect	Salt-retaining effect	Equivalent dose
Cortisol (Hydrocortisone)	+	+	100 mg
Cortisone	+	+	125 mg
Prednisolone	++	+	25 mg
Prednisone	++	+	25 mg
Methyl-prednisolone	++	(+)	20 mg
Betamethasone	++	0	4 mg
Dexamethasone	++	0	4 mg
Triamcinolone	++	0	20 mg
Fludrocortisone	(+)	++	—

alternate days. Evening dosage should be avoided as this may keep the patient awake at night.

Replacement therapy. In these circumstances steroid hormones are used to replace the normal secretions of the adrenal glands because the adrenals have either been destroyed by disease (Addison's disease) or removed at operation.

When this occurs, the kidneys are no longer able to retain sodium, which is excreted in the urine and the body thus becomes depleted of sodium. This in turn leads to collapse with vomiting and low blood pressure. A curious feature of Addison's disease is widespread pigmentation, particularly characteristic in the mouth.

The aim of treatment in this disorder is to replace the missing hormones. In an acute Addisonian crisis with a collapsed and severely ill patient, cortisol (hydrocortisone) is given intravenously in doses of 100 mg and repeated as required. Saline and glucose are infused and any concurrent infection is treated vigorously.

For maintenance treatment it is important to use a steroid with sodium-retaining properties. Cortisol (hydrocortisone) 20 mg in the morning and 10 mg at night is satisfactory and may be combined with fludrocortisone 50–200 micrograms daily to further reduce salt loss. A rough check of adequate replacement can be achieved by measuring the blood pressure supine and erect. If inadequate, there will be a large postural fall in blood pressure. Other indications are the weight and well-being of the patient.

Any stress such as an acute infection will increase the requirements of steroids by these patients and the dose should be *increased* over the period of the acute episode.

Topical steroids (see p. 330)

Steroids may be applied to the skin in the treatment of various dermatological conditions. The best vehicle for the drug is soft white paraffin and between 5 and 10% of the applied dose is absorbed through the skin. The most active steroids for this purpose include betamethasone, triamcinolone, beclomethasone and fluocinolone. Prolonged application can produce atrophy of the skin and a tendency to bacterial or fungal infection.

Nursing point

Nurses should wear gloves when applying topical steroids otherwise they will absorb the drug.

Adverse effects of steroid therapy. These hormones produce some potentially dangerous side-effects when given in suppressive as against physiological doses. They are summarized in the following (Fig. 14.6):

1. *General appearance.* With large doses the patient may develop a moon face and acne and oedema may be troublesome. The skin becomes atrophic and purpura may occur.
2. *Blood pressure.* This may become raised and should be measured at regular intervals.
3. *Blood electrolytes.* These may become deranged, particularly in those with renal disease and should be measured with particular attention to sodium retention and potassium loss. Occasionally, supplementary potassium or sodium restriction is required.
4. *Urine.* Rarely these drugs precipitate *diabetes* and the urine should be tested for glucose.
5. *Symptoms of peptic ulcer* may rarely occur and require the withdrawal of the drug and NSAIDs should be avoided, if possible.
6. Any infective disease may spread rapidly and yet produce minimal signs in these patients.

Such an infection requires prompt treatment with antibiotics, together with an *increase* in the dose of steroid. *Chickenpox, which is usually a mild disease, may become life-threatening in patients taking steroids if they have no immunity from a previous attack. Such patients should avoid contact with chickenpox or herpes zoster. A similar risk applies to measles.*

7. With large doses *decalcification of bone* occurs and vertebrae may collapse.
8. *Avascular necrosis of bone*, producing severe pain and usually affecting the hips, is a very troublesome complication.
9. *Psychological disturbances* can occur.
10. The *eyes* may be affected with the development of cataracts or glaucoma.
11. *Growth is retarded* in children.
12. *Adrenal cortical atrophy.* Prolonged treatment with steroid hormones causes atrophy of the adrenal cortex. If this treatment is stopped suddenly or if the requirement is increased by stress or infection the adrenal cortex cannot produce adequate amounts of cortisol and a shock-like state develops. It may take the adrenal cortex 2 years to recover after prolonged steroid treatment.

Drugs reducing steroid action

Spironolactone blocks the action of *aldosterone* on the kidney and may be used as a diuretic (see p. 217).

Nursing points

1. Patients receiving long-term steroids will require double their usual dose if they develop a moderate illness and treble their usual dose for a severe illness. They must be taught to recognize stress situations.
2. Before an operation the surgeon and anaesthetist must be informed if the patient is receiving steroids. Patients must also inform their doctor and dentist if they are receiving steroids.
3. If treatment with steroids lasts more than 10 days, withdrawal must be gradual as adrenal suppression will have occurred. Patients must be taught not to stop taking steroids suddenly.
4. All patients receiving long-term steroids should carry a card detailing their treatment.
5. Careful monitoring of adverse effects (see Fig. 14.6) is important.

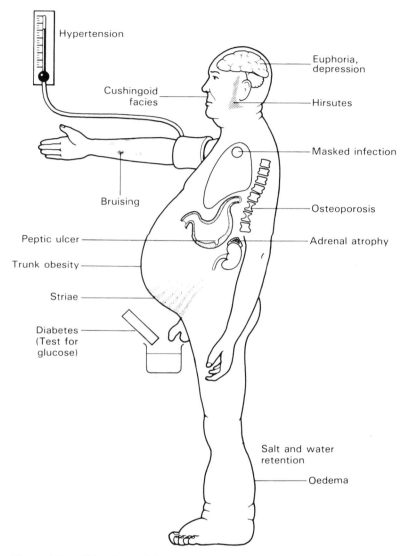

Figure 14.6 Side-effects of the steroids.

THE ADRENAL MEDULLA

The adrenal medulla produces both epinephrine and norepinephrine which are released into the circulation. The properties of these substances are discussed on page 38.

Tumours of the medulla occur rarely and may produce both these substances in excessive amounts.

THE PARATHYROID GLANDS AND CALCIUM

The parathyroid glands are situated in the neck in close relationship with the thyroid gland. They are concerned with the levels of calcium and phosphorus in the blood and their excretion by the kidney. A fall in the level of blood calcium concentration stimulates the parathyroids to produce more hormone, which mobilizes calcium from bone and decreases its loss through the kidney, thus returning the blood calcium level to normal.

Deficiency in parathyroid hormones results in an increase in blood phosphorus and a decrease in blood calcium levels. Lowering of the blood calcium causes a disorder known as *tetany*, which is characterized by increased irritability of muscles with spasm of the hands and feet (carpo-pedal spasm) and of the larynx. A decrease in blood calcium may result from parathyroid deficiency, from a lack of calcium in the diet, particularly if the patient is also deficient in vitamin D, and from alkalosis. The latter disorder, although not necessarily associated with low blood calcium, causes a decrease of ionized calcium in the blood and it is the ionized fraction which is important in preventing tetany.

In cases of tetany due to parathyroid deficiency, several drugs are available to treat the disorder.

Calcium. Acute attacks of tetany due to low blood calcium may be quickly relieved by giving calcium salts. They are usually administered as the gluconate or chloride. Calcium gluconate 10 ml of a 10% solution given slowly intravenously (2 ml/minute) produces rapid but short-lived relief. Calcium salts can also be given orally, not only to relieve tetany, but to prevent chronic calcium deficiency developing, particularly in those who absorb calcium poorly. This occurs in rickets (vitamin D deficiency), following gastrectomy, in steatorrhoea and in elderly subjects. Calcium is also required in those with excessive loss due to lactation. Prolonged calcium deficiency may lead to decalcification of bones which may become bent or may fracture. Calcium supplements in *deficiency states* should contain 20 mmol of calcium. This could be obtained from:

- 2 tablets of Sandocal 400, an effervescent preparation
- 8 tablets of calcium gluconate effervescent daily.

For pregnancy supplements lower doses are used.

Nursing point

Calcium salts should never be mixed with sodium bicarbonate in a syringe or infusion as the calcium will precipitate. Note that they may both be used intravenously in cardiac arrest.

Parathyroid hormone is obtained from the parathyroid of animals. It is destroyed in the intestinal tract and should be given by injection. Its maximum effect appears about 6 hours after injection.

It causes a rise in the blood calcium and a decrease in blood phosphorus levels. It is not satisfactory for long-term treatment, as increasing doses are required to produce the desired effect and it may cause allergic reactions.

Vitamin D (see also p. 265). The plasma calcium level can also be raised by vitamin D which increases the absorption of calcium from the intestine. Vitamin D may be required if the diet is deficient in the vitamin, in various disorders in which resistance to the action of Vitamin D occurs and in parathyroid hormone deficiency.

Vitamin D (calciferol) itself can be used or substances which have a similar action such as **dihydrotachysterol** or **alfacalcidol**. These drugs are considered on page 266.

Calcitonin. Calcitonin is a hormone which is produced in the thyroid gland but is concerned with calcium balance. It lowers the concentration of calcium in the blood and increases its deposition in bone. It is used in disorders where there is a rapid breakdown of bone, such as Paget's disease, or to control malignant deposits in bone where they release excessive amounts of calcium into the blood causing hypercalcaemia. It is prepared from either pig or salmon and is given by injection.

Salcatonin (calcitonin (salmon)) is given by subcutaneous or intramuscular injection. The dose and frequency of administration depend on the disorder being treated.

Adverse effects include nausea, vomiting and flushing after the injection and pain at the site of injection.

The bisphosphonates can be taken orally but should not be combined with food. They are absorbed onto the calcium-containing crystals in bone and slow both their rate of formation and dissolution. It must be realized that bone is not an inert structure, but is always being broken down and reformed. In Paget's disease and in malignant disease involving bone, this process accelerates, resulting in pain and in the release of calcium into the blood with consequent hypercalcaemia.

Bisphosphonates, by slowing bone 'turnover', relieve pain and control hypercalcaemia. They can also be used in post-menopausal osteoporosis.

Disodium etidronate is given orally in the treatment of Paget's disease. Food should not be taken for 2 hours before and after treatment.

It is sometimes used in the treatment of vertebral osteoporosis.

Alendronic acid increases the mineral content of bone and shows promise in the treatment of osteoporosis. It is given orally and can cause oesophagitis and ulcers. It should therefore be taken half an hour before breakfast, in the upright position, washed down with a full glass of water and the patient should remain upright for the next half hour.

Disodium pamidronate is given by intravenous infusion to treat bone pain or hypercalcaemia due to secondary malignant deposits in bone.

Sodium clodronate is similar but can be given orally.

Adverse effects include nausea and diarrhoea.

Treatment of hypercalcaemia due to malignancy

Malignant disease involving bone can cause a dangerous rise in the plasma calcium concentration which can be a medical emergency. It is treated as follows:

1. 0.9% sodium chloride solution is infused to correct the loss of water and salt through the kidney.

2. When this deficiency has been corrected, frusemide can be given to increase calcium excretion.

3. Disodium pamidronate is infused to prevent further bone breakdown.

Other drugs which can be given are steroids and calcitonin.

Prevention of calcium absorption

Sometimes it is necessary to lower a raised blood calcium concentration, which is dangerous, by reducing calcium absorption from the gut. This is achieved by giving phosphate in the form of **Phosphate-Sandoz**, which binds to calcium in the intestine and prevents its absorption.

Osteoporosis

In this condition the rate of bone resorption exceeds that of bone replacement so there is a loss of bone mass resulting in a tendency to fractures, particularly of the vertebrae, the upper end of the femur and the lower end of the radius. It is responsible for a great deal of morbidity and some mortality among elderly people. With increasing age, bone mass diminishes and there is a markedly rapid loss in women after the menopause (Fig. 14.7). Members of this group are especially prone to fractures. Osteoporosis can also result from various endocrine disorders, malabsorption, rheumatoid arthritis and the prolonged use of steroids.

Prevention and control. This is achieved by using drugs which decrease resorption and/or increase bone formation. In women, hormone replacement therapy is very effective in preventing bone loss (see p. 201). It should be continued for at least 5 years. Other preventive measures include regular exercise, an adequate intake of calcium (20 mmol daily) and Vitamin D and giving up smoking.

Bisphosphonates also prevent and control osteoporosis. *Alendronate*, given daily, considerably reduces the risk of fractures and increases bone density.

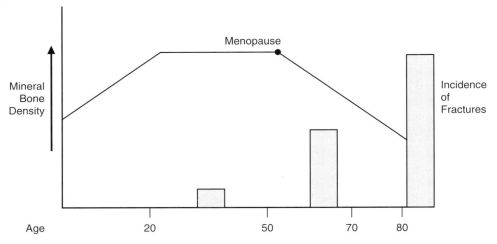

Figure 14.7   Bone density and the incidence of fractures related to age for women. (Based on a figure first published in the *BMJ*: Peel N & Eastell R 1995 ABC of rheumatology: osteoporosis. British Medical Journal 310: 989.)

THE PANCREAS

The pancreas is a relatively large gland lying across the upper part of the posterior abdominal wall. It produces a number of digestive enzymes which drain into the duodenum and help digestion.

Scattered throughout the gland are small collections of tissue known as the islets of Langerhans. These islets contain two types of cell called alpha and beta cells and from the beta cells is produced the important hormone called insulin.

INSULIN AND DIABETES MELLITUS

Insulin (Fig. 14.8) is a hormone which lowers the concentration of glucose in the blood by:

1. Stimulating the uptake of glucose by the tissues.
2. Converting glucose to glycogen in the liver where it is stored.
3. Increasing the production of fat and protein.

In *diabetes mellitus* there are two types of insulin deficiency. The first type is known as *insulin-dependent diabetes* (IDDM) or Type I in which there is a true deficiency of insulin due to atrophy of the islets of Langerhans and which

occurs predominantly in young people. This deficiency leads to a rapid rise in the blood glucose concentration with subsequent loss of large amounts of glucose with water and salt in the urine. In addition, fats in the body are broken down, releasing ketoacids which cause acidosis. Protein is also lost and weight loss may be marked. If not treated, the patient will lapse into a coma (*hyperglycaemic ketoacidosis*).

The second type of diabetes, known as *non-insulin-dependent* (NIDDM) or Type II, occurs in middle-aged or elderly people who are frequently overweight. In this type there appears to be resistance to the action of insulin rather than a true deficiency. The blood glucose concentration is raised with glycosuria, but ketoacidosis is not common and the symptoms are often those of the late complications of diabetes.

These complications occur with both types of diabetes. Disease of the small arteries leads to damage to the retina of the eye, declining renal function and serious interference with the circulation to the legs, sometimes requiring amputation, and various peripheral nerves may be damaged. Patients with diabetes are particularly prone to infection and these infections may, in turn, exacerbate the diabetes, sometimes leading to ketoacidosis and coma. Good control of the diabetes reduces the severity of the complications but does not entirely prevent them.

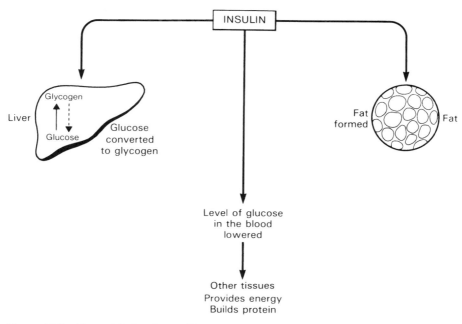

Figure 14.8   The metabolic effects of insulin.

Sources of insulin

Insulin is available in many preparations which vary in both their duration of action and their purity. Until recently insulin was extracted from the pancreas of cows (bovine) or pigs (porcine). Bovine insulin differs in its structure from human insulin and is thus inherently immunogenic. Porcine insulin is very similar to human insulin and is not much more liable to produce immunological reactions.

It is now possible to produce *human insulins* either by modifying porcine insulin or by a recombinant method involving bacteria. The code for synthesizing human insulin can be inserted into bacteria (*Escherichia coli*), which then multiply and produce human insulin.

Purification

All insulins are now highly purified to remove traces of other substances and make them less immunogenic. Non-human insulins can, however, stimulate the production of anti-insulin antibodies (AIA), which occasionally give rise to local and systemic allergic reactions and to insulin resistance.

Short-acting insulins (soluble insulins)

These are available as human or purified animal insulins. They are used in the treatment of diabetic coma (ketoacidosis), to cover operations and illnesses in patients with diabetes and sometimes in the long-term control of diabetes, combined with a longer-acting insulin. They are the only insulins suitable for intravenous injection. Following subcutaneous injection their action starts after about 30 minutes and continues for 8 hours. After intravenous injection their onset is more rapid, but only lasts for about half an hour. They include Humulin S; Human Actrapid; and Velosulin (porcine).

Insulin lispro is a modified form of human insulin which is very rapidly mobilized from the subcutaneous injection site. It acts even more quickly than soluble insulin (15 minutes against 30 minutes) and its duration of action is only 4 hours. Its place in the management of diabetes is not settled but it may be useful, if given immediately before a meal, in controlling the rise in blood sugar and thus mimicking more closely the response of the normal pancreas.

Intermediate-acting insulins

These insulins act for varying periods depending on the mix of rapid and slow-acting components. The blood glucose starts to fall in 1–2 hours after injection and this effect continues for 16–24 hours. They are usually given once or twice daily and may be combined with soluble insulin.

Insulin zinc suspension (IZS). It was found that if insulin was buffered with acetate its action was prolonged, and a further two types of insulin could be prepared: amorphous, in which the particles were small, and a crystalline form with larger particles. The action of amorphous insulin is rapid and short-lived, but that of crystalline insulin is more prolonged. By using a mixture of these insulins a smooth and prolonged effect can be achieved. Among those available are Human Monotard (30% amorphous, 70% crystalline); and Human Ultratard (crystalline).

Biphasic isophane insulins consist of insulin complexed with protamine. This can then be mixed with varying amounts of soluble insulin to produce an immediate and a longer effect. These include Human Mixtard 30/70 and Humulin M1, M2, M3, M4 (varying proportions of soluble and isophane insulin).

Long-acting insulins

Protamine zinc insulin (PZI). This is produced by adding protamine and zinc to insulin. Its action is prolonged, starting after 6 hours and lasting for 24–30 hours. It is a bovine insulin and may give rise to skin rashes and painful lumps at the site of injection. If soluble and PZI insulin are mixed in the syringe before injection, some of the soluble insulin becomes PZI insulin. To minimize this, the soluble insulin should be drawn up first and the mixture of insulins injected immediately. Alternatively, the crystalline form of human insulin zinc suspension (Human

Ultratard) also has a prolonged action and is not immunogenic.

TREATMENT OF DIABETES MELLITUS

Management of patients with insulin-dependent diabetes (IDDM)

These patients require insulin replacement and the object of treatment is to give them a diet suited to their lifestyle and work, then give enough insulin to replace the deficiency and maintain them in good health as judged by their subjective feelings, their weight (which should be kept at the correct level for their age and height) and keep their blood glucose levels near normal (Fig. 14.9).

There are many dietary schemes and with changing fashions it is too lengthy a subject to discuss here in detail. Briefly, about 50% of the calories in the diet should be from carbohydrate in forms which are slowly absorbed such as wholemeal bread, potatoes and various vegetables, but not rapidly digestible sugars such as sweets and cakes. About 35% of the calories may come from fat and the rest from protein.

Because they are at special risk from atheroma, patients with diabetes should avoid foods which have a deleterious effect on plasma lipids. Hypertension, if present, should be treated, exercise encouraged and smoking avoided.

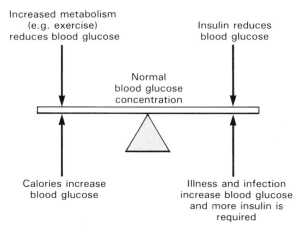

Figure 14.9 Balancing patients with diabetes.

Choice of insulin

If a patient is satisfactorily controlled on a certain type of insulin, that preparation should usually be continued. Human insulin is the least immunogenic and it should be used in the following circumstances.

1. For patients starting treatment.
2. If the patient develops generalized allergies to an unpurified insulin.
3. If injection causes severe local reactions.
4. If very large doses are required, a situation which suggests that antibodies have been produced by the impure insulin and are interfering with its action.
5. If the patient is pregnant because impurities in the older types of insulin can cross the placenta and affect the islet tissue of the fetus.

If a change is made from animal to human insulin it should be remembered that human insulin acts a little more rapidly and its effect lasts a shorter time so that some readjustment of dosage may be necessary. Also, only 80–90% of the previous dose may be needed.

Giving insulin

Because insulin is broken down in the stomach it has to be given by injection. One regime is to give a short-acting insulin 15–30 minutes before the three main meals and an intermediate-acting insulin at night; alternatively, a short- and intermediate-acting insulin can be given before breakfast and the evening meal. In some patients, provided the dose is small, a single injection of an intermediate-acting insulin is adequate. The type of insulin, dosage and frequency of administration are modified in the light of the patient's response until optimum control is obtained.

Strength of insulin preparations. The introduction of U100 insulin has greatly simplified insulin dosage. All insulins are now of standard strength—100 units in 1 ml. The U100 syringes are marked in units of insulin and so it is only necessary to draw up the required number of units (Fig. 14.10).

Insulin should be stored in the refrigerator (not

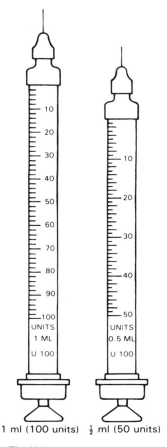

1 ml (100 units)   ½ ml (50 units)

Figure 14.10   The U100 syringe marked in units of insulin.

the freezing compartment), but the bottle in current use can safely be kept at room temperature.

Injection of insulin. Most patients receiving insulin are instructed how to inject themselves and this instruction is usually given by the nurse.

The best sites for injection are the front of the thighs, the abdomen and the outer side of the upper arm and the insulin is given subcutaneously. A different site should be used each time, but it must be remembered that the rate of absorption of insulin into the circulation varies with different parts of the body. Therefore, it is better to use the same area, but not exactly the same site, at the same time of day: for example, the morning dose into the thigh and the evening dose into the arm. Other points of note about injecting insulin are:

1. A microfine i.v. needle and syringe or a 25 G × $\frac{5}{8}$ inch should be used. The skin should be pinched up and the needle introduced at an angle of 90°.

2. No spirit should be used for skin cleaning as it hardens the skin and the injection site should not be massaged after injection.

3. Special syringes are available for those with poor eyesight or other infirmities.

Insulin pens are devices which contain a cartridge of insulin which is automatically injected. A wide range of insulins are available in cartridges and they may be more convenient for the patient.

Syringe pumps give a continuous subcutaneous infusion of insulin. The pump is worn by the patient and the rate of infusion modified to the patient's needs, thus producing a very fine control of the diabetes.

Monitoring treatment

Patients should be taught to monitor their response to treatment by measuring glucose levels in the blood or urine.

In normal subjects the blood glucose concentration varies from 3 to 7 mmol/l. The object of treatment is to keep the blood glucose as near as possible to these levels. In patients receiving insulin this is best achieved by measuring the blood glucose using the drop of blood from a finger prick which is applied to a special indicator strip. The resulting colour change can be read against a colour chart or by a meter. This enables patients to measure their own blood glucose levels and is usually carried out once daily at different times of day. The blood glucose concentration should be kept between 4 and 9 mmol/litre.

The proportion of haemoglobin in the red cells which is glycosylated (i.e. combined with glucose) provides an index of the blood glucose concentration over a period of time. Ideally, the HbA1 should be kept below 8.8% and this can be used to monitor treatment.

In patients not on insulin or for whom strict control is not considered practical, the urine is tested for glucose before breakfast, before the midday meal, before retiring, using some dipstick method or Clinitest tablets. This gives a less precise picture of how the blood glucose level is being controlled as glucose does not appear in the urine until the blood level is about 10 mmol/litre, which is higher than normal. Also it gives no indication if the blood glucose is too low. Nevertheless, it is easy to perform and adequate for some patients, particularly those with NIDDM.

If the diabetes is seriously out of control, the urine will show the presence of ketones as well as glucose. This means a dangerous situation is developing and immediate treatment is required (see later).

Hypoglycaemia. Overdosage with insulin causes an undue decrease in the blood sugar. This leads to faintness, dizziness, tremor, sweating and abnormal behaviour, which may be mistaken for drunkenness. If no treatment is given convulsions, coma and death may occur. It can quickly be relieved by giving sugar or glucose, 4 teaspoonfuls or lumps of sugar in half a glass of fruit juice followed by two biscuits being effective. Glucagon (see p. 198) by injection is also effective and is useful if the patient is too drowsy to swallow.

About a quarter of patients with long-term diabetes may not be aware that they are becoming hypoglycaemic. Alcohol and β blockers may aggravate this and it has been suggested that it is more likely to occur when human insulin is used, but proof is lacking.

Driving a car. The danger is that the patient may lose control of the vehicle as a result of hypoglycaemia, due to excess insulin. Special care is therefore necessary, and patients who are being treated with insulin should check their blood sugar before setting out and at 2-hourly intervals during a long journey. Sugar should always be available in the car.

Insulin in special circumstances

Details of the methods used under these

circumstances vary, but the general principles are the same.

Pregnancy. Human insulin is preferable (see p. 191). It is necessary to control the diabetes as well as possible, usually giving insulin two or three times daily. Poor control increases the incidence of fetal abnormality and perinatal problems. After delivery of the placenta, insulin requirements fall and dosage adjustment will be necessary.

Serious intercurrent illness. The patient's insulin requirement will rise and this situation is a potent cause of diabetic coma; therefore, it is important not to reduce insulin dosage. It may be necessary to change the regime to 1–6 units/hour of soluble insulin given by intravenous infusion or by multiple small intramuscular injections, together with fluid and glucose as determined by blood glucose estimations.

Major surgery. It is easiest if the patient is first on the morning operating list. The morning dose of insulin is not given, but at least an hour before surgery an infusion of 5% glucose with 10 mmol of potassium in each 500 ml is started at 100 ml/hour. Human Actrapid is commenced at the same time at a rate of 1–4 units/hour. The rate of insulin infusion is subsequently adjusted depending on the blood glucose levels.

Diabetic coma (hyperglycaemic ketoacidosis). Patients with diabetes who are not treated, or develop some infection during treatment, may pass into a diabetic coma. These patients have not only a very high blood and urinary glucose level, but are producing large quantities of ketone bodies which can be detected in the urine and which, being acids, lead to an acidosis. The excessive diuresis produced by the glucose in the urine leads to severe depletion of sodium, potassium and water.

Soluble human insulin (Humulin S or Human Actrapid) is given *intravenously* by an infusion pump. It is diluted to 1 unit/ml and infused at the rate of 6 units/hour for an adult. The rate is adjusted to produce a fall in the blood glucose concentration of about 5 mmol/hour. The aim is to reduce the level to about 11 mmol/litre and maintain it until oral feeding and subcutaneous injection of insulin can be introduced. If no pump is available, 20 units can be given *intramuscularly* followed by 6 units per hour. At the same time water and electrolyte imbalance is corrected by giving an infusion of normal saline containing 20 mmol of potassium chloride per litre. Restoration of electrolyte and water balance is usually sufficient and the kidneys will correct the acidosis by secreting an acid urine. Occasionally, however, the acidosis is so severe that it is necessary to infuse sodium bicarbonate until the degree of acidosis is improved. Frequent examination of the urine for sugar and ketones and of the blood sugar hourly and of the electrolytes is important in controlling treatment. Subsequent doses of insulin are determined by the blood glucose concentration.

The possibility of infection as a cause of diabetic coma should not be forgotten, and if this is found it is treated by the appropriate antibiotic.

Deep vein thrombosis is a common complication and prophylactic subcutaneous heparin is often given.

Management of patients with non-insulin-dependent diabetes (NIDDM)

The main objective in treating NIDDM is to prevent the development of the late complications of the disease—myocardial infarction, vascular disease, renal failure, retinopathy and neuropathy. This is best achieved by controlling plasma glucose, lipids and blood pressure (if raised) and by avoiding risk factors such as smoking and obesity. Seventy-five per cent of these patients will be overweight and initially the treatment of choice is diet, which should contain 750 kcal daily—aiming to reduce the patient's weight to the ideal level. Sucrose and glucose should be largely avoided and most carbohydrate taken in the form of polysaccharides (vegetables, cereals, pasta, etc.). The intake of saturated animal fat should be low. When the appropriate weight has been reached the diet may be increased to maintain it at that level (see p. 198). Regular exercise, tailored to the abilities of the patient, is beneficial by increasing insulin sensitivity.

This regime is intended to keep the fasting blood sugar below 9 mmol/litre and the plasma cholesterol below 6.5 mmol/litre. Blood pressure control is important and, if the blood pressure is raised, it should be reduced to 145/85, if possible. ACE inhibitors are the preferred hypotensive drugs as they decrease renal damage. In elderly patients the requirements may be relaxed a little.

If, after 6 months, these objectives are not achieved treatment with oral agents will be necessary. Most patients are given one of the sulphonylureas, although if obesity is a problem metformin may be preferred. Adherence to the diet is still important as the sulphonylureas may cause some weight gain. A number of patients may still fail to attain the desired objectives, in which case the two types of drug may be combined. Finally, if this fails injections of insulin will be needed. There is a group of NIDDM patients for whom insulin is the only way to control the disease.

ORAL HYPOGLYCAEMIC AGENTS

The sulphonylureas

This group of drugs is related to the sulphonamides. They lower blood glucose levels by increasing insulin production by the pancreas.

They are all given orally and differ largely in their duration of action. They are used in patients with NIDDM who are usually middle-aged or elderly and obese, and supplement, but do not replace, treatment by diet. They have no place in the treatment of the young patient with diabetes who requires insulin or of diabetic coma. There are several drugs in the group which are in common use.

Tolbutamide has been used for many years and is very safe and satisfactory if used correctly. Its duration of action is about 6 hours and for this reason it is particularly recommended in elderly patients as the risk of hypoglycaemia is reduced and it is given orally two or three times daily. The dose is 0.5–1.5 g/day and if no satisfactory response is achieved with this dose, larger amounts are unlikely to be successful.

Chlorpropamide is similar to tolbutamide, but

its action lasts a full 24 hours so once daily dosage is appropriate. Because of adverse effects it should only be used for patients who have been successfully treated with it for some time.

With both these drugs gastrointestinal upsets, rashes or rarely blood dyscrasias and fluid retention can occur. Both tolbutamide and chlorpropamide can produce hypoglycaemia, but it is much more common after chlorpropamide because of its longer action and because accumulation can occur with impaired renal function. It usually follows a prolonged fast while taking the drug or may occur at night. It is especially dangerous in elderly patients. In some patients chlorpropamide can cause flushing after taking alcohol.

Glibenclamide has been widely used. Its action lasts about 12 hours and it can be given once daily. With a large single dose, hypoglycaemia can occur and in these circumstances it is best to split the dose and give it twice daily. The initial dose is 5 mg (2.5 mg for the elderly) taken with breakfast and increased as required to a maximum dose of 15 mg daily. However, because of its lengthy action with the attendant risk of hypoglycaemia, its use should now be restricted to patients who have already been successfully treated with it and it should not be used in elderly patients or those with renal impairment.

Glipizide has a shorter action (6 hours) and serious hypoglycaemia is less likely. The initial dose is 2.5–5.0 mg before breakfast and the dose adjusted. Doses above 15 mg daily should be divided and the maximum is 40 mg daily.

Other sulphonylureas

	Single dose	Duration of action
Gliquidone	15–60 mg	3 hours
Gliclazide	40–80 mg	12 hours
Tolazamide	100–250 mg	20 hours

At present the choice usually lies between tolbutamide, which is relatively cheap, and glipizide.

Interactions. NSAIDs, including aspirin, enhance the effect and thiazide diuretics reduce the effect of sulphonylureas.

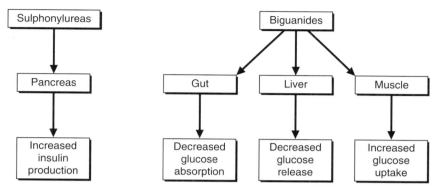

Figure 14.11   Comparison of the actions of sulphonylureas and biguanides.

Repaglinide is an oral hypoglycaemic agent which stimulates insulin release from the pancreas. It is rapidly absorbed and very short-acting. Given before a meal, it reduces the postprandial rise in blood sugar and can be used to improve control of NIDDM. Its place in treatment is not yet clearly defined.

The biguanides

This group differs from the sulphonylureas (Fig. 14.11) both in chemical structure and mode of action. Biguanides reduce glucose absorption from the intestine and may also stimulate the uptake of glucose by muscles by direct action; they do not, however, prevent the production of ketone bodies. Their main use is combined with one of the sulphonylureas when the patient is not responding satisfactorily to diet or to these drugs alone. The biguanides are also occasionally used combined with insulin in patients with IDDM whose disease is proving difficult to control. They decrease appetite and this may be useful in treating obese patients with diabetes. They do not cause hypoglycaemia.

Metformin is the only biguanide in common use at present. The dose is 500 mg three times daily, with or after food.

Adverse effects. Anorexia and nausea are troublesome and may lead to the abandonment of this form of treatment. More serious but rare is *lactic acidosis* with drowsiness, abdominal pain, vomiting and shock. The mechanism of this side-effect is not understood, but it is more liable to occur in alcoholics and those with liver, renal and cardiac failure. It was particularly likely to occur with the biguanide phenoformin which has now been withdrawn.

Acarbose

Taken orally before meals, this agent inhibits the digestion of complex carbohydrates such as sucrose and starches, thus preventing their absorption, but it does not interfere with glucose absorption. The postprandial rise in the blood sugar is reduced. However, the unabsorbed carbohydrates in the bowel may cause flatulence and diarrhoea. The role of this drug in diabetes is not yet determined, but it may be a useful adjunct to treatment in NIDDM.

Troglitazone

In NIDDM the major defect is a resistance to the action of insulin in the peripheral tissues, and thus, a failure of glucose uptake. Troglitazone reduces this resistance with subsequent lowering of blood glucose levels. It can be used as a single agent or combined with insulin or oral hypoglycaemic agents and shows considerable promise. Unfortunately, disturbances of liver function occur in about 2% of patients and, rarely, serious liver disease develops. It is not licensed in the UK but is available in Europe.

Glucagon

Glucagon is a substance which mobilizes the liver glycogen and thus releases glucose into the blood. It is used to raise the blood sugar in patients who are hypoglycaemic: for instance, after an overdose of insulin. The dose is 0.5–1.0 units i.m. and the effect is seen in about 10 minutes.

The nurse and the patient with diabetes at home

The management of patients with diabetes is a team activity involving the patient, the doctor, the nurse, the dietician and often laboratory staff. Patients with diabetes may be managed by a hospital diabetic clinic, but may also be stabilized and controlled in the community. Nurses are trained to supervise treatment in the home with the back-up of the hospital or family doctor. This has the advantage that treatment can be geared to the patient's lifestyle and, most importantly, the family can be involved particularly in planning meals, etc.

Education is very important for the patients who must realize as far as possible the implications of their illness and its treatment.

APPETITE SUPPRESSION AND OBESITY

Obesity is a serious health hazard and is increasingly common throughout the Western World. 15% of the population of the UK are obese (i.e. they have a body mass index (BMI) of over 30). It is strongly associated with heart disease, hypertension, NIDDM and arthritis of weight-bearing joints.

The essential cause is an imbalance between calorie (food) intake and energy expenditure (exercise). Normally, various mechanisms within the body keep these in balance but, even a small disturbance in this balance can lead to increasing deposition of fat. This is particularly liable to occur with a sedentary occupation and the consumption of energy-rich foods which are features of modern lifestyles. Genetic factors play a part in maintaining the calorie intake/ energy expending balance and obesity often runs in families.

Management. The definitive treatment is to decrease calorie intake and increase energy expenditure. In spite of extensive literature on all types of diet, it remains essential to eat less. The actual composition is less important than its calorie content, and a normal, mixed diet, low in fat and sugar is adequate. The diet should be combined with a programme of exercise related to the age and health of the patient to increase energy expenditure.

For the average adult, not doing heavy work, a daily intake of 750 kcal will result in the loss of 1.0 kg/week which is ideal. The aim should be to reduce the weight to the correct BMI, given as:

$$BMI = \frac{\text{Weight in kilograms}}{(\text{Height in metres})^2}$$

which should be between 20 and 25.

The waist/hip circumference ratio should not exceed 1.0 as central obesity is especially associated with increased morbidity.

As yet there is no entirely satisfactory or safe drug to suppress appetite, but the use of thyroid hormones or amphetamine-like drugs should be avoided.

Orlistat has recently been introduced to treat obesity. It inhibits the action of lipase in the intestine, thus reducing fat absorption. It has been shown, in trials, to reduce weight but it causes steatorrhoea. Orlistat will not enable those who wish to lose weight to eat what they like but, combined with a low fat diet, it could be an adjunct to treatment.

FURTHER READING

Boyle I, Ralston S 1990 The treatment of hypercalcaemia. Prescribers Journal 30: 180
Brownlow I 1992 Transformed by thyroxine. Nursing Times 88 (8): 40
Compston J E 1994 The therapeutic use of biphosphonates. British Medical Journal 309: 711
Eastell R, Peel N 1998 Osteoporosis. Journal of the Royal College of Physicians, London 32: 14
Editorial 1990 Corticosteroids—Getting replacement right. Prescribers Journal 28: 71

Editorial 1990 Insulin injection technique. British Medical
    Journal 301: 3
Editorial 1991 Hypoglycaemia and diabetic control. Lancet
    338: 853
Editorial 1991 Treating obesity. British Medical Journal 302:
    803
Editorial 1997 Humalog—a new insulin analogue. Drug and
    Therapeutics Bulletin 35: 8: 57
Editorial 1998 Combined blood pressure and glucose in
    Type 2 diabetes. British Medical Journal 317: 693
Editorial 1998 Appetite suppression and valvular heart
    disease. New England Journal of Medicine 339: 765
Fernez R E, Alberti K G 1989 Sulphonylurea treatment of
    non-insulin dependent diabetes. Quarterly Journal of
    Medicine 73: 987
Franklyn J A 1994 The management of hyperthyroidism.
    New England Journal of Medicine 330: 1731
Jordan J, White J 1998 Hyperthyroidism. Nursing Times 94:
    24: 46
Lebovitz H E 1995 Diabetic ketoacidosis. Lancet 345: 767
Thomas B 1994 Manual of diabetic practice, 2nd edn.
    Blackwell, Oxford
Toft A D 1994 Thyroxine therapy. New England Journal of
    Medicine 331: 174
Wang P H 1993 Tight glucose control and diabetic
    complications. Lancet 342: 129
Wilding J 1997 Obesity treatment. British Medical Journal
    315: 997
Williams G 1994 Management of non-insulin-dependent
    diabetes mellitus. Lancet 343: 95

SECTION III: HORMONES AFFECTING REPRODUCTION

THE FEMALE SEX HORMONES

It is important to understand the hormone background of the normal menstrual cycle and of pregnancy before considering the individual hormones.

At the commencement of the menstrual cycle, the *follicular stimulating hormone* (a gonadotrophin) from the pituitary causes ripening of the ovarian follicle which releases *estrogenic* hormones. The estrogens in turn cause proliferation of the mucosa lining the uterus. Ovulation occurs about halfway through the menstrual cycle and the pituitary now releases *luteinizing hormone* (a gonadotrophin), which helps the development of the corpus luteum when the ovum has been discharged from the ovary. The corpus luteum produces the hormone *progesterone*, which causes further thickening of the endometrium. If

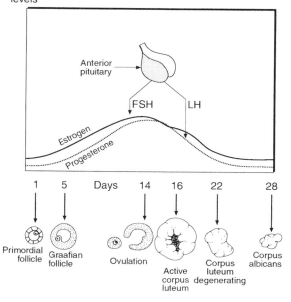

Plasma hormone levels

Figure 14.12   Events of the 'average' menstrual cycle. Reproduced from *Nursing Care of Women* with permission from Prentice Hall.

implantation of the fertilized ovum does not occur, the corpus luteum regresses and the superficial part of the endometrium breaks down and is discharged as the menstrual flow (Fig. 14.12).

If a fertilized ovum is implanted in the uterus the corpus luteum does not immediately regress. Throughout pregnancy large quantities of progesterone and estrogens are produced, probably by the placenta, and can be recovered from the urine. Gonadotrophic hormone is also produced by the human placenta during the early months of pregnancy and its presence in the urine forms the basis of various tests for pregnancy.

Just before parturition the production of progesterone ceases and this may be concerned with the start of labour.

Both estrogens and progesterone are used therapeutically and are considered in detail on page 201.

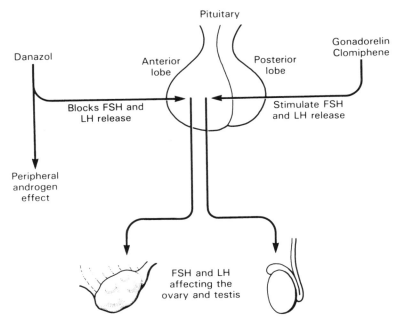

Figure 14.13 Drugs modifying the release of FSH and LH and thus modifying gonadal activity.

GONADOTROPHINS

These pituitary hormones are used therapeutically and will be considered in detail (Fig. 14.13).

Follicular stimulating hormone (FSH) is available as *urofollitrophin* and as *follitropun alfa and beta*. In the female it causes ripening of the ovarian follicles and the production of estrogen, and in the male it is necessary for the production of spermatozoa. It is given by injection.

Luteinizing hormone (LH) is available as *chorionic gonadotrophin*. In the female it produces the corpus luteum and in the male it stimulates the interstitial cells of the testis to produce androgens. It is given by injection.

Human menopausal gonadotrophins (HMGs) are a combination of FSH and LH.

Therapeutics. In female infertility these hormones are given by injection to induce normal ovarian function. FSH is given first to produce an ovarian follicle followed by LH to induce ovulation, or they may be given together as HMG. They will only be successful if infertility is due to lack of normally secreted gonadotrophins and not if there is primary ovarian failure.

Clomiphene *stimulates increased secretion* of gonadotrophins and is used in the treatment of infertility due to failure of ovulation; 50 mg is given daily for 5 days early in the menstrual cycle. It may be so successful that it results in twins, but multiple pregnancies can be avoided by careful dosing.

Adverse effects include flushing, headaches, nausea, weight gain and visual disturbances.

Gonadorelin *releases* gonadotrophins and induces ovulation. It is given as a pulsed injection every 90 minutes.

Gonadorelin analogues

Buserelin and goserelin increase the release of gonadotrophins initially, but this is followed by a falling off of secretion so the action of gonadotrophins on the ovary and testis is reduced resulting in decreased activity of the male and female gonads. They are used in the treatment of endometriosis and carcinoma of the prostate.

Danazol and gestrinone *inhibit* gonadotrophin release. They are used in treating endometriosis and various benign breast disorders.

Adverse effects reflect that they are androgen derivatives and cause abnormal hair growth, greasy skin, acne, fluid retention and nausea.

Cyclical breast pain

This is due to swelling and tenderness of the breasts which occurs during the second half of the menstrual cycle and is associated with the corpus luteum. If the symptoms are severe, danazol is effective in prevention, but its side-effects are troublesome.

Gamolenic acid extracted from evening primrose, may decrease the sensitivity of the breasts to hormones and may thus also be effective, but relief is delayed for about 3 months.

THE ESTROGENS

The estrogen hormones have a variety of effects, the most important being proliferation of the endometrium, sensitization of the uterine muscle to certain stimulating agents, increase in duct tissue in the breast and inhibition of production of prolactin by the pituitary. They are also concerned with the development of the female secondary sex characteristics.

Estradiol 17β and estrone are secreted by the ovary, but there is a number of estrogens which are used therapeutically.

Natural estrogens	Estradiol
	Estrone
Synthetic estrogens	Ethinylestradiol
	Diethylstilbestrol
Conjugated estrogens	Premarin, which is similar to natural estrogens

Therapeutic uses. Estrogens are used for

1. Replacement therapy
2. Controlling cancer of the prostate and breast
3. Oral contraception.

Hormone replacement therapy (HRT)

A woman is considered to be postmenopausal 1 year after her last menstrual period and the menopause may be associated with a number of disorders.

Menopausal symptoms. These fall into two groups:

1. Those due to estrogen deficiency include some atrophy of the uterus and dryness of the vagina which may cause dyspareunia.

Osteoporosis. Loss of protein from bone, with subsequent risk of fracture, is a serious problem in postmenopausal women. Estrogen treatment is the most effective way of preventing this. In addition, HRT appears to give some protection against coronary artery disease, stroke and possibly, Alzheimer's disease.

Hot flushes. Their cause is unknown, but they respond to treatment with estrogen.

2. Vague emotional symptoms of varying and ill-defined aetiology.

Symptoms in group 1 respond to HRT with an estrogen, but in group 2 the response is variable.

Most patients receiving HRT will have an intact uterus. The unopposed action of estrogens stimulates the endometrium and may ultimately cause a carcinoma of the uterus. To prevent this happening, the estrogen is combined with a progestogen to mimic the normal menstrual cycle, with regular shedding of the endometrium. A monthly course consists of an estrogen given daily and a progestogen for the last 10–14 days of the cycle. Withdrawal bleeding may occur. A convenient preparation is Prempak C in which an estrogen is given throughout the cycle and a progestogen (norgestrel) for the last 12 days. It is presented in a more or less foolproof pack. Other similar preparations are available.

Tibolone is a synthetic hormone which will control postmenopausal symptoms and limit osteoporosis without stimulating the endometrium, and thus eliminate the risk of causing uterine cancer. There is therefore no need for a progestogen and no monthly bleeding.

Raloxifene has effects similar to estrogens on blood and lipids, but blocks estrogen action on the breast and uterus. It reduces osteoporosis and its use is not associated with menstrual bleeding. Its effect on breast cancer and heart disease is not known. It may cause hot flushes; and there is an increased risk of thrombosis.

Estrogens can also be given as a patch applied to the skin. The patch available in the UK contains estradiol, which diffuses through the skin and is effective for 3–4 days when the patch is replaced. Cyclical progestogen treatment causing monthly bleeding is still required.

If the patient has had a hysterectomy the progestogen is not needed and replacement can be with an estrogen alone, e.g. conjugated estrogens (Premarin) 625 micrograms daily orally.

On balance, HRT is indicated in post-menopausal women if they have symptoms (vaginitis, flushing) or are at special risk of osteoporosis or cardiovascular disease. Many practitioners consider that HRT should be used by most women, provided there are no contra-indications. However, possible problems, which must be weighed against the benefits, are:

1. There may be a slightly increased risk of carcinoma of the breast, particularly in older women and those taking hormones for more than 5 years.

2. Adverse effects include nausea, weight gain, headache and fluid retention. Breast swelling may occur early in treatment but usually subsides within 3 months.

3. There is a slight risk of venous thrombosis.

4. Before starting treatment a full examination is necessary to exclude cancer, gynaecological abnormalities and thrombotic disease which may be made worse by HRT, and the patient should be given a full explanation of the implications of the treatment.

Duration of treatment depends on the therapeutic objectives. To relieve menopausal symptoms, 5 years is usually adequate. To prevent arterial disease, stroke and osteoporosis, lifelong treatment might be desirable, but 10 years is perhaps more practical because of the slight risk of breast cancer which is related to the duration of treatment. For preventing osteoporosis, HRT may be delayed as it is still effective late in life.

Menstrual disturbances. In patients who are deficient in natural ovarian hormones it is possible to produce uterine bleeding by giving estrogens for a time and then stopping the hormone. This is, of course, not a normal menstrual cycle, and it is difficult to see any real therapeutic use in the manoeuvre except for its psychological value.

Nursing point

HRT patches should be replaced every 3–4 days. They should be applied to clean, dry, unbroken skin on the trunk below the waist and not near the breasts.

Neoplastic disease. Estrogens have been used with some success in two types of neoplasm.

In *carcinoma of the prostate* estrogens probably act by suppressing the production of male hormone which stimulates the neoplasm. Large doses are required. Stilboestrol 1–3 mg daily is given by mouth or pellets of the hormone may be implanted subcutaneously. Some patients report nausea and hypertrophy of the breasts with pigmentation of the nipple. Fluid retention may be troublesome and there is an increased risk of venous thrombosis. An alternative is *cyproterone* which directly blocks the action of androgens on the prostate or gonadorelin analogues, which reduce androgen secretion.

A proportion of patients with advanced *carcinoma of the breast* obtain temporary, but sometimes striking remission of their disease with estrogens. They are most successful in postmenopausal patients.

Estrogens can also be applied locally. They are used in atrophic vaginitis which occurs in post-menopausal women due to estrogen deficiency. Dienestrol cream (0.01%) applied daily for 1 week and then reduced, is satisfactory.

PROGESTERONE AND PROGESTOGENS

Progesterone which is the natural hormone and is produced mainly in the ovary, causes further thickening and development of the secretory phase in the endometrium which has been induced by estrogen and 'damps down' the excitability of the uterine muscle. It probably plays a large part in maintaining the fetus in the uterus until the time is ripe for labour to commence.

In addition to progesterone several *progestogens* are available. These are synthetic substances which have the same general actions as progesterone, although they differ in detail.

The older progestogens altered plasma lipids and increased the possibility of vascular disease. Most of those in common use at present (*norethisterone, norgestimate, gestodene, desogestrel*) have little or no adverse effect on lipids.

Therapeutics. The main uses of progestogens are:

1. In the combined or progestogen—only contraceptive pill where they make the cervical mucus impenetrable to sperm. *Medroxyprogesterone* given intramuscularly, can also be used as a contraceptive.

2. In HRT where they prevent the development of intrauterine cancer by causing cyclical shedding of the endometrium.

3. In various menstrual disorders and endometriosis which is due to ectopic areas of endometrium.

Adverse effects include fluid retention, weight gain, breast discomfort and acne.

ORAL CONTRACEPTIVES

The combined oral contraceptive pill is very widely used and is the most effective method of preventing conception. It is a combination of an estrogen and a progestogen and acts in several ways.

1. By inhibiting ovulation—this is the consequence of reducing the output of pituitary gonadotrophins.

2. By changing the character of the mucus of the uterine cervix, and making penetration to the uterus by sperms more difficult.

3. By making the endometrium less suitable for implantation of the ovum.

The estrogen used is usually *ethinylestradiol* and the usual progestogens are *norethisterone, levonorgestrel, desogestrel or gestodene*. Usually the composition of the pill is unaltered throughout the full monthly course, but there are a few preparations in which pills of varying composition are given sequentially—the biphasic and triphasic preparations. Of the many preparations now available the most effective and widely used are those in which both an estrogen and a progestogen are given throughout the course, with a failure rate of less than 0.5 per 100 women years.

Table 14.2 shows the estrogenic and progestogenic content of some of the preparations in use at the time of writing.

It is also possible to give preparations which only contain a progestogen, but although they impair fertility, they only prevent ovulation in about half the menstrual cycles so are less efficient as contraceptives.

If used correctly, the combined pill provides the most effective contraceptive available and failure rarely occurs.

Using the combined pill

1. It is usual to start with the lowest dose formulation because the risk of thrombosis (see later) is related to the estrogen content. Preparations containing 20–35 micrograms of ethinylestradiol are usually prescribed.

2. The 'Pill' is started on the first day of the menstrual cycle (first day of bleeding) and continued for 21 days, then stopped for 7 days during which bleeding occurs. The regime is then repeated.

3. The 'Pill' must be taken regularly. If the dose is taken 12 hours late, other contraceptive precautions should be used for the next 7 days.

4. If a low-dose combination 'Pill' fails· to control the cycle after 3 months, alternatives such as triphasic preparations should be tried.

5. After childbirth, the 'Pill' should be started 3 weeks postpartum if the woman is not breast-feeding. If she is breast-feeding a progestogen-only 'Pill' or a different method of contraception is advised.

Table 14.2 Oral contraceptives

Progestogen only			
Norethisterone	Micronor	350 micrograms	} oral
Levonorgestrel	Microval	30 micrograms	
Medroxyprogesterone		150 mg	} depot
Norethisterone		200 mg	

Combined preparations		
	Estrogen	Progestogen
	micrograms	micrograms
Ethinylestradiol + norethisterone		
Loestrin 20	20	1000
Ovysmen	35	500
Brevinor	35	500
Norimin	35	1000
Ethinylestradiol + levonorgestrel		
Microgynon 30	30	150
Ovranette	30	150
Eugynon 30	30	250
Ovran 30	30	250
Ovran	50	250
Ethinylestradiol + desogestrel		
Mercilon	20	150
Marvelon	30	150
Ethinylestradiol + gestodene		
Femodene	30	75
Minulet	30	75
Ethinylestradiol + norgestimate		
Cilest	35	250

Triphasic preparations			
Ethinylestradiol + norethisterone			
Trinovum	(7 days)	35	500
	(7 days)	35	750
	(7 days)	35	1000
Ethinylestradiol + levonorgestrel			
Trinordiol	(6 days)	30	50
	(5 days)	40	75
	(10 days)	30	125
Logynon	(6 days)	30	50
	(5 days)	40	75
	(10 days)	30	125
Ethinylestradiol + gestodene			
Triadene	(6 days)	30	50
Tri-minulet	(5 days)	40	70
	(10 days)	30	100

Nurses working in family planning clinics and health centres have an important role in teaching women about taking oral contraceptives and allaying anxieties. If concerned, women should be advised to seek medical advice. Stopping the 'Pill' may result in an unplanned pregnancy.

Using progestogens only

This method which inhibits ovulation and changes the character of the cervical mucus is less safe than the combined pill, but has virtually no risk of thrombotic disease (see later) and may be preferred in older women or those at special risk from thrombosis.

The 'Pill' is started on day 1 of the cycle and taken at the *same time* each day throughout the cycle with no break.

Progestogens can also be given as depot injections lasting 2–3 months or as capsules containing a progestogen which is slowly released (*Norplant*). These capsules are inserted into the upper arm under a local anaesthetic and are effective for about 5 years.

The main side-effects of the progestogen-only 'Pill'

Amenorrhoea is common in women taking this form of the 'Pill' and it is essential to teach them the early signs and symptoms of pregnancy to avoid anxiety.

Spotting—slight blood loss—may occur through much of the cycle.

Postcoital contraception (Yuzpe method)

The risk of pregnancy after unprotected sexual intercourse is about 1 : 20. It is possible to reduce the risk of pregnancy by using the oral contraceptive as a 'morning after' pill. Two tablets of Schering PC 4, a high estrogen preparation, are taken immediately and repeated after 12 hours. These measures must be instituted within 72 hours of intercourse. Nausea may be a problem. Postcoital contraception can be obtained in family planning clinics.

The patient should be told that a barrier method of contraception will be required until the next period.

An alternative is to give levonorgestrel (a progestogen) 750 micrograms repeated after

12 hours. It is acceptably effective if given up to 48 hours after exposure.

The main side-effects of the combined 'Pill'

Nausea is probably related to the estrogen dosage and can usually be relieved by changing to a preparation with less estrogen.

Weight gain usually settles after a few cycles.

The menstrual cycle is induced to be more regular and menstrual loss is often decreased.

Thrombosis. There is now clear evidence that taking oral contraceptives carries an increased risk of venous and cerebral thrombosis. Taking the 'Pill' makes it more likely that the subject will be admitted to hospital with an episode of thrombosis. In addition, there is a slightly increased risk of cerebral arterial disease. The overall mortality is about 2 per 100 000. Older women who smoke heavily are especially at risk from thromboembolic complications. Heavy smokers in the 40–44 age group have an excess mortality of 54 per 100 000 women, and they should therefore use some other form of contraception. Thrombosis is believed to be due to the estrogen in the 'Pill'. For this reason the estrogen content of these preparations is kept as low as possible.

The associated arterial disease is due to the progestogen fraction of the 'Pill' which alters the blood lipids.

The new progestogens desogestrel and gestodene were introduced as they are less likely to cause changes in plasma lipids and, therefore, might be expected to reduce the risk of vascular disease (e.g. coronary thrombosis and strokes). However, evidence has emerged that they may actually increase the incidence of *venous thrombosis* in the legs and, thus, the risk of pulmonary embolism.

The incidence of venous thrombosis is approximately:

5 per 100 000 women per year—no contraceptive

15 per 100 000 women per year—with older progestogens

25 per 100 000 women per year—with desogestrel or gestodene (third-generation 'Pill')

60 per 100 000 women per year—in pregnancy

In view of this very small risk of thrombosis with the third-generation 'Pill', which is considerably less than that of pregnancy, they can be prescribed after a discussion with the patient. However, there is a case for avoiding contraceptives containing desogestrel or gestodene in those who are overweight, immobile or have a history of thrombosis.

Occasionally patients taking oral contraceptives develop *hypertension*. This is common in older women, but usually improves on stopping the 'Pill'.

Many studies have been undertaken to determine whether oral contraceptives could cause cancer.

Breast. In those who are taking the 'Pill' there may be a slightly increased risk of breast cancer. This appears to be related to the age at which it is stopped rather than to the duration of exposure. After stopping the 'Pill', the risk diminishes over 10 years.

Cervix. There is some evidence that cancer of the cervix is more common in those taking oral contraceptives. There are many complicating factors and the case is not proven. However, women who have taken oral contraceptives for more than 5 years should have an annual cervical smear.

Ovary/uterus. The use of oral contraceptives reduces the risk of endometrial and ovarian cancer.

Gall stones are more common in those taking the 'Pill'.

Older women may find that conception is delayed after stopping the 'Pill'.

Other side-effects, real or imaginary, of oral contraception must be set against the fact that many women feel better while taking these preparations, and also the potential reduction in abortion and unwanted and uncared-for children.

Ten years after discontinuation of the 'Pill' there appear to be no long-term ill effects.

*Contraindications to the use of oral contraceptives**

- Thromboembolic disease, past or present
- Carcinoma of the breast or uterus
- Severe liver disease or recent viral hepatitis, previous cholestatic jaundice of pregnancy
- Pregnancy
- Hypertension (diastolic pressure > 100 mmHg)
- Porphyria
- Herpes gestationis (previous)
- Focal migraine
- Progressive otosclerosis in pregnancy.

In addition to these contraindications the following may be made worse:

- Migraine
- Epilepsy
- Depression.

Drugs which interfere with oral contraceptives

Certain drugs when taken with oral contraceptives will increase the rate of breakdown of the estrogen they contain and thus decrease their efficiency and may occasionally lead to unwanted pregnancy. The most troublesome drug in this respect is *rifampicin* but *phenobarbital, carbamazepine phenytoin, isoniazid* and *griseofulvin* have also been implicated. In addition, *broad-spectrum antibiotics* may interfere with estrogen absorption. The occurrence of breakthrough bleeding may give a warning that the contraceptive is ineffective. If this occurs a preparation containing 50 micrograms of estrogen can be tried or an alternative contraceptive method used.

The efficacy of antihypertensive treatment is reduced by the 'Pill'.

THE PROSTAGLANDINS

These interesting substances are formed by most cells of the body and are released as a result of a number of stimuli. They usually produce their effects locally rather than at distant sites in the body, and many of them are removed from the circulation when they pass through the lung.

Prostaglandins have been implicated in a number of pathological processes:

1. *Inflammation.* It seems probable that prostaglandins of the E series are the mediators in some of the changes (swelling, redness and pain) which are seen in inflammation. This is important as drugs which block the production of prostaglandins, such as aspirin, and other NSAIDs reduce the symptoms and signs of inflammation.

2. *Thrombosis.* Two types of prostaglandins appear to be involved in thrombosis. Thromboxanes stimulate clumping of platelets and constriction of blood vessels and thus encourage thrombosis, whereas prostacycline has the reverse effect. It seems possible therefore that increasing the availability of prostacycline and decreasing that of thromboxanes would guard against thrombosis and a great deal of research is being done in an attempt to achieve this effect.

3. *Effects on uterine muscle.* Prostaglandins cause contraction of the uterine muscle and are concerned with both menstruation and childbirth. Prostaglandin E_2 can be used to induce labour or terminate pregnancy by causing the uterus to contract (see later).

4. *Effects on the stomach.* Prostaglandins increase mucous secretion by the cells lining the stomach and thus protect the mucosa against ulcer formation.

ERGOMETRINE AND OTHER DRUGS AFFECTING UTERINE MUSCLE

Ergometrine is rapidly absorbed either from the intestinal tract or from the site of injection. Its chief action is to cause contractions of the uterus. With small doses these contractions are rhythmic, but with larger doses they become very powerful and more or less continuous. They are brought about by a direct action of ergometrine on the uterine muscle. The uterus is especially sensitive to ergometrine at the time of

---

*The reader is referred to the *British National Formulary* for a full list of contraindications.

childbirth. It has little effect on other plain muscle throughout the body.

Therapeutics. Ergometrine is given after childbirth to cause the uterus to contract and thus prevent bleeding. It should not be given before delivery, even if the uterus is sluggish, as it may produce such powerful contractions that the uterus is ruptured, or the fetus asphyxiated. The usual dose is 500 micrograms orally or by intramuscular injection or 250 micrograms intravenously. The increased contractions of the uterus are seen within 5 minutes of intramuscular injection.

A number of other drugs cause the uterus to contract.

Oxytocin causes contraction of the muscle of the uterus. This effect is not marked until the later stages of pregnancy, and at parturition, when extremely small amounts will cause powerful uterine contractions.

Therapeutics. Oxytocin is used to induce labour. For this purpose it is usual to use synthetic oxytocin (Syntocinon), for the naturally prepared oxytocin contains a small amount of vasopressin. The oxytocin is given by intravenous infusion in saline and the rate of infusion is regulated according to the response of the patient. There is a risk of rupture of the uterus with oxytocin and it should only be used to induce labour under expert supervision. Oxytocin is also used after delivery of the placenta to cause uterine contraction, but its effects are not as prolonged as those of ergometrine. For this reason it is sometimes combined with ergometrine as *Syntometrine* (see later). Whole posterior pituitary extract should not be used, because of its vasopressor effects.

Adverse effects. In addition to producing powerful uterine contractions, which may be inappropriate in certain circumstances, oxytocin can cause a rise in blood pressure and water retention. It should not usually be combined with prostaglandins to induce labour.

Syntometrine is a mixture of ergometrine 500 micrograms and oxytocin 5 units in 1 ml. It is given intramuscularly in doses of 1 ml, and combines the rapid action of oxytocin on the uterus with the prolonged contraction caused by ergometrine. It is commonly used after the expulsion of the placenta to prevent bleeding.

Prostaglandins (see p. 206) may also activate the uterus.

Dinoprostone (prostaglandin E$_2$) is used to terminate pregnancy and to induce labour. It can be given by several routes.

1. Extra-amniotic injection to terminate pregnancy
2. Vaginal tablets or gel to induce labour.

Gemeprost (Prostaglandin E$_1$ analogue) pessaries are inserted into the vagina to soften the cervix and thus facilitate abortion during the first 2 months of pregnancy.

Adverse effects include nausea, vomiting, diarrhoea, headache and fever.

Interactions. Dinoprostone increases the effects of oxytocin and these drugs should never be given together.

The bladder should be emptied before insertion and the patient should lie down for 15 minutes after insertion.

Carboprost is given by intramuscular injection. It is used to treat postpartum haemorrhage when ergometrine and oxytocin have failed to control bleeding. It should only be used in specialist units.

Mifepristone is a progesterone antagonist. In pregnancy, the uterus is prevented from contracting before term by progesterone. If this inhibition is blocked the uterus can be induced to contract and thus abort the fetus.

Therapeutics. Mifepristone is used for the medical termination of pregnancy up to 63 days from the start of the last period. A single dose of 600 mg is given orally, followed after 48 hours by a gemeprost vaginal pessary. This procedure must be under medical supervision.

Nursing point

Dinoprostone sterile solutions for intravenous or extra-amniotic administration must be diluted before use.

Gemeprost pessaries should be warmed to room temperature for 30 minutes before insertion and kept away from direct heat or sunlight.

Termination of pregnancy

Most terminations of pregnancy are carried out in the first trimester.

First 9 weeks — Mifepristone, as above, or vacuum aspiration. Both are equally effective.

9–13 weeks — Vacuum aspiration preceded by the insertion of a gemeprost pessary to soften the cervix.

There is a risk of infection after termination; this can be reduced by prophylactic antibiotics.

Drugs inhibiting uterine contractions (Tocolytic agents)

Stimulation of β_2 receptors in the uterine muscles will diminish uterine activity. The β_2 agonists *salbutamol*, *terbutaline* and *ritodrine* are used in the management of premature labour between 24 and 33 weeks of pregnancy and are usually given by intravenous infusion for this purpose. There is a real risk of fluid overload.

Menorrhagia

Excessive bleeding during a period is quite common and may sometimes be serious enough to require a hysterectomy. The majority of patients have no underlying pelvic disease but a very small proportion have a mild inherited bleeding disorder. It is believed to be due to a functional defect in the mechanism which normally controls uterine bleeding.

Mefenamic acid, a weak NSAID, used in doses of 500 mg three times daily is widely used, with some success, to control pain and reduce bleeding. Iranexamic acid, which inhibits the breakdown of fibrin, is more effective. It is given orally when bleeding has started and continued for 3–4 days.

Dysmenorrhoea

Dysmenorrhoea is experienced by most women at some time, but occasionally periods become so painful and heavy that they disrupt everyday

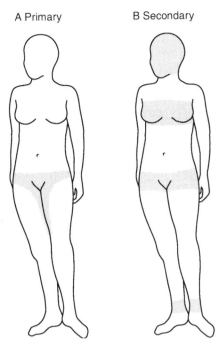

Figure 14.14 **A** Primary, **B** secondary sites of discomfort in primary and secondary dysmenorrhoea. Reproduced from *Nursing Care of Women* with permission of Prentice Hall.

life. Most women manage with a hot water bottle and mild analgesics. However, a nurse may be approached for advice so the type of dysmenorrhoea must be established (Fig. 14.14).

Primary dysmenorrhoea is common in young women whose usual symptoms are low backache and colicky pain in the pelvic area. This is due to the cyclical release of prostaglandins in the uterus, leading to contraction of the uterine muscle and constriction of the arteries supplying the muscle, with consequent ischaemia. Other symptoms include nausea, vomiting, diarrhoea and faintness. NSAIDs (p. 124), e.g. ibuprofen or mefenamic acid, by inhibiting prostaglandins, relieve pain in most cases. They should ideally be taken after menstrual bleeding has commenced to avoid the ingestion of drugs by a possibly pregnant subject. If this fails, oral contraceptives (estrogen + progestogen) are frequently effective.

Secondary dysmenorrhoea affects women in their late 20s and 30s, causing a dragging pain often preceded by headaches. As its name implies, this occurs in response to some pathological condition (fibroids, endometriosis) and treatment is by removal of the cause.

Premenstrual syndrome (PMS)

The cyclical appearance of a cluster of symptoms in the second half of the menstrual cycle which terminate abruptly with the onset of menstruation is known as the premenstrual tension syndrome (PMS). Although PMS is very common, only about 5% of women experience symptoms severe enough to disrupt their lives.

The symptoms are legion and are both emotional and physical.

Emotional	Physical
Depression	Headache
Tension	Breast swelling and discomfort
Crying	Bloating
Aggression	Backache
Failure to concentrate	

The range of these symptoms suggests that there is more than one cause and, in keeping with this theory, women respond differently to prescribed treatments, but its relationship with the menstrual cycle indicates that it is probably related to the hormonal and metabolic changes which occur.

A selection of possible aetiological factors and treatments is given below.

1. *Changes in water and salt balance.* Although feelings of bloating and swelling are frequent symptoms, there is little evidence that fluid retention actually occurs. Diuretics are often prescribed, but are rarely beneficial.

2. *Elevated prolactin levels.* Prolactin is released from the anterior pituitary and stimulates lactation. When a women is not lactating its secretion is suppressed by a hormone inhibitor. Some women with PMS have raised prolactin levels. *Bromocriptine*, which inhibits prolactin release, has been found useful for some symptoms, especially breast discomfort, but adverse effects may be troublesome.

3. *Diminished progesterone levels* have been suggested as an aetiological agent, but injection of progesterone or of a synthetic substitute has not been shown to be beneficial.

4. *Changes in prostaglandin E_1 levels.* This appears important in hormone balance and it has been suggested that PMS is a manifestation of deficiency. *Gamolenic acid* (evening primrose oil) is converted into prostaglandin E_1 and, given as Efamol, it has been shown to be effective sometimes. Conversely, prostaglandin synthesis inhibition by *mefenamic acid* can improve headaches and aches and pains.

5. Attention is now directed to the relationship between ovarian hormones and neurotransmitters in the brain. It is thought that progesterone or, more probably one of its metabolites, interacts with the GABA or serotonin (5-HT) systems and a disorder of these interactions is responsible for PMS.

These ideas receive support from:

a. The relief of symptoms by alprazolam (a GABA agonist) and by 5-HT re-uptake inhibitors such as fluoxetine.
b. The therapeutic efficacy of suppressing ovarian estrogen and progesterone secretion by the gonadotrophic-releasing hormone, goserelin (see p. 200) which, in the long term, reduces ovarian activity.

6. *Various dietary modifications* have been tried. Fluctuation in blood glucose levels can be avoided by giving a high starch diet every 3 hours, which may relieve symptoms, but weight gain can be a problem. *Pyridoxine* has been used, but with high doses there is a danger of neuropathy.

In summary, there is no overall regime to control PMS. In patients with mild symptoms it is probably best to employ self-help measures combining symptomatic treatment and dietary modifications, or gamolenic acid can be tried. With more severe symptoms, fluoxetine, alprazolam, an oral contraceptive or goserelin may be used.

Self-help measures

The nurse can do much to help the individual to gain insight into her problem. Keeping a diary of the menstrual cycle with daily accounts of the main symptoms and when they occur is useful. It can be used to predict the appearance of PMS in subsequent months, confirm a physical basis for the symptoms and exclude suggestions of neuroticism. It can also allow the patient to plan her life so that PMS does not clash with events such as holidays.

MALE SEX HORMONES

The male hormone *testosterone* is produced by the interstitial cells of the testis. It is responsible for the secondary male sex characteristics, including distribution of hair, deepening of the voice and enlargement of the penis and seminal vesicle.

It can be isolated from the testis, but is usually prepared synthetically.

Its release from the testis is controlled by the luteinizing hormone (LH) of the pituitary.

Therapeutics. Testosterone is used in the treatment of testicular hormone deficiency. This may be of an unknown origin or due to injury, or disease of the testis or may be secondary to lack of gonadotrophic hormone following pituitary gland disease.

Mesterolone, which is similar to testosterone, is given orally. Unlike testosterone it does not cause jaundice or depress spermatogenesis.

Esters of testosterone (Sustanon) can be given intramuscularly every 3 weeks and are released slowly from the injection site.

Testosterone is effective in about 30% of premenopausal patients with advanced carcinoma of the breast in relieving symptoms and causing temporary regression of secondary deposits. When given to women, testosterone causes the growth of facial hair, deepening of the voice and acne.

Sex hormone antagonists

Cyproterone acetate and flutamide block the action of testosterone at the cell receptor. They are used in various endocrine disorders where there is overproduction of male hormone caus-ing hirsutism in the female (when it may be combined with an estrogen) and hypersexuality in the male. They are also used in treating carcinoma of the prostate.

Finasteride interferes with the action of testosterone on the prostate gland, causing it to decrease in size and is used to treat benign enlargement of the prostate.

Carcinoma of the prostate

The prostate depends to some extent on continued stimulation by testosterone and this also applies to carcinomatous tissue.

When widespread deposits have developed the disease can be controlled by interfering with hormone stimulation of these secondaries. This can be achieved by giving an estrogen (usually stilbestrol), but adverse effects (feminization and fluid retention) can be troublesome. Alternatively, a gonadorelin analogue may be used. This initially causes increased testosterone activity, which can be controlled by cyproterone, but after about 2 weeks, LH release (see p. 260) is inhibited, resulting in a fall in testosterone levels and a regression of the tumour.

ANABOLIC HORMONES

The structure of these male sex hormones has been modified so that they have little masculinizing effect, but have considerable anabolic action and are capable of building up protein in bone and other tissues. They are used occasionally to hasten convalescence and in senile osteoporosis, which is due to lack of protein in bone. Their effectiveness in these conditions is not proven.

They also produce an increase in muscle bulk and have been used by athletes to improve their performance. This is undesirable as it is not only dishonest, but also carries the possibility of adverse effects.

MALE ERECTILE DYSFUNCTION (IMPOTENCE)

Impotence is a common disorder. Its incidence increases with age and it may have a considerable effect on the well-being of the individual. The cause can be psychological, physical or a combination of both.

Erection depends on the relaxation of the penile smooth muscle, with subsequent engorgement with blood following psychological or tactile stimulation. The autonomic nervous system is involved and it is believed that nitric oxide is an important mediator in the vascular relaxation.

There are two aspects which involve drugs:

1. Drugs may interfere with sexual performance. Among those implicated are various centrally acting drugs (alcohol, tricyclic antidepressants, neuroleptics), antihypertensives (particularly thiazides) and cimetidine (due to its estrogen-like action).

2. Performance can also be improved by drugs. An effective method is the intracavernosal injection of *papaverine* or *prostaglandin* E_1, which relaxes smooth muscle and produces a very satisfactory erection. After preliminary training the drug can be self-administered. The erection should not be allowed to continue for more than 4 hours. Alternatively, a small pellet of prostaglandin E_1 can be inserted into the urethra and enough is absorbed to achieve an erection in a proportion of subjects.

Sildenafil (Viagra) is an oral preparation which is a specific inhibitor of phosphodiesterase 5 in the blood vessels of the penis, leading to vasodilation and enhanced erection when taken an hour or two before intercourse. It is effective in the majority of subjects with impotence, whatever the cause, and will probably largely replace other methods.

Adverse effects are rarely serious and include headache, flushing and occasional disturbances of colour vision. It should not, however, be combined with nitrates.

In addition to drugs, various mechanical treatments are available.

FURTHER READING

Beral V et al 1997 Breast cancer and hormone replacement therapy. Lancet 350: 1047

Beral V et al 1999 Mortality associated with oral contraceptive use. British Medical Journal 318: 96.

Berga S L 1998 Understanding premenstrual syndrome. Lancet 351:465

Catalona W J 1994 Management of cancer of the prostate. New England Journal of Medicine 331: 996

Dunn N et al 1999 Oral contraception and myocardial infarction. British Medical Journal 318: 1579

Editorial 1990 Medical termination of pregnancy. British Medical Journal 301: 352

Editorial 1992 New gonadotropins for old? Lancet 340: 1442

Editorial 1993 Gonadotrophin releasing hormone analogues for endometreosis. Drugs and Therapeutics Bulletin 31: 21

Editorial 1994 Oral contraceptives and cancer. Lancet 344: 1378

Editorial 1995 Advising women on which pill to take. British Medical Journal 311: 1111

Editorial 1996 Hormone replacement therapy. Drug and Therapeutics Bulletin 34: 11: 81

Editorial 1999 Replacing testosterone in men. Drugs and Therapeutics Bulletin 37: 1: 3

Editorial 1998 Termination of first trimester pregnancy. Drug and Therapeutics Bulletin 36: 2: 13

Glasier A 1997 Emergency postcoital contraception. New England Journal of Medicine 337: 1058

Goldstein I et al 1998 Oral sildenafil in the treatment of erectile dysfunction. New England Journal of Medicine 338: 1397

Greendale G A, Lee N P, Arriola E R 1999 The menopause. Lancet 353: 571

Hillard A 1998 Managing the menopause. Nursing Standard 12(27): 49

Holleman F, Hoekstra JBL 1997 Insulin lispro. New England Journal of Medicine 337: 176

Kirby R S 1994 Impotence. Management of male erectile dysfunction. British Medical Journal 308: 957

Knowledon H A 1990 The Pill and cancer. Journal of Advanced Nursing 15: 1016

Mills A M et al 1996 Guidelines for prescribing combined oral contraceptives. British Medical Journal 312: 121

O'Brian P M S 1993 Helping women with premenstrual syndrome. British Medical Journal 307: 1471

Rittmaster R S 1994 Finasteride. New England Journal of Medicine 330: 120

Spitzer WO 1997 Balanced view of the risks of oral contraceptives. Lancet 350: 1566

Wagner G, de Tejeda IS 1998 Update on male erectile dysfunction. British Medical Journal 316: 678

15

Drugs affecting renal function

DIURETICS

Diuretics are drugs which cause increased secretion of urine by the kidneys. They are useful in patients who are suffering from retention of water and sodium chloride (salt) which usually accumulates in the tissue spaces and is called oedema. Diuretics are not used in patients who cannot empty their bladders; this is called urinary retention.

Oedema occurs most commonly in heart failure, the nephrotic syndrome and cirrhosis of the liver. Ankle oedema may also develop in those sitting with their legs dependent—a common example being elderly people who are confined to their chairs for long periods. It can also complicate the use of calcium channel blockers (see p. 69).

The factors which cause fluid retention are various and depend on the underlying disease. They include:

1. Lowered cardiac output and underfilling of the vascular system (hypovolaemia), which activates the renin–angiotensin system with increased secretion of *aldosterone* by the adrenals leading to salt and water retention by the kidney. This occurs in *heart failure, cirrhosis of the liver* and the *nephrotic syndrome.*

2. Raised pressure in the veins and capillaries. This leads to increased exudation of fluid from the blood to the tissue spaces, and occurs in *heart failure, liver cirrhosis* and oedema due to prolonged immobility with legs dependent.

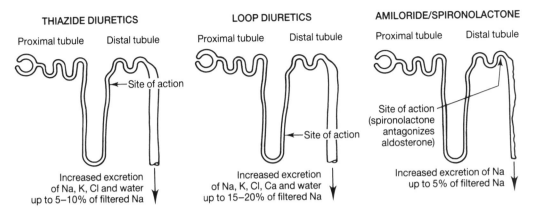

Figure 15.1 Sites of action of diuretics.

3. Low plasma proteins. This is found in the *nephrotic syndrome* where it is due to protein loss in the urine and *cirrhosis of the liver* where there is a failure to make protein.

Renal function

The role of the kidney is to excrete the waste products of metabolism, drugs, etc., and maintain the correct amounts of water and electrolytes in the body by getting rid of any excesses which may be absorbed or produced by the body.

This is effected in two stages (Fig. 15.1):

1. At the glomeruli, water along with soluble substances is filtered from the blood. The volume of this filtration is about 100 litres of water per day and it contains glucose, electrolytes, urea and other substances.

2. In the renal tubules a selective reabsorption occurs. Glucose is normally completely reabsorbed. Water and electrolytes (including sodium, potassium, chloride and bicarbonate) are partially reabsorbed, whereas urea is almost entirely excreted. The exact amount of each substance finally excreted in the urine is controlled so that the composition of the body fluids remains constant.

DIURETIC DRUGS

All diuretic drugs produce their effect by decreasing the reabsorption of water and electrolytes by the renal tubules and thus allowing more water and electrolytes to be excreted.

Water

It is common experience that in a normal person, increased ingestion of water results in an increased urine flow. When water is absorbed, it causes the plasma to become more dilute and this in turn decreases the release of antidiuretic hormone (ADH) by the posterior lobe of the pituitary gland (see p. 176). Less ADH reaches the kidney and this causes the tubules to reabsorb less water, so that more is excreted as the urine. In those with fluid retention, for example in heart failure, the normal response to water disappears and so it is no use as a diuretic in these circumstances.

OSMOTIC DIURETICS

Any substance which passes through the glomeruli and is not reabsorbed by the renal tubules will increase the concentration of the urine within the tubules. This prevents the reabsorption of salt and water from the tubule back into the blood and the water is then passed out and produces a diuresis. Osmotic diuretics are now little used in treating oedema.

Mannitol is sometimes used to lower raised intracranial pressure after a head injury or in a patient with a cerebral tumour or to reduce the intraocular pressure in glaucoma. It is given intravenously as a 10% or 20% solution.

THIAZIDE DIURETICS

There are several diuretics in this group and although there are marginal differences in their actions, the general pattern of their effects is the same and they will be described together.

They are all absorbed from the intestinal tract and are therefore effective orally.

Their actions on the kidney are:

1. They interfere with the reabsorption of salt and water by the tubules; thus more fluid passes out of the tubules and causes a diuresis.
2. There is an increased excretion of potassium by the kidney.

Therapeutics:

1. *Cardiac failure.* The thiazides are used in treating the oedema of cardiac failure. They are not very powerful diuretics and their use is usually confined to mild failure. They are given in the morning as the diuresis lasts throughout the day.

2. *Hypertension.* The thiazides have some blood pressure lowering action and may be used for this purpose, either alone or with other hypotensive drugs. This is not only due to their diuretic action and they also act as mild vasodilators. For this purpose, *small doses of thiazides are required*; for example, cyclopenthiazide 250 micrograms or bendroflumethiazide (bendrofluazide) 2.5 mg once daily are adequate. Potassium supplements are not usually required.

3. *Cirrhosis of the liver with ascites.* The thiazides will produce a diuresis in this disorder with reduction in the ascites and oedema. Care is required, however, as their use may be followed by mental changes with disorientation which it is believed is due to the potassium deficiency produced by these drugs.

4. *Nephrotic syndrome.* The thiazides can be used to treat the oedema found in this disorder. Frequently, however, a more powerful diuretic will be required such as frusemide.

The following table gives some members of the group, with their relative strengths:

Preparation	*Dose*
Chlorothiazide	0.5–1 g
Hydrochlorothiazide	25–75 mg
Bendroflumethiazide (Bendrofluazide)	2.5–10 mg
Cyclopenthiazide	0.25–1.0 mg
Polythiazide	0.5–4.0 mg
Xipamide	20–80 mg

Chlortalidone is very similar to the thiazides but it has a more prolonged action. The dose is 50–200 mg on alternate days.

Metolazone is a thiazide which generally has no advantage over others in the group but it will sometimes produce a diuresis when other thiazides have become ineffective or it may be combined with a loop diuretic, particularly in patients with impaired renal function.

LOOP DIURETICS

This group of diuretics is more powerful than the thiazides. Loop diuretics act at a different site in the renal tubule (see Fig. 15.1) and interfere to a greater extent with the reabsorption of salt and water. Like thiazides these diuretics also increase renal excretion of potassium.

Furosemide (Frusemide) has a short duration of action; if given by mouth the diuresis lasts about 6 hours. It can also be given intravenously when there is an almost immediate massive diuresis which is finished in about 2 hours.

Therapeutics. Furosemide is particularly useful in:

1. Acute left ventricular failure with oedema of the lungs. In doses of 20–50 mg intravenously, furosemide rapidly clears the oedema and pulmonary congestion. In these circumstances it also has a vasodilating action which relieves the load on the heart.

2. Patients with congestive heart failure which is no longer responding to other diuretics. Furosemide is often effective when given orally in doses of 40–80 mg daily or more.

3. In oedema associated with the nephrotic syndrome, especially if there is some degree of renal failure, oral furosemide is particularly useful. In these cases very large doses are sometimes used.

4. Large doses may be given when acute renal failure is developing to try and jolt the kidneys into resuming normal function.

Bumetanide. This powerful diuretic is similar to furosemide in its pharmacological action, although it is distinct chemically. It is given orally in doses of 1–4 mg daily and produces a rapid diuresis lasting about 3 hours. For an even more immediate effect it may be given intravenously. Its therapeutic uses and adverse effects are similar to those of furosemide.

NSAIDs and steroids reduce the efficacy of these diuretics.

Adverse effects of thiazide and loop diuretics

1. Hypokalaemia—this is due to increased potassium loss by the kidneys and is more marked with high doses of diuretics. It is considered below.
2. Uric acid retention by the kidney, causing gout.
3. Decreasing glucose tolerance which may make control of diabetes more difficult and even lead to a diabetic-like state which, however, usually recovers when the drug is stopped. There may also be a temporary rise in plasma cholesterol concentration.
4. Sodium depletion—with large doses of loop diuretics, particularly when given intravenously, the patient's blood volume may be reduced rapidly, causing hypotension and collapse. This can also occur with prolonged oral treatment.
5. A large and rapid diuresis can precipitate acute retention in those with prostatic enlargement.

Large doses of furosemide can cause transient deafness.

Interactions. Thiazide and loop diuretics can cause:

1. Lithium retention (see p. 164)
2. Renal damage when combined with gentamicin
3. Increase digoxin toxicity due to hypokalaemia
4. Hypotension with ACE inhibitors.

DIURETICS AND POTASSIUM DEPLETION

Both the thiazides and loop diuretics cause loss of potassium through the kidneys and if the plasma potassium is lowered excessively (<3.0 mmol/litre) there is a risk of dangerous cardiac arrhythmias. This rarely occurs in patients receiving small doses of diuretics for hypertension or heart failure and it is adequate to check the plasma potassium level 1–2 months after the start of treatment. However, the following risk factors may require more careful monitoring and some form of potassium replacement:

1. Large doses of diuretics.
2. Poor diet—the elderly.
3. Concurrent use of digitalis—the toxicity of digitalis is increased by potassium deficiency.
4. Immediately following myocardial infarction—low plasma potassium is associated with an increased risk of dangerous arrhythmias.
5. Patients with cirrhosis of the liver are particularly sensitive to potassium depletion.
6. Concurrent use of steroids increases potassium loss.

In all these patients the plasma potassium should be monitored and replacement started if depletion occurs. This may be achieved by:

1. **Potassium supplements.** These should be given in the form of potassium chloride. Unfortunately, this substance is nauseating and can cause ulceration of the gut if given in tablet form. It is therefore formulated as *effervescent potassium chloride tablets* (Sando-K) containing 12 mmol K or as *slow-release potassium chloride tablets* (Slow-K) containing 8 mmol K. The amount of potassium required for replacement varies but is usually between 30 and 60 mmol per day orally.

Potassium can also be given by intravenous infusion if depletion is severe. *This can be a dangerous procedure as hyperkalaemia from too rapid infusion can cause cardiac arrest.* The rate of infusion depends on the degree of depletion and should not normally exceed 20 mmol of potassium in two hours and the blood potassium and ECG should be monitored.

Certain diuretics are made up as combined diuretic + potassium chloride, e.g. cyclopenthiazide + potassium chloride (Navidrex K), but are not recommended as they contain too little potassium to be useful.

2. **Potassium-sparing** diuretics. These substances have a diuretic action of their own, and if combined with a thiazide or loop diuretic prevent excessive loss of potassium.

POTASSIUM-SPARING DIURETICS

Triamterene This drug increases the excretion of salt and water and reduces potassium excretion. It is thought that this is probably due to a direct action on the renal tubules.

Amiloride antagonizes the action of aldosterone on the renal tubule and thus increases sodium and water excretion with some potassium retention.

Therapeutics. Triamterene is usually combined with a thiazide diuretic to increase its efficacy and at the same time to prevent potassium loss. Amiloride can be used alone or in combination. The usual dose is 10–20 mg daily if used alone.

Adverse effects. Hyperkalaemia can occur in patients with impaired renal function and those taking ACE inhibitors or supplemental potassium.

Combinations. A thiazide or a loop diuretic can be combined with a potassium-sparing diuretic in one tablet to prevent potassium loss. Among the preparations available are:

- Co-amilozide—hydrochlorothiazide + amiloride
- Dyazide—hydrochlorothiazide + triamterene
- Co-amilofruse—frusemide + amiloride.

These preparations are effective and reduce potassium loss but it must be remembered that they have the adverse effects of both constituents and with co-amilozide both sodium depletion and potassium retention can occur, particularly in elderly patients.

Spironolactone. Overproduction of aldosterone by the adrenal glands is a factor in maintaining oedema in patients with cardiac failure, the nephrotic syndrome, and particularly in cirrhosis of the liver. The aldosterone causes increased retention of sodium and water by the kidneys.

Spironolactone blocks the action of aldosterone on the kidney and thus leads to less sodium and water retention and a diuresis. It will also cause some fall in blood pressure.

Therapeutics. Spironolactone is given orally. It is usually reserved for those patients who have not responded to the usual diuretic drugs. It is more effective when combined with other diuretics.

It is not usually given in the long term (e.g. in treating hypertension) as there is a remote risk of carcinogenicity.

Adverse effects appear rarely, but rashes, gynaecomastia and menstrual disorders limit its use.

Interactions. Supplementary potassium or potassium-sparing diuretics should not normally be combined with ACE inhibitors as this causes potassium retention by the kidneys and can be dangerous.

Potassium canrenoate is similar to spironolactone but can be given intravenously.

Diuretics in cirrhosis of the liver

In such cases diuretics carry serious risks of hypokalaemia and hypotension leading to renal failure. It is best to start with spironolactone and then add a thiazide or loop diuretic cautiously a few days later. All drugs causing fluid retention (e.g. NSAIDs) should be avoided.

Diuretics in elderly patients

For various reasons, not always sound, one in five people over 65 take diuretics and they are the commonest cause of adverse reactions in

---

Nursing point

Swollen ankles in the elderly do not necessarily call for a diuretic — they may be due to sitting in a chair all day.

If an elderly person taking diuretics develops diarrhoea and/or vomiting it is sometimes wise to stop the diuretic temporarily to prevent undue water and salt loss.

Nursing point

The best way to monitor the efficiency of a diuretic is to weigh the patient regularly. Fluid balance charts are not always accurate but can be improved with the cooperation of the patient. Before leaving the hospital the timing of diuretic dosage must be tailored to the patient's daily programme. It is distressing to have a diuresis while stuck in your car in a traffic jam!

---

elderly people. These adverse effects are the same as those which occur in younger subjects, but are more severe and may have serious consequences.

Most important is sodium depletion leading to a marked fall in blood pressure, particularly on standing, and causing faints, falls and confusion. As in other age groups disturbances of potassium and uric acid metabolism occur.

MISCELLANEOUS DIURETICS

Acetazolamide suppresses the activity of the enzyme carbonic anhydrase which is present in the renal tubule and the eye. In the kidney this prevents the reabsorption of sodium and water from the tubule and thus causes a diuresis. It is a poor diuretic as its effect is short-lived and is not now used for this purpose. In the eye, however, it reduces the formation of aqueous humour and is useful in lowering the intraocular pressure in glaucoma. It will also help relieve mountain sickness. Overbreathing which occurs at altitude 'washes out' carbon dioxide from the lungs and causes increased alkalinity of the blood. By increasing the excretion of bicarbonate (alkali) by the kidneys, acetozolamide helps to correct this disorder.

DRUGS CHANGING THE REACTION OF URINE

Drugs making urine alkaline

Sodium citrate is the substance most commonly used to make the urine alkaline. It is usually given every 2 or 4 hours. The correct dose is that which keeps the urine alkaline. Sodium bicarbonate is often combined with sodium citrate and acts in a similar fashion.

Therapeutics. Occasionally urinary tract infections are treated by making the urine alkaline as this prevents the multiplication of certain bacteria. Some drugs are more rapidly eliminated by the kidney in an alkaline urine, particularly aspirin, and this may be useful in overdose.

FURTHER READING

Brater D C 1998 Diuretic therapy. New England Journal of Medicine 339: 387

Editorial 1988 Diuretics in the elderly, how safe? British Medical Journal 296: 1551

Editorial 1990 Thiazides in the 1990s. British Medical Journal 300: 168

Editorial 1991 Routine use of potassium sparing diuretics. Drug and Therapeutics Bulletin 29: 85

Editorial 1994 Diuretics for Heart Failure. Drug and Therapeutics Bulletin 32: 83

16

Chemotherapeutic agents and antibiotics

Ever since it was realized that bacteria cause many diseases, humans have been seeking a substance to kill the bacteria without harming the host.

The first advance was the preparation of neoarsphenamine, an organic compound containing arsenic, by Ehrlich and his co-workers in 1910. This would kill the bacterium *Treponema pallidum*, which caused syphilis, without untoward effects on the patient. Ehrlich hoped to eradicate the disease with a single injection, but this proved inadequate and a long course was required.

In 1935 Domagk in Germany synthesized the first of the sulfonamide group of drugs and during the next 20 years several more were added. Before and during the Second World War the discoveries by Fleming, Florey and Chain led to the isolation of penicillin from the fungus *Penicillium notatum* and this was the first of the antibiotics. These are substances (produced by living organisms) which either kill or inhibit the growth of bacteria, fungi or viruses. Since then a large number of antibiotics have been produced from various sources. Further, their structure has been modified in the laboratory to improve their efficacy and these drugs are known as semisynthetic antibiotics.

Antibacterial drugs have revolutionized the treatment of infection and many diseases such as bacterial meningitis which previously were often fatal are now usually curable, but it must be realized that the battle against pathogenic bacteria is by no means over. Many organisms have become resistant to antibacterial drugs and this requires a continuing search for new drugs and modification of those already in use. It also means that *they should not be used unnecessarily.*

It should be remembered that even with powerful antibacterial drugs the patient's natural resistance plays an important part in combating infection. The nurse will note that those with impaired immunity, due to prolonged illness, old age or perhaps the use of cytotoxic or immuno-suppressive drugs, respond poorly to antibacterial drugs and the infection is much harder to eradicate.

How antibacterial substances work

Antibiotics exert their effects in two main ways:

1. Bactericidal agents kill bacteria rapidly (e.g. aminoglycosides, polymixin)
2. Bacteriostatic agents prevent bacteria from replicating, but do not kill them (e.g. sulfonamides, tetracyclines, chloramphenicol).

The distinction between these two categories is not clear. Many antibiotics which operate principally as bacteriostatic agents can become bactericidal under favourable circumstances. Factors affecting the mode of action include concentration of the drug and the number and type of organisms. When modest numbers are present and the drug is given in high doses to highly sensitive organisms, a normally bacteriostatic agent such as penicillin may become bactericidal.

Each of the main groups of antibiotics has a different molecular structure and this is the factor which determines its mode of action. Many antibiotics exert their effects directly on the bacterial cell wall or must pass through it before disrupting bacterial metabolism at the intracellular level. The cell walls of all bacteria are composed of layers of protein molecules bound together by cross-linkages, resulting in a large, complex chemical aggregate, but their fine structure depends on whether they are Gram-positive or Gram-negative. The fine structure of the cell wall influences susceptibility to the different groups of antibiotics. For example, erythromycin is able to penetrate the cell walls

of Gram-positive bacteria and is effective in the treatment of some staphylococcal or streptococcal infections, but has no effect on Gram-negative bacteria. Some of the diverse ways in which the different groups of antibiotics exert their effects are illustrated in Fig. 16.1.

Gram-positive and Gram-negative bacteria

With few exceptions bacteria may be classified as Gram-positive or Gram-negative according to a staining technique used in laboratory identification. Generally Gram-positive bacteria are able to withstand dessication better than Gram-negative bacteria and many form spores which resist drying. Gram-negative species multiply rapidly in the presence of moisture even when provided with minimal nourishment. Several Gram-positive and Gram-negative bacteria have had a long association with hospital infection and, because they can be carried on the hands, may be spread by cross-infection in any health care setting.

Gram-positive	*Gram-negative*
Staphylococcus aureus	*Haemophilus (H.) influenzae*
Streptococcus pyogenes	*Neisseria (N.) gonorrhoea (Gonococcus)*
Streptococcus viridans	*Neisseria (N.) meningitidis (Meningococcus)*
Streptococcus pneumoniae (Pneumococcus)	*Escherichia (E.) coli*
	Proteus
	Pseudomonas
	Klebsiella

Anaerobes

This term refers to bacteria which can live and multiply in the absence of free oxygen. In the laboratory they require special conditions before they will grow in culture, but they are able to cause severe infections given the correct circumstances. Anaerobic bacteria naturally inhabiting the gut may cause severe sepsis following abdominal surgery. If *Clostridium tetani* gains

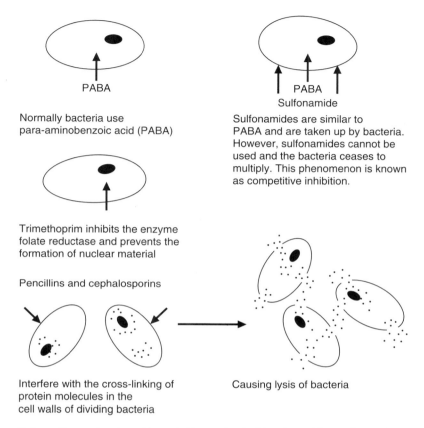

Normally bacteria use para-aminobenzoic acid (PABA)

Sulfonamides are similar to PABA and are taken up by bacteria. However, sulfonamides cannot be used and the bacteria ceases to multiply. This phenomenon is known as competitive inhibition.

Trimethoprim inhibits the enzyme folate reductase and prevents the formation of nuclear material

Pencillins and cephalosporins

Interfere with the cross-linking of protein molecules in the cell walls of dividing bacteria

Causing lysis of bacteria

Tetracycline, aminoglycoside and chloramphenicol interfere with protein synthesis within the cell. In normal cells RNA is bound to ribosomes which are essential for protein synthesis. This group of antibiotics binds onto the ribosomes, excluding the RNA and preventing protein synthesis. Thus bacteria do not multiply.

Figure 16.1 Some of the modes of action of antibacterial drugs.

access to a penetrating wound which is free of oxygen, it multiplies and produces a toxin which causes tetanus.

Choosing an antibiotic

When faced with a patient with an infectious disease, the first consideration is whether an antibiotic is required. Many infections (e.g. a mild sore throat) get better quickly without specific treatment.

If antibiotic treatment is needed the following points should be considered:

1. The infecting organism. This if often suspected from the nature of the disease and initial treatment is usually based on this guess. If possible, the nature of the organism should be confirmed by culture of blood, sputum, urine, etc., though in practice this is not always possible and may not be necessary.

2. The correct antibiotic to eradicate the infection.

3. The ability of the antibiotic to penetrate the site of infection (for example, in meningitis not all drugs enter the cerebrospinal fluid).

4. The route of administration. Some antibiotics are ineffective orally and injection may also be required for rapid action.

5. *A drug history is essential (as always)* to ensure that the patient has not previously had

an adverse reaction to the chosen antibiotic.

6. Possible complicating factors such as pregnancy, renal or hepatic failure.

7. In these difficult times—the cost of the drug.

THE SULFONAMIDES

This is one of the oldest groups of antibacterial agents. They differ to some extent in the range of organisms which they attack, but most of their pharmacological properties are similar. They have been largely replaced because of the development of bacterial resistance and adverse side-effects and most have disappeared from use. They are, with few exceptions, well and rapidly absorbed from the intestinal tract. They circulate widely in the body fluids and cross the meningeal barrier to enter the cerebrospinal fluid (CSF).

After absorption the liver begins to acetylate the sulfonamides. The acetylated drugs together with unaltered sulfonamide are excreted in the urine. The acetylated sulfonamides are very poorly soluble and therefore there is a danger that they will precipitate in the urine unless an adequate flow is maintained.

Most of the sulfonamides are effective against a fairly wide range of bacteria. Unfortunately, certain of these bacteria have become resistant.

Table 16.1 gives a number of available sulfonamides.

Therapeutics. **Sulfadimidine** is still used occasionally in urinary infections provided that the infecting organism is susceptible. The dose is 2 g initially followed by 1 g every 6 hours. **Sulfasalazine** is given in doses of 0.5–1.0 g

every 6 hours in the long-term treatment of ulcerative colitis and Crohn's disease (see p. 99). Sulfasalazine can also be used in the treatment of rheumatoid arthritis (see p. 129).

Adverse effects:

1. *Nausea* can be troublesome and with sulfasalazine may be relieved by giving small and more frequent doses.

2. *Rashes* of various types, sometimes with fever.

3. *Blood dyscrasias.*

4. *Sperm count* is reduced by sulfasalazine, but recovers on stopping the drug.

5. *Precipitation in the urinary tract* causing obstruction. The patient should be given 2–3 litres of fluid daily to maintain a good urinary flow when receiving sulfadimidine.

Co-trimoxazole–trimethoprim and sulfamethoxazole

Sulfonamides affect bacteria by interfering with their use of para-aminobenzoic acid (PABA), a precursor of folic acid which is ultimately essential in cell division (see Fig. 16.1). Trimethoprim also interferes with folic acid metabolism, at the phase when folic acid is changed to folinic acid to build up the cell nucleus. This requires the action of an enzyme and, by combining with that enzyme, trimethoprim stops the reaction and the cell dies. The combination of a sulfonamide with trimethoprim is particularly effective in preventing bacterial cell division and is also bactericidal. Co-trimoxazole is effective against *S. pyogenes, S. pneumoniae, E. coli, H. influenzae,* salmonella and *Pneumocystis carinii* (in large doses).

Therapeutics. Each combined tablet of co-trimoxazole contains 80 mg of trimethoprim plus 400 mg of sulfamethoxazole, and has been widely and successfully used in exacerbations of chronic bronchitis and in urinary infections. It also has a place in treating the more severe salmonella and other infections. Unfortunately, its adverse-effect profile has led to its use being largely confined to pneumocystis pneumonia.

Table 16.1 Available sulfonamides

Drug	Important features
Sulfadimidine	Well absorbed orally
Sulfasalazine	Used in ulcerative colitis. It is particularly useful for long-term maintenance treatment
Silver sulfadiazine	Applied locally as a cream to prevent infection in severe burns

In large doses it is used to treat *pneumocystis* infection of the lung, a disease which occurs in patients whose immunity has been suppressed, often as a result of cancer chemotherapy or AIDS.

Adverse effects are largely those of the sulfonamides, namely nausea and vomiting, and occasionally blood disorders. More serious is the occasional development of the *Stevens–Johnson syndrome* with a bullous rash, mouth ulceration and fever which can be fatal.

Trimethoprim can also be used alone. At present it is largely used to treat urinary infection, the dose being 200 mg twice daily for an acute infection and, for long-term use, 100 mg daily. It can also be used to treat bronchitis.

Adverse effects include nausea, rashes and rarely, depression of the blood count and it should not be used in the first 3 months of pregnancy.

THE NITROFURANS

This group of chemotherapeutic agents has been investigated sporadically for over 30 years. The only one currently used is nitrofurantoin.

Nitrofurantoin has a fairly wide antibacterial spectrum and is considerably concentrated in the urine. It is used in the treatment of urinary tract infections; the oral dose is 50–100 mg four times a day or once daily as a prophylactic. Nausea sometimes occurs but can be minimized by giving the drug after food. Other adverse effects include rashes and fever. It should not be used in patients with renal failure as accumulation will occur.

THE QUINOLONES

This group of antibacterial drugs is increasingly important; several are available already and more will probably be introduced in the next few years. They interfere with an enzyme which is necessary for the cell division of bacteria.

Ciprofloxacin acts against a wide range of organisms, but is not very effective against some Gram-positive organisms, *particularly pneumococci*.

It is given orally in doses of 250–750 mg twice daily or by infusion, which is very expensive. At present, its use should be confined to patients for whom older antibacterial drugs are unsatisfactory, particularly for typhoid, urinary infection and gonorrhoea. It is the preferred drug in adults as a prophylactic for close contacts of meningococcal meningitis.

Adverse effects include gastrointestinal upsets and rashes. It should be avoided, if possible, in patients with epilepsy as it has a potential to cause fits, and in children it may cause damage to developing weight-bearing joints. It can also cause pain and inflammation of tendons, especially in older people.

Interactions. It raises the blood levels of theophylline. The action of warfarin is increased.

Ofloxacin is similar to ciprofloxacin **Grepafloxacin** and **levofloxacin** are more active against *S. pneumoniae* and can be used in community acquired pneumonia but offer no real advantage over the usual antibiotics.

Norfloxacin is effective only in urinary tract infections because it is concentrated in the urine and is used when the infecting organism is resistant to the older antibacterial drugs. For uncomplicated infection a 3-day course is adequate, but prolonged treatment is required for severe or recurrent infections. It should be avoided in children and pregnancy.

Cinoxacin is similar.

THE ANTIBIOTICS

β LACTAM GROUP

The β lactam antibiotics all contain the β lactam ring, which is a chemical structure essential for their antibacterial activity. The group contains (Fig. 16.2):

- The penicillins
- The cephalosporins
- Others.

PENICILLINS

The penicillins were the first of the antibiotics to be isolated. Over the years their structure has been modified repeatedly to deal with the prob-

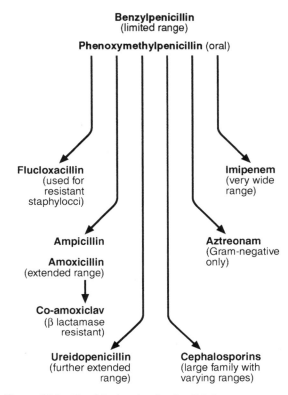

Figure 16.2 The β lactam family of antibiotics.

lem of resistance to penicillin and to extend their antibacterial range. They are still probably the most widely used family of antibiotics.

Benzylpenicillin was the first penicillin to be used clinically. It is usually given by deep intramuscular injection, which is painful, and if a single dose of more than 1.8 g (3 mega units) is needed it should be given intravenously. It rapidly enters the circulation and spreads through the body; it does not, however, cross into the cerebrospinal fluid in any great quantity, although this may be increased if the meninges are inflamed.

All penicillins are excreted by the kidneys, partially through the glomeruli but the major part via the renal tubules. The excretion is rapid and blood levels nearly fall to zero 4 hours after injection.

If benzylpenicillin is given orally it is partially broken down by the gastric acid and is not now given by this route.

Benzylpenicillin is effective against a fairly wide range of organisms. The following are the most common:

Organisms	*Disease*
Streptococcus pyogenes	Tonsillitis, scarlet fever, septicaemia
Streptococcus viridans	Subacute bacterial endocarditis
*Staphylococcus aureus	Carbuncles, osteomyelitis, septicaemia, boils
S. pneumoniae	Pneumonia
N. gonorrhoeae	Gonorrhoea
N. meningitidis	Meningococcal meningitis
Treponema pallidum	Syphilis
Clostridium perfringens	Gangrene
Clostridium tetani	Tetanus
Actinomyces	Actinomycosis

Penicillins are bacteriostatic and in higher doses are bactericidal. When treating infection it is ideal to maintain the blood level of penicillin continually at bactericidal levels, and this requires injections every 4 hours. In milder infections, however, it is often adequate to give less frequent injections, for even when the blood levels of penicillin drop below bactericidal or bacteriostatic levels, the organism may take some time to recover and by that time the blood level of penicillin has risen again following a further injection.

Numerous attempts have been made to prolong the action of benzylpenicillin after injection by slowing down its release from the injection site. A successful method is to combine benzylpenicillin with procaine. The combination is called **procaine benzylpenicillin** and will maintain a satisfactory blood level for at least 12 hours. This preparation is, however, rather slow at producing a satisfactory blood level, so that if a rapid effect is required, benzylpenicillin should be given as well.

---

*Note that a high proportion of staphylococci found in hospital are now resistant to benzylpenicillin.

The action of penicillin can be augmented and prolonged by slowing down its excretion. This can be done by giving *probenecid*, a drug which blocks the tubular secretion of penicillin, thus allowing the drug to accumulate in the body.

Certain organisms develop resistance to the action of penicillin. Organisms which were originally sensitive appear to adapt themselves to the penicillin by producing a substance *penicillinase* which inactivates penicillin by attacking part of the penicillin molecule known as the *β lactam ring*. This structure is an essential part of penicillins and cephalosporins and the family of enzymes involved is sometimes known as the *β lactamases*. This is particularly so in the case of staphylococci and strains of this organism which are resistant to penicillin and other antibiotics are a serious clinical problem.

Other penicillins

1. There are a number of penicillins which are similar to benzylpenicillin but are effective by mouth. The example given below is not destroyed by the acid in the stomach and is fairly well absorbed from the intestinal tract. It maintains an adequate blood level for 6 hours and is therefore given four times daily.

Phenoxymethypenicillin — usual dose 500 mg four times daily.

Adequate absorption with a satisfactory therapeutic response usually occurs with oral penicillin but it is important that it is taken *30 minutes before a meal*. The patient must be carefully observed in case the drug is ineffective due to vomiting or inadequate absorption. Penicillin must then be given by injection.

2. The elucidation of the structure of the penicillin nucleus has made it possible to produce penicillins which are not broken down by penicillinase and are therefore effective against organisms (particularly staphylococci) which have become resistant to benzylpenicillin. In common use is:

Flucloxacillin — 250–500 mg every 6 hours orally or by injection.

It is used almost exclusively for treating staphylococcal infections. Strains of staphylococci are emerging which are even resistant to flucloxacillin. They are named *methicillin-resistant Staphylococcus aureus (MRSA)* and respond only to vancomycin (see p. 232).

3. Broad-spectrum penicillins. **Ampicillin** is an entirely new departure in that it is effective against a number of bacteria, including salmonellae, *E. coli*, shigellae and *H. influenzae* which are little affected by benzylpenicillin. It has proved particularly useful in chronic bronchitis, urinary infections and typhoid. The dose is 250–500 mg every 6 hours by mouth. It can also be given by injection.

Amoxicillin is very similar to ampicillin, but is better absorbed so a smaller dose is required. For this reason it is perhaps to be preferred to ampicillin. The dose is 250–500 mg every 8 hours.

Pivampicillin consists of ampicillin linked to another moiety. As it passes through the gut wall it is split and ampicillin is released. It therefore has no advantage over ampicillin except that it is better absorbed.

Some of the bacteria produce β lactamases which are capable of breaking down both ampicillin and amoxycillin together with other antibiotics. Antibiotics can be combined with a substance called **clavulanate** which prevents this breakdown and thus enables it to destroy β-lactamase-producing bacteria. The combined preparation of amoxicillin and clavulanate is called **co-amoxiclav**.

4. There is a further group of extended-spectrum penicillins (*ureido penicillins*) which have much the same antibacterial spectrum as ampicillin but are also effective against *Pseudomonas aeruginosa* and *Proteus morgani*. They are, however, inactivated by some β lactamases and are not therefore active against penicillin-resistant staphylococci and, in addition, are not very effective against other Gram-positive organisms (e.g. *S. pneumoniae*). They are not absorbed from the gut and must be given by injection. They are reserved for serious infections with pseudomonas or when the causative organism is not known, in which case, due to deficiencies in their antibacterial spectrum, they

Table 16.2 Extended-spectrum penicillins

Drug	Dose	Special features
Azlocillin	15 g daily	The most effective agent against pseudomonas. Not quite so effective against other organisms
Piperacillin	4 g every 6–8 hours	Good all-round activity
Ticarcillin		Available combined with clavulanic acid

are usually combined with an aminoglycoside but must not be mixed in the same infusion or syringe. They are very expensive. Some are shown in Table 16.2.

As these drugs are excreted via the kidney, the dose should be reduced in renal failure.

Adverse effects of penicillins

Considering the wide use of penicillin, it is remarkably free from toxic effects. Pain and rarely abscess formation may be seen at the site of injection. More commonly sensitization rashes occur either as a result of contact with the drug during or after systemic administration. The rash is often urticarial and is sometimes resistant to treatment. With ampicillin or amoxicillin the rash is sometimes erythematous and is particularly liable to occur if they are given to a patient with glandular fever or lymphoma. It may also appear after they have been stopped. Rarely penicillin causes an acute anaphylactic reaction with collapse which can be fatal.

Nursing point

Always ask about previous drug reactions before giving a patient a penicillin, cephalosporin, or for that matter, any other drug.

Other adverse effects include diarrhoea and penicillins may reduce the efficacy of the contraceptive pill. Co-amoxiclav can cause jaundice.

THE CEPHALOSPORINS

This is a large group of antibiotics which struc-turally bear some relationship to the penicillins in that they both contain a β *lactam ring*. They have a wide spectrum of antibacterial activity, although there are differences in this respect between the older cephalosporins and the newer introductions. Most of them can only be given by injection.

Although they are efficient antibiotics they are rarely the drug of first choice as for many infections there are cheaper, effective substitutes.

They can be divided into three groups:

1. The older cephalosporins
2. The recently introduced cephalosporins
3. Oral cephalosporins.

The older cephalosporins (Table 16.3)

These are active against:

- *Staphylococcus aureus* (including some strains resistant to penicillin)
- *Streptococcus pyogenes*
- *Streptococcus pneumoniae*
- *E. coli* (most strains)
- *Klebsiella* (most strains)
- *Proteus* (most strains)
- *H. influenzae* (variable)

They may be inactivated by β lactamases and are excreted by the kidneys.

The newer cephalosporins

These are an improvement on the older members of the group. They are more β lactamase-stable and therefore effective against some resistant strains. In general they act against:

- *Streptococcus pyogenes*
- *Staphylococcus aureus*
- *H. influenzae*

Table 16.3 The older cephalosporins

Drug	Important features
Cefazolin	Some biliary excretion so used before surgery on the bile duct
Cefradine	Fairly β lactamase-stable

This group is being superseded.

Table 16.4 The newer cephalosporins

Drug	Important features
Cefuroxime	Good all-round activity
Cefamandole	Effective against staphylococci
Cefoxitin	Active against *B. fragilis*
Cefotaxime	Good all-round activity against Gram-negative organisms
Ceftizoxime	Similar to cefotaxime
Ceftazidime	Useful in pseudomonal infection
Ceftriaxone	Long-acting
Cefpirome	Good all-round activity

- *N. meningitidis*
- *E. coli*
- *Proteus*.

Some of them also have activity against pseudomonas and *Bacillus fragilis*—important organisms in abdominal infection.

The latest introductions do, however, show some falling off in their activity against certain Gram-positive organisms.

There are now so many of this group available that only a selection is shown in Table 16.4.

The main uses for these new cephalosporins:

1. To treat severe infection (septicaemias, etc.) when the causative organism is not known or other antibiotics are contraindicated.

2. Cefotaxime and ceftriaxone penetrate well into the cerebrospinal fluid and are effective in meningo-coccal meningitis.

3. Possibly in hepatobiliary or abdominal sepsis.

4. Very rarely in resistant urinary infections.

5. Cefuroxime is effective in most chest infections even by Gram-positive organisms, i.e. *Strep. pneumoniae*.

Most of this group are expensive.

Oral cephalosporins

Cefadroxil is given in doses of 500 mg every 12 hours and has a similar antibacterial range to the older cephalosporins. It can be used in urinary and respiratory infections.

Cefixime is similar but rather long-acting and more effective against *H. influenzae*.

Although cefuroxime is ineffective if given orally a compound of it (**cefuroxime axetil**) is absorbed from the gastrointestinal tract and is now available.

Cefpodoxime is used in respiratory infections.

Cross-sensitivity to penicillin

Approximately 10% of patients who are allergic to penicillin will also be allergic to a cephalosporin. In general, this excludes the use of cephalosporins in penicillin-sensitive patients although exception may be made in special circumstances.

OTHER β LACTAMS

Aztreonam has a relatively narrow spectrum of antibacterial action. It can be used against infections caused by *N. gonorrhoeae* and *H. influenzae*, but is ineffective against the common Gram-positive organisms. It is given by injection.

Imipenem has the widest antibacterial range of any antibiotic, including not only the usual Gram-positive and Gram-negative bacteria, but also *pseudomonas* and *anaerobes*. The dose is 250 mg–500 mg every 8 hours via an intravenous infusion, or 500–750 mg every 12 hours by deep intra-muscular injection. It is excreted via the kidney and is inactivated in the renal tubule by an enzyme; the urinary concentration is therefore very low. This is prevented by combining it with *cilastatin* which inhibits the enzyme. At present its use is confined to patients in whom older antibiotics are contraindicated or ineffective.

Both these drugs can show cross-sensitivity with penicillin.

Moropenem is similar to the above but is not broken down by the kidneys and does not therefore need to be combined with cilastatin. It is given by injection.

THE AMINOGLYCOSIDES

This group of antibiotics interferes with protein synthesis in the bacteria and is bactericidal (i.e. they kill the bacteria rather than preventing them from multiplying). They have a fairly wide anti-bacterial range and one of them (streptomycin) is effective against the tubercle bacillus.

They have a number of common properties:

1. They are all given by injection if a systemic effect is required.

2. They are all excreted by the kidneys and accumulation occurs with impaired renal function.

3. They are all, to a greater or lesser degree, ototoxic and nephrotoxic.

Their antibacterial spectrum differs a little, but they are generally active against a fair range of organisms.

Organism	Disease
Staphylococcus aureus	Septicaemia, abscesses
S. viridans	Endocarditis
H. influenzae	Pneumonia, meningitis
Brucella abortus	Abortus fever
E. coli	Renal and other infections
Proteus	Various infections,
Pseudomonas	largely abdominal
Klebsiella	Chest infection
*Myobacterium tuberculosis	All forms of tuberculosis they are not particularly effective against S. pneumoniae or S. pyogenes.

Gentamicin

This antibiotic is widely used, especially in treating severe infection by staphylococci and by various Gram-negative organisms. It is given intravenously or intramuscularly. Excretion, which is via the kidneys, is fairly rapid so that it is usually given three times daily.

It is important to maintain a correct blood level, which should be measured every 48 hours or more often if necessary. The peak level (half an hour after injection) should be between 5 and 10 mg/litre and the trough level (just before injection) should be below 2 mg/litre. The dose is adjusted to produce these levels. If the blood level is too low the antibiotic may not be effective, but if it is above 10 mg/litre for long, ototoxicity will result. It should be remembered that toxicity depends not only on the blood level, but also upon the length of treatment.

The initial dose for patients with normal renal function is usually 1 mg/kg body weight three times daily. This may be too little for severe infections, when it is better to give 1.5 mg/kg/body weight. Elderly patients usually require reduced dosage.

Increasing interest is being shown in the once daily administration of aminoglycosides, the initial dose being in the region of 5 mg/kg/day. Blood levels are measured once or twice daily and the dose adjusted accordingly.

Gentamicin is excreted via the kidneys and *accumulation and toxicity will occur if the drug is given to patients with impaired renal function.* In these circumstances a lower dosage will be required and information is available which relates the dose necessary to the degree of impairment of renal function.

Nursing points

1. It is essential to monitor the blood levels of gentamicin, etc. Renal function may deteriorate in the course of a serious illness and, if impaired, accumulation and toxicity will occur.

2. Gentamicin reacts with many drugs in vitro, therefore it should be given as a bolus or separate injection.

Interactions and adverse effects. Renal damage may occur if gentamicin is combined with furosemide or cephaloridine. Gentamicin is ototoxic, causing disorders of balance and hearing, which are dose-related. Gentamicin augments the action of curare-like neuromuscular blocking agents. It should be avoided during pregnancy as it is ototoxic to the fetus.

Tobramycin, amikacin and netilmicin are very similar to gentamicin; however, they are sometimes effective against Gram-negative organisms which are resistant to gentamicin. They should only be used in this situation as they offer no other advantage. Side-effects are similar, except that netilmicin is perhaps a little less toxic.

---

*Streptomycin only.

Spectinomycin has only one use, the treatment of gonorrheal infection due to organisms which have become resistant to penicillin.

Adverse effects include rashes and vomiting.

Neomycin is an antibiotic which is bactericidal against a wide range of Gram-positive and Gram-negative organisms and against the tubercle bacillus. It is very poorly absorbed from the intestinal tract and because of toxicity is not given systemically. It is chiefly used to sterilize the gut in doses of 1 g every 4 hours for a day or two. It can also be applied locally as ear or eye drops.

Extensive local application to areas such as burns should be avoided as enough absorption can occur to cause ototoxicity.

Streptomycin is derived from one of the actinomyces group of fungi.

Streptomycin is usually given by intramuscular injection. The maximum concentration in the blood is reached after about 1–2 hours and excretion is not completed for 24 hours or more. Streptomycin is excreted in the urine. It is not absorbed after oral administration so this route is not used except for treating gut infections.

Resistance. The development of resistance to streptomycin is relatively common. This may be largely prevented by combining the streptomycin with some other chemotherapeutic agent or antibiotic to which the organism is sensitive; under such treatment the development of resistance is delayed or even prevented altogether.

Streptomycin is now rarely used for infections other than drug-resistant tuberculosis. It may be combined with doxycycline in the treatment of brucellosis.

TETRACYCLINES

Following the discovery of penicillin and streptomycin, a large-scale investigation was carried out into substances that were produced by various fungi.

Three important antibiotics which were discovered are known as the tetracyclines. They are very similar in chemical structure and toxic effects and are effective against the same wide range of organisms. They are: **chlortetracycline**, **oxytetracycline** and **tetracycline**.

The properties of these drugs are so similar that they may be considered together.

They are usually given orally and are quite well absorbed from the intestinal tract and 6-hourly dosage is satisfactory. Tetracycline hydrochloride may also be given by intravenous injection. It is, however, very irritating to the vein and is best given by continuous intravenous infusion.

After absorption the tetracyclines spread widely through the body. The penetration across the meningeal barrier into the cerebrospinal fluid is variable, being greatest in the case of tetracycline itself. The greater part of these drugs is excreted in the urine; the fate of the remainder is unknown.

The tetracyclines have a very wide antibacterial range, which includes not only true bacteria but some of the larger viruses.

However, with some bacteria resistant strains have emerged which limit their use. The main uses for the tetracyclines at present are:

Organism	*Disease*
H. influenzae	⎫
Streptococcus pneumoniae	⎬ Bronchitis
Mycoplasma	Pneumonia
Chlamydia	Non-specific urethritis
Rickettsia	Typhus, Q fever, etc.
Brucella abortus	Abortus fever

They are also used over long periods in the treatment of acne. Whether their efficacy in this disorder is due to their antibacterial action or is due to some other factor is not known. The dose is 250 mg every 6 hours. Chlortetracycline is now only available as an ointment.

Nursing point

Tetracycline tablets should be swallowed whole with the patient sitting or standing and washed down with plenty of water. Absorption is reduced by concurrent administration of iron, calcium or magnesium compounds (including milk).

Demeclocycline is similar to the others in the group, but rather smaller doses are required and its action is more prolonged.

Doxycycline is similar to the older tetracyclines, but is excreted slowly so that only one dose is required daily. The other important difference is that, unlike tetracycline, it can be used when renal function is impaired (see below). It is also used in the prevention of malaria.

Adverse effects. A certain amount of nausea, vomiting and epigastric disturbance due to a direct irritant effect often follows administration of the tetracyclines.

Because of their wide antibacterial spectrum the tetracyclines cause considerable changes in the bacterial flora both in the intestine and elsewhere. This often results in diarrhoea, which usually recovers quickly when the drug is stopped. Occasionally, they may cause a serious enteritis due to the multiplication of a resistant organism, usually a staphylococcus. *Candida* is the other troublesome organism which may emerge in those receiving tetracyclines, causing 'thrush' in the mouth or vaginal candidiasis.

Tetracyclines damage and discolour developing teeth and should be avoided if possible from the fourth month of pregnancy until the child is 12 years old. Other toxic effects are rare, but include skin rashes and other sensitization phenomena.

Tetracyclines (except doxycycline) should not be given when renal function is impaired as they cause increased tissue breakdown with a subsequent rise of breakdown products in the blood, and exacerbation of the renal failure.

CHLORAMPHENICOL

Chloramphenicol is a broad-spectrum antibiotic closely related in its action to the tetracyclines; it has, however, serious but rare toxic effects on the bone marrow which limit its use to those patients who cannot obtain benefit from any other form of treatment.

It is given by mouth and is rapidly absorbed from the intestine. It diffuses widely and crosses the meningeal barrier into the cerebrospinal fluid. It is excreted via the kidneys. Like the tetracyclines it is effective against a wide range of organisms with the important addition of *Salmonella typhi* and the *paratyphoid* group.

Therapeutics. Bone marrow toxicity limits its use but it can be used for meningitis and acute epiglottitis due to *H. influenzae*. It is also very effective in typhoid and paratyphoid fevers, though resistant strains are emerging and ciprofloxacin may be preferred. The dose for adults is 50 mg/kg daily, divided into doses every 6 hours. It is also commonly used in solution as eye and ear drops.

Adverse effects. The most serious toxic effects of chloramphenicol are on the bone marrow. Although they are rare (perhaps about 1 in 40 000 treatment courses), they are nearly always fatal when they occur. The most common effect is aplastic anaemia—the other reported change being depression of white cells and platelets.

Toxic effects are more common after prolonged or repeated courses of chloramphenicol and their appearance may be delayed for up to 2 months after receiving the drug.

In newborn infants, chloramphenicol is less rapidly broken down so that accumulation may occur, producing the '*grey syndrome*' with circulatory collapse and shock.

THE MACROLIDES

Erythromycin

Erythromycin was first introduced in 1952. It is absorbed rather erratically after oral administration and diffuses widely, but does not enter into the cerebrospinal fluid very well. It is bacteriostatic and acts against a wide range of organisms, including *Streptococcus pyogenes*, *Staphyloccus aureus, Mycoplasma pneumoniae* and *Legionella pneumophila* (causing legionnaires' disease). It is not, however, always effective against *H. influenzae*, a common cause of respiratory infection.

Resistance. Bacteria fairly readily become resistant to erythromycin, but do not show cross-resistance to other antibiotics.

Therapeutics. Erythromycin has a similar range of activity to penicillin and is used instead of that drug in those who are sensitive to penicillin.

Table 16.5 The antibacterial activity of antibiotics and chemotherapeutic agents

Organism	Diseases	Macrolides	Benzyl-penicillin	Gentamicin	Ampicillin, Amoxicillin	Others
Staphylococcus aureus	Purulent infection	++	++†	++	++†	Vancomycin ++ Erythromycin ++ Flucloxacillin ++ Sodium fusidate ++
Streptococcus pyogenes	Tonsillitis, scarlet fever	++	++	0	++	
Streptococcus viridans	Infective endocarditis	++	++	+	++	
Streptococcus pneumoniae	Pneumonia	++	++	0	++	
N. meningitidis	Meningitis	0	++	0	++	Newer cephalosporins ++
N. gonorrhoeae	Gonorrhoea	0	++	++	++	Spectinomycin ++, 4-quinolones ++
E. coli	Urinary tract infection	0	0	++	++	Trimethoprim Nitrofurantoin ++ Ciprofloxacin ++
Shigella	Dysentery	0	0	+	++	Chloramphenicol ++ Trimethoprim ++
Salmonella typhi	Typhoid	0	0	+	++	Chloramphenicol ++
Haemophilus influenzae	Meningitis and pneumonia	+	0	+	++	
Treponema pallidum	Syphilis	++	++	0	0	
Pseudomonas aeruginosa	Various infections, septicaemia	0	0	++	0	Ureido penicillins ++ some new Cephalosporins +
Chlamydia	Non-specific urethritis	++	0	0	++	Doxycycline ++

Very effective, ++; sometimes effective, +; little or no action, 0.
† Owing to resistance — flucloxacillin, ++

It is used for various respiratory diseases including *Mycoplasma pneumoniae* and legionnaires' disease. The usual dosage is 2 g a day divided into doses every 6 hours. To reduce nausea it is best taken with food. Erythromycin can be given by infusion as the preparation erythromycin lactobionate.

Adverse effects are rare and include diarrhoea and vomiting and rarely jaundice, if injected.

Intravenous administration is liable to cause thrombophlebitis.

Clarithromycin has a similar antibacterial spectrum to erythromycin, but higher concentrations are found in the tissues and it has a greater effect against *H. influenzae* than erythromycin. It is also used for the eradication of *Helicobacter pylori* (see p. 98). Gastrointestinal upsets are less frequent.

Azithromycin appears to be similar, but with a long half-life; one daily dose is adequate.

The precise place of these new macrolides in treatment is still not settled, but they appear to be an improvement on erythromycin. They are, however, considerably more expensive at present.

Interactions. Erythromycin and clarithromycin interfere with the breakdown of certain drugs. They should not be combined with terfenadine, astemizole (antihistamines) or cisapride.

MISCELLANEOUS ANTIBIOTICS

Clindamycin is effective against many Gram-positive organisms and can be used to treat infections by anaerobic organisms, particularly those which complicate bowel surgery. It is well absorbed when taken orally and appears to penetrate into bone. This makes it particularly useful for treating infection in bone. The dose is 150 mg four times daily.

Adverse effects are not common; diarrhoea

may be a problem and rarely takes the form of a serious colitis (*pseudomembranous colitis*).

Polymixin is effective against a wide range of Gram-negative organisms. It is particularly useful when applied locally for resistant infections by such organisms as pseudomonas; for example, otitis externa.

Sodium fusidate is effective against resistant *staphylococci*. Its main use is combined with other antibiotics in the treatment of severe staphylococal infections. It is given orally in doses of 1–2 g daily and is relatively free of side-effects, though high doses may cause jaundice which recovers when the drug is stopped.

Vancomycin is particularly useful in treating severe staphylococcal infections which are resistant to other antibiotics. It is given by slow intravenous infusion and the dose is controlled by measuring blood levels. It is ototoxic and nephrotoxic and is often given into a central vein as it can cause venous thrombosis. It is also given orally in the treatment of pseudo-membranous colitis which occasionally follows the use of antibiotics and is due to infection of the colon with *C. difficile*.

Teicoplanin is similar, but with considerably less adverse effects and a longer action.

Linezolid is a new type of antibiotic which interferes with protein synthesis in the bacteria. Early testing shows that it is effective against *Staph. aureus* and *Strep. pneumoniae*, and in the treatment of pneumonia and soft-tissue infections. It is given orally or intravenously and has a relatively short half-life. So far, adverse effects do not appear to be serious.

It is still under trial and not, at the time of writing, generally available in the UK but, if early promise is fulfilled, it should be a valuable addition to the range of antibiotics, particularly in the treatment of infections by antibiotic-resistant Gram-positive organisms (e.g. *Staph. aureus* and *Strep. pneumoniae*).

TUBERCULOSIS

In former times tuberculosis was a common and frequently fatal disease. In the last 50 years its incidence has declined rapidly in the UK due to improved living conditions and effective drug treatment. However, where the resistance of the population is lowered by poverty, malnutrition and, more recently, by AIDS, it is still a dangerous and lethal disease.

Drugs used in tuberculosis

Isoniazid. This drug is bacteriostatic and possibly bactericidal to tubercle bacilli. It is rapidly absorbed from the intestine and largely excreted by the kidneys. It diffuses widely through the body; it enters cells and it crosses the meningeal barrier to the cerebrospinal fluid in amounts adequate to inhibit the growth of the tubercle bacillus. The usual dose for an adult is 300 mg/day by mouth in divided doses.

Isoniazid is metabolized in the liver. It is possible to divide people into two groups: those who break isoniazid down rapidly and those who break it down slowly. As a result of this the rapidly inactivating group will have lower concentrations of the drug in their blood than the slow inactivators. In the dosage schemes used in the UK this is of no importance, but in less developed countries where the drug may be given less frequently to save cost, rapid in-activators are in danger of getting less than a full therapeutic effect from the drug.

Adverse effects. Neuropathy can develop in slow inactivators who are given large doses and in those at special risk of nerve damage (patients with diabetes, alcoholics). This can be prevented by giving pyridoxine 10 mg daily.

Rifampicin. Rifampicin is effective against several Gram-positive and Gram-negative organisms and in particular against the tubercle bacillus. Its use is largely confined to tuberculosis but it can also be used in *legionnaires' disease* and to prevent infection in subjects who have had close contact with meningococcal meningitis. It is well absorbed orally, the dose being 450–600 mg once daily before breakfast. It is mainly excreted in the bile. It is useful in the treatment of tuberculosis, but must be combined with other antituberculous drugs to prevent resistance developing.

Adverse effects are uncommon, but it should

not be used in patients with liver disease as it can cause changes in liver function tests and, rarely, causes severe liver damage. It may cause red discoloration of the urine and sputum and by increasing the rate of breakdown of estrogen may reduce the effectiveness of oral contraceptives.

Rifabutin is similar to rifampicin.

Ethambutol is usually satisfactory, but is now rarely used unless there is a possibility of resistance to other antituberculous drugs. It is given in doses of 15 mg/kg body weight. The most important side-effect is damage to the optic nerve, leading to deterioration of visual acuity and colour vision. Correct dosage reduces this risk, but vision should be tested before starting treatment and at 6-monthly intervals.

Pyrazinamide is powerful and effective with good penetration into tuberculous lesions and the CSF. Its use is limited by adverse effects but is justified, particularly in tuberculous meningitis, provided that the correct dose is given and the course lasts no longer than 2 months. During treatment liver function tests should be performed and alcohol avoided. The usual dose is 20–30 mg/kg/body weight daily by mouth.

Adverse effects include liver damage with jaundice, light sensitization (use a barrier cream) and attacks of gout.

Combined preparations

Preparations which combine isoniazid, rifampicin and pyrazinamide are available and they improve compliance.

Streptomycin is very effective against the tubercle bacillus, but resistant strains develop in about 6 weeks if it is used alone. This is prevented if it is combined with other antituberculous drugs. It is given by injection once daily, the dose being 1 g. In older or small patients this may be reduced to 0.75 g to decrease toxicity. *Because it has to be injected and adverse effects can be troublesome, it has now been largely replaced by other drugs.*

Adverse effects are not uncommon with streptomycin. The most important are those affecting the eighth nerve. The symptoms include high-pitched tinnitus and vertigo. This may be followed by varying degrees of deafness.

Sensitization phenomena also occur with streptomycin. These may affect not only the patient, but the person injecting the drug. Swelling of the eyelids is an early sign. Care should be taken when giving the drug to avoid contamination of the hands and face, which may occur when the syringe is held at eye level to measure the exact dose. The wearing of plastic gloves and a mask is advisable in those who handle large quantities of it.

Drug regimes for tuberculosis

There are now a number of drugs which are effective against the tubercle bacillus. It is important, however, that:

1. At least two drugs are used at the same time to prevent the emergence of resistant organisms.

2. Treatment is continued for a long time to eradicate the infection completely. The choice of drugs is determined by the sensitivity of the infective tubercle bacillus. However, the regimes commonly used are:

Pulmonary tuberculosis

Rifampicin 450–600 mg ⎫
                       ⎬ once daily before
Isoniazid 300 mg   ⎪ breakfast for 2 months
Pyrazinamide 1.5–2.0 g ⎭

followed by

Rifampicin ⎫
Isoniazid ⎬   for a further 4 months.

Ethambutol is only used if resistance is a possibility.

Variation in the drugs used is due to their differing penetration of tissue, their effectiveness against dividing organisms and their ability to sterilize a lesion. The excellent penetration of isoniazid and pyrazinamide into the CSF makes them particularly useful in meningeal tuberculosis. Resistance by the tubercle bacillus to one or other drug may require a change of regime.

Although the discovery of these drugs has revolutionized the treatment of tuberculosis, it must be realized that they form only part of the treatment. The basic measures of rest, good food and good nursing are as important as ever.

Multidrug resistance

In recent years the problem of patients infected with tubercle bacilli which are resistant to one or more antibiotics has emerged in some countries, but, as yet, not seriously in the UK. This happens most often in patients who have relapsed as they may have received inadequate treatment. Patients with AIDS have poor resistance to infection; this makes treatment difficult and may add to the number of resistant organisms. Such patients require individually designed combinations of drugs and the treatment is prolonged. Among the drugs used are streptomycin, capreomycin, cycloserine and clarithromycin.

Special points for patient education

It is very important that patients realize the importance of taking their medication regularly as directed. Poor compliance or failure to finish the course of treatment is common in tuberculosis and is a major factor in the emergence of resistant strains.

Nursing point

Patients with tuberculosis should cease to be infectious after 1 week of treatment provided that the organism is sensitive.
When nursing patients with open tuberculosis nurses must be careful to avoid infection. This is particularly important if the patient has a multidrug-resistant infection, when the infective period may be prolonged.

ANTIFUNGAL AGENTS

Nystatin. This antibiotic binds to the wall of the fungus disrupting its integrity. It is very poorly absorbed after oral administration and is therefore used to treat infections of the intestinal tract or is applied locally. It is particularly used in *Candida* infection. Oral infections respond to nystatin pastilles (100 000 units) dissolved in the mouth four times daily. It is very effective in treating vaginal candidiasis, one pessary being inserted daily for 14 days. Nystatin cream should be applied to the penis of the sexual partner over the same period.

Clotrimazole and miconazole are most effective if applied locally as pessaries in the treatment of vaginal candidiasis. Miconazole is available as a gel for treating oropharyngeal infection. Both can be applied to the skin as a 1% or 2% ointment for dermatophytoses.

Ketoconazole is largely used in severe candidiasis and other systemic fungal infections. It can be given orally and is well absorbed, the dose being 200–400 mg daily.

Adverse effects. The most important is jaundice when the drug must be stopped. Others include nausea, drowsiness and rarely, adrenal suppression.

Itraconazole is used in systemic candidiasis and dermatophyte infections. The dose is variable and the capsules should be taken immediately after food to ensure maximum absorption. It should not be used in patients with liver disease.

Fluconazole is effective in candidiasis and cryptococcus and serious adverse effects, particularly liver damage, have not been reported. For vaginal candidiasis a single oral dose of 150 mg is adequate and for oropharyngeal infection 50 mg daily for 7–14 days is required.

Griseofulvin is administered orally in the treatment of various fungal infections. It is used in most types of fungal infection of the skin, particularly in ringworm of the scalp where local treatment is inadequate. It is slow-acting and may be continued for several weeks.

Adverse effects. Gastrointestinal upsets may occur when it is used and griseofulvin may enhance the action of alcohol taken at the same time as the drug.

Terbinafine is given orally for tinea infections of the skin or nails.

Tioconazole is applied locally over long periods (6–12 months) for fungal infection of the nails.

Amphotericin. This is used in systemic infection with fungal organisms, namely systemic *candidiasis, cryptococcul meningitis* and *histoplasmosis*. After an initial test dose, it is given by intravenous infusion, the dose being increased gradually. Amphoteracin B is now available enclosed in liposomes for use intravenously. This renders it easier to use and less toxic. It is also used in lozenges containing 10 mg of amphotericin B, which are given four times daily in the treatment of oral candidiasis.

Adverse effects which may limit the dose are nausea, vomiting and fever. Some renal damage may occur.

Flucytosine is an antifungal agent which is effective against *Candida albicans* and *Cryptococcus*. It is given orally, four times daily. It is excreted by the kidney and therefore reduced dosage may be required in patients with impaired renal function. Side-effects are rare, but depression of the blood count has been reported.

Candidiasis

This is a common and troublesome problem. It can occur for no apparent reason but is particularly common in ill or immunocompromised patients, particularly those receiving broad spectrum antibiotics, those receiving drugs which suppress immunity (i.e. cytotoxic drugs and steroids), patients with AIDS, patients with diabetes and infants. It may affect the mouth (thrush), the vagina or other mucous membranes. Rarely, it enters the bloodstream and becomes a systemic infection.

Treatment

Oral candidiasis

Acute	Nystatin 100 000 unit pastilles or amphotericin B 10 mg tablets sucked every 6 hours after food.
Oropharyngeal	Fluconazole 50 mg daily or itraconazole 100 mg daily for up to 14 days.
Children	Miconazole gel.

Oesophageal, intestinal or systemic candidiasis

Fluconazole 50–400 mg daily.

Vaginal candidiasis

Fluconazole, a single oral dose of 150 mg or itraconazole 200 mg twice daily for 1 day. Clotrimazole vaginal pessaries 500 mg, one inserted at night as a single dose.

Nursing points

1. In oral candidiasis remove dentures (if any) during treatment. They should be soaked in 1% sodium hypochlorite overnight and rinsed before being worn again.
2. In vaginal candidiasis do not forget to treat the partner (if any) with a cream preparation.

Systemic fungal infections

These are an increasing problem because of the large number of immunocompromised subjects due to AIDS, cancer chemotherapy and other causes. Until fairly recently amphotericin and flucytosine were the only drugs available, but recent introductions including fluconazole and itraconazole are equally, and sometimes more, effective. The correct drug for a particular fungal infection is still being studied and the choice of treatment requires expert guidance.

TRICHOMONACIDES

Trichomonas vaginalis is a small mobile parasitic protozoan which frequently causes vaginitis and occasionally urethritis in men.

Metronidazole. Metronidazole given orally in doses of 200 mg three times daily for 1 week will eradicate trichomonas in about 90% of patients. It is relatively free of *adverse effects*, but may cause nausea, headaches and skin rashes. *It interacts with alcohol, producing headaches and flushing, and with prolonged use can cause nerve damage*.

Metronidazole is also used in treating infections by anaerobic organisms such as bacteroides. Such infections frequently complicate abdominal operations involving the intestines. It may be used prophylactically before operation, a suppository containing 1 g being given 4 hours before operation and repeated every 8 hours until oral medication with 400 mg every 8 hours can be started. For established infection 400 mg every 8 hours is satisfactory. It is highly effective orally in amoebiasis and giardiasis (see p. 254).

It is advised that metronidazole is not used in the first 3 months of pregnancy, although there is no evidence that it causes fetal damage.

ANTIVIRAL AGENTS

Viruses cause a number of diseases, some of which are serious and potentially fatal, although most are of minor importance (e.g. the common cold). In subjects who are immunosuppressed (e.g. by AIDS or treatment with cytotoxic drugs), relatively benign viral infection may become virulent.

It is difficult to produce effective antiviral agents for several reasons. Viruses live within human cells and use processes in those cells to multiply; they are not therefore readily accessible. They are relatively simple structures and not easy to kill; furthermore, a great deal of virus replication occurs before the patient develops symptoms.

Aciclovir. This agent is effective against the herpes viruses. It enters the infected cells where it is changed into a powerful antiviral agent.

Therapeutics.

1. It can be applied as a 3% ointment five times daily to treat ulceration of the cornea due to the herpes simplex virus and should be continued for 3 days after healing.

2. Given orally in doses of 200 mg five times daily for 5 days it accelerates the healing of genital herpes. Very severe attacks may require parenteral treatment.

3. A 5% cream of aciclovir is only effective in labial herpes if used in the prodromal period when there is only a local burning sensation.

4. In generalized herpes simplex infection in immunosuppressed patients or in herpes meningo-encephalitis it is given by intravenous infusion,

5 mg/kg over 1 hour, every 8 hours for five days. This may cause an apparent deterioration of renal function which should be monitored. Patients with impaired renal function will require smaller doses.

5. Aciclovir is not usually needed in herpes zoster (shingles), but if the ophthalmic branch of the trigeminal nerve is affected, this may be followed by prolonged neuralgia and damage to the eye and aciclovir 800 mg five times daily should be given for 7 days. It should be started within 48 hours of the onset of symptoms.

It also shortens the course of varicella (chickenpox), but its use in this disorder should be confined to those at special risk (i.e. immunosuppressed patients).

Adverse effects include rashes, nausea and vomiting.

It is contraindicated in pregnancy.

Famciclovir and **valaciclovir** are similar and are given orally to treat herpes simplex and herpes zoster. They have the advantage of only needing to be administered two or three times daily.

Amantadine (see also p. 173) has some action against the influenza virus. A daily dose of 100 mg for 5 days may prevent an attack in those at risk.

Ganciclovir is used specifically for the treatment of serious infections by the cytomegalovirus. The disease is usually mild except in immunosuppressed patients (e.g. those with AIDS) and as a risk to the fetus in pregnancy. It is given by intravenous infusion.

The most serious *adverse effect* is suppression of the white cell count and of the platelets, which usually recover when the drug is stopped.

Foscarnet is reserved for cytomegalovirus infection in immunocompromised patients. It is given by intravenous infusion and is highly nephrotoxic.

Tribavirin is used in the treatment of respiratory tract viruses, particularly respiratory syncytial virus, which causes bronchiolitis in infants. It is given by nebulizer or aerosol inhalation.

ACQUIRED IMMUNODEFICIENCY SYNDROME (AIDS)

There are about 12 million people worldwide who are infected with the human immuno-deficiency virus (HIV), at present, and this number is likely to rise. So far, no cure is available but treatment is becoming more successful.

After infection there is a latent period when the patient is symptom-free. During this time the virus enters the cells of the immune system (CD4 T cells) and, using the host cells' metabolic processes, multiplies and finally kills the cells, releasing further viruses. When the immune system has been sufficiently depleted of T cells, the patient becomes susceptible to a variety of infections which ultimately prove fatal. The AIDS syndrome refers to the terminal stage (Fig. 16.3).

Treatment

The use of single agents against the HIV leads to the emergence of resistance and failure of treatment. It is now apparent that using several antiviral agents, particularly if they affect different phases in the viral life cycle, is more effective.

Two main groups of antiviral drugs are available:

1. Nucleoside analogues. On entering the cells, these drugs are modified and then interfere with viral reverse transcriptase and thus, with the production of viral DNA which is an essential step in the formation of further viral particles.

Zidovudine is the most widely used drug of this group and can be given orally or intravenously.

Adverse effects include nausea, headache and muscle pains and, rarely, bone marrow suppression.

Similar drugs are lamivudine, didanosine and zalcitabine.

2. Protease inhibitors. These drugs act at a later stage in the formation of virus particles by inhibiting viral proteases which are necessary for the formation of viral proteins.

They are given orally and include indinavir, ritonavir and saquinavir.

Adverse effects include nausea, vomiting and diarrhoea. Patients taking indinavir should have a high fluid intake as there is a risk of renal stone formation.

Two or three drugs are given together (nucleoside analogue + protease inhibitor) and most experts believe that it is best to start treatment when the infection is first diagnosed rather than when symptoms develop. Although it is too early to talk of a cure, active life can be prolonged and complications minimized.

Antiviral agents are expensive and considering the widespread nature of HIV infection, much of it in the Third World, the cost of treatment will be enormous. In addition, when the disease is controlled, some maintenance treatment may be necessary to prevent relapse.

Needle stick injuries. Accidental infection of health professionals is rare but the possibility of becoming HIV positive after a needle-stick injury is about 1:400. For those thought to be seriously at risk, a recommendation is to give zidovudine + lamivudine + indinavir for 4 weeks and treatment should be started within 2 hours

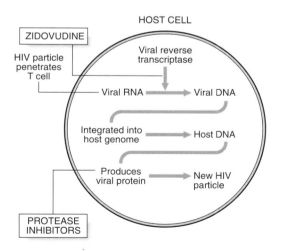

Figure 16.3 Intracellular cycle of an HIV virus particle and site of action of zidovudine which inhibits the enzyme reverse transcriptase and protease inhibitors which prevent the formation of new viral particles.

of exposure. This will greatly reduce the chance of infection. Many hospitals will have their own guidelines.

Mother-to-infant transmission of HIV from an infected mother to the fetus during pregnancy can be considerably reduced by treating both the pregnant mother and the newborn infant with zidovudine.

Monitoring treatment

It is important to measure the extent of HIV infection in a patient in order to decide on optimal treatment and to assess progress. This can be achieved by:

a. Counting the number of CD4 T cells in the blood—the lower the count, the more advanced the disease.

b. Measuring the concentration of RNA derived from the HIV in the plasma (viral load)—the higher the load (which is a measure of viral multiplication), the more active the disease.

Complications of HIV infection

Pneumocystis carinii pneumonia is common and is treated by high-dose co-trimoxazole or by intravenous pentamidine.

Relapse can be prevented by long-term treatment with co-trimoxazole, inhaled pentamidine or dapsone.

Patients with AIDS are also susceptible to various fungal and viral infections and to tuberculosis.

THE INTERFERONS

This is a family of protein-like substances produced by various cells in the body in response to viral infections. Interferons have the ability to act on cells and increase their resistance to viral infections and may also modify the immune response. In addition, they control the growth and differentiation of certain cells.

Interferons can now be produced synthetically and have been used in both neoplastic and infective disease in humans. Their main success has been in treating leukaemias, particularly the hairy-celled types, and to a lesser degree in some other forms of cancer. In the control of viral infections their usefulness is limited but they are used with some success in hepatitis B and C infections.

Interferon B is now being used in the relapsing/remitting form of multiple sclerosis with some benefit. It is given by intramuscular injection.

Adverse effects are fever and nausea.

BACTERIAL RESISTANCE TO ANTIBIOTICS

It has been realized since the time of Ehrlich that organisms might become resistant to treatment with antibacterial drugs. This has now become a worldwide problem and includes *Staph. aureus*, *Strep. pneumoniae*, *N. meningitides*, enterococci, *E. coli*, *P. aeruginosa* and *M. tuberculosis*. Penicillin-resistant strains of staphylococci first became significant in the 1950s, especially in the hospital environment. For a time these strains were still sensitive to methicillin and flucloxacillin but, more recently, strains have emerged which are resistant to both drugs (methicillin-resistant *Staphylococcus aureus*; MRSA). Outbreaks of infection by these organisms are very difficult to control and when an infection by a sensitive organism has been controlled by antibacterial drugs, cross-infection by resistant organisms may ensue.

Resistance may be produced in several ways. In any population of bacteria there may be a few organisms which are resistant to an antibiotic and when all the sensitive organisms have been killed off, the resistant ones are left to flourish and multiply. These resistant organisms have often been produced by mutations (changes in their genetic make-up). It has also been shown that certain bacteria can transmit resistance to each other, and even to different types of bacteria by incorporating foreign DNA which induces resistance. It follows therefore that wherever antibiotics are widely used (as in hospitals), resistant strains will appear. To reduce resistance to a minimum certain precautions should be taken.

1. Antibiotics should only be used when really necessary.

2. Antibiotics should be given in adequate doses.

3. The use of antibiotics prophylactically is generally to be deplored as it breeds resistant strains. There are exceptions to this rule, i.e. the use of penicillin to prevent tonsillitis in patients who have had rheumatic fever and to prevent endocarditis when those with damaged heart valves have dental treatment or before certain operations.

4. In certain circumstances, i.e. the treatment of tuberculosis, the use of several antibiotics together may prevent resistant strains developing.

The use of antibiotics by farmers to promote animal growth should be strictly controlled as it has led to the emergence of resistant strains of bacteria.

Antibiotic policies

Policies have been developed to encourage the efficient, safe and economical use of antibiotics. One of their chief aims is to reduce the emergence of antibiotic-resistant strains. In most hospitals a local formulary is drawn up to reserve the use of particular drugs. Most local policies adopt the following general format:

1. A section which includes a single member of each of the main groups of antibiotics. Each of these can be prescribed without formality. These drugs are held as ward stock.

2. A reserve section containing alternatives, including the most newly developed antibiotics. These are not usually prescribed without liaison with the infection control team and are not held as ward stock.

Policies need regular updating and reviewing to take account of new drugs and changing patterns of microbial behaviour.

ANTIBACTERIAL DRUGS IN THE TREATMENT OF SOME COMMON INFECTIONS

The common cold

The treatment of the common cold is the relief of symptoms with NSAIDs, paracetamol, antihistamines and inhalations. The value of vitamin C is still undecided. Although antibiotics are often prescribed, they are usually of no value in healthy adults; they are expensive and increase the risk of resistant organisms emerging.

Various antiviral agents have been tried, including interferons, but as yet there is no evidence that they are of special benefit.

Sore throat

Minor sore throats are usually viral and do not require antibiotic treatment, but streptococcal throat infection should be treated with phenoxymethylpenicillin 250 mg four times daily for 10 days. If vomiting is a problem, benzylpenicillin should be given by injection. This drug is also used in smaller doses over long periods to prevent throat infection in those who have had rheumatic fever and thus decrease the chance of recurrence.

Bronchitis

A mild attack of acute bronchitis in an otherwise healthy adult does not usually require antibiotic treatment and is frequently due to a viral infection. A severe attack or an acute exacerbation of chronic bronchitis is best treated with amoxicillin 250 mg three times daily or doxycycline as the infection in these circumstances may be due to *H. influenzae, S. pneumoniae* or *Moraxella catarrhalis*.

Pneumonia

The problem with pneumonia is that it may be caused by various bacteria with different antibiotic sensitivities. Table 16.6 is a guide but is by no means definitive.

Table 16.6 Types of pneumonia and their treatment

Type of pneumonia	Usual organism	Antibiotic
Lobar	*S. pneumoniae*	Amoxicillin 500 mg orally every 8 hours
Severe in previously healthy	*S. pneumoniae* *Staphylococcus*	Erythromycin 1 g i.v. every 6 hours + cefuroxime 1.5 g i.v. every 8 hours Modify antibiotic when pathogen is known
Bronchopneumonia often in chronic bronchitics	*S. pneumoniae* *H. influenzae*	Amoxicillin 500 mg orally every 8 hours or co-amoxiclav
Postinfluenzal	*Staphylococcus* (often)	Ampicillin 500 mg i.v. + flucloxacillin 500 mg i.v. every 6 hours. If *Staphylococcus* proved, add sodium fusidate 500 mg every 8 hours
Primary atypical	*Mycoplasma*	Erythromycin 500 mg every 6 hours
Legionnaires' disease	*Legionella*	Erythromycin up to 1.0 g every 6 hours + rifampicin 600 mg i.v. daily
Aspiration pneumonia (postoperative)	Mouth organisms	Ampicillin 500 mg i.v. every 6 hours + metronidazole 400 mg every 8 hours

Sputum and blood cultures may help the *correct choice of antibiotic when results are available.*

In parts of the world, penicillin-resistant *Strep. pneumoniae* have appeared and, in the future, this may alter the choice of antibacterial treatment.

Urinary infections

Urinary infections are usually due to *E. coli* and respond satisfactorily to trimethoprim 200 mg every 12 hours for 5 days. It should, however, be avoided in the first 3 months of pregnancy. A 3-day course of cefadroxil can also be used.

In some areas the organism has become resistant to these antibacterial drugs and norfloxacin twice daily is an alternative. In serious infections cefuroxime can be added to the regime.

It is sometimes necessary to use antibacterial drugs prophylactically, particularly in children. Trimethoprim 100 mg or less at night or on alternate days is usually adequate.

Meningitis

Meningitis may be caused by a variety of organisms and its treatment is complicated because certain antibiotics penetrate poorly into the CSF. Drugs which penetrate poorly have been given intrathecally.

Good penetration	Poor penetration
Sulfonamides (particularly sulfadiazine)	Penicillin Streptomycin
Chloramphenicol	
Tetracycline	
The newer cephalosporins	

Meningococcal meningitis

This should be treated with benzylpenicillin 2.4 g intravenously, every 4–6 hours. Enough penicillin will diffuse through the inflamed meninges to eradicate the infection. If the bacterial diagnosis is in doubt, ceftriaxone should be used as it has a wider antibacterial spectrum. Immediate treatment is important as, sometimes, a very dangerous state of shock develops.

Prevention. Close contacts of patients with meningococcal meningitis should be given rifampicin twice daily for 2 days for children, or ciprofloxacin as a single dose for adults.

Meningitis in neonates

This is usually due to Gram-negative organisms and is treated either with gentamicin and ampicillin, or with a new cephalosporin such as ceftriaxone or cefotaxime.

Streptococcus pneumoniae meningitis

This does not usually respond so well as meningococcal infection. The usual treatment is with cefotaxime as some strains of *S. pneumoniae* are penicillin-resistant.

Haemophilus influenzae meningitis

Ceftriaxone 4.0 g i.v. followed 24 hours later by 2.0 g i.v. daily for 5 days.

Infective endocarditis

This is an infection of damaged heart valves, usually with *Streptococcus viridans*. Because the organisms are buried in the thick vegetation on the valves, they are difficult to reach and kill with antibiotics, so that prolonged treatment with high doses is needed. Usually, benzyl-penicillin and gentamicin are given together for 2 weeks and penicillin continued for another 2 weeks. If the organism is less sensitive, benzyl-penicillin and gentamicin should be continued for 4 weeks. Other organisms may require other regimes and the management should be worked out with a microbiologist.

If a 'butterfly' needle is used to give the antibiotics intravenously, it is necessary to change the site of the cannula regularly or local infection will occur.

Prevention. The trauma of dental treatment often releases microorganisms into the blood. If the patient has damaged heart valves, the organism settles on the valve and sets up an infection. This can be prevented by giving an antibiotic to cover dental treatment. A single oral dose of 3 g of amoxicillin given 1 hour before treatment is easy to give and most satisfactory. For children from 5 to 10 years the dose is 1.5 g and for those under 5 years it is 750 mg. For people who are sensitive to penicillin, clindamycin 600 mg orally 1 hour before treatment can be used.

Staphylococcal infections

These cover a wide range, including simple boils and carbuncles and extending to severe and sometimes fatal septicaemias, pneumonias and osteomyelitis. Mild infections usually respond to phenoxymethylpenicillin, but the severe infections are often due to organisms which have become resistant to penicillin. In these circumstances flucloxacillin 250–500 mg four times daily by mouth or by injection is given. Other useful antibiotics in staphylococcal infections are gentamicin, erythromycin, clindamycin, sodium fusidate and vancomycin or teicoplanin. One or other of these is often combined with flucloxacillin.

Infection due to *methicillin-resistant Staphylococcus aureus (MRSA)* will require isolation and vigorous action to eliminate the organism. A high degree of hygiene should be maintained, including the use of antibacterials in bathing and to eradicate nasal infection. Wounds will require cleaning and the local application of antibacterial agents such as Iodosorb. In addition, an appropriate antibiotic (usually vancomycin) will be employed.

Many hospitals will have their own protocols to deal with this difficult problem.

Chlamydial infection

Organisms of the chlamydia group can cause various infections. *Chlamydia trachomatis* is responsible for most cases of non-specific urethritis and cervicitis, which are the most common sexually transmitted diseases in the Western world. Acute infections may lead to chronic pelvic sepsis in women and prostatitis in men. Treatment is with doxycycline 100 mg twice daily for 2 weeks or azithromycin 1 g as a single dose. Both sexual partners must be treated.

Intestinal infections

Intestinal infections can be caused by various organisms, the most common in the UK being *salmonellae* and *shigellae*. Although these organisms are sensitive to a number of antibiotics it has been found that their use does not hasten recovery and may lead to an increased number of chronic carriers of these infections. Antibiotic treatment is not indicated, therefore, except in the dangerous systemic infection by *Salmonella typhi* (typhoid or paratyphoid fever) or severe gut infection which is treated with ciprofloxacin.

Septicaemias

Septicaemias are becoming common, particularly in ill and/or immunosuppressed patients. Various bacteria may be implicated and initial treatment aims at a wide antibacterial effect until the nature of the infection becomes clear as a result of blood cultures. Gentamicin combined with flucloxacillin and metronidazole is frequently used, but there are many other possibilities.

Gram-negative septicaemia in particular affects those who have undergone extensive surgery or have depressed immunity. It is a very dangerous infection, leading rapidly to organ failure. It should be treated as early as possible with a combination of antibiotics.

Accidental viral infections (see also p. 237)

Two other viral infections to which nurses and other health care workers may be exposed in their occupation are of particular concern:

1. Hepatitis B virus (HBV)
2. Hepatitis C virus (HCV).

Transmission is usually by blood or blood products, though other body fluids may be involved. Infection occurs most commonly by needle-stick injury; rarely, it may be through a break in the skin or via a mucous membrane. It does not occur through intact skin.

Prevention and management

The most important preventative is avoidance of risk and scrupulous techniques when dealing with possible sources of infection. Active immunization is available against HBV, but not against HCV.

If exposure to the virus has occurred the following steps are advised, though it is possible that advances may alter these procedures.

Hepatitis B. Determine the immune status of the exposed subject—if susceptible, give HBV hyperimmune globulin and immunize with vaccine.

Hepatitis C. There is no effective protection yet, but the subject must be followed up for evidence of infection as there is a chance of developing chronic active hepatitis.

PREVENTION OF SURGICAL SEPSIS

Antibacterial agents are now commonly given before operations to prevent postoperative sepsis. Opinions differ as to the best drugs to use, but the following are popular. Prophylaxis is most effective if antibiotics are given within 2 hours before surgery.

Acute appendicitis (anaerobes, coliforms)	Metronidazole suppository inserted 2 hours before surgery. Cefuroxime i.v. at induction.
Large bowel surgery (anaerobes, coliforms)	Metronidazole as above + cefuroxime at induction followed by doses at 8 and 16 hours.
Biliary surgery	Not required in elective surgery, otherwise cefuroxime as above at induction and then at 8 and 16 hours.
Amputation of ischaemic limb (staphylococci, clostridia)	Metronidazole as above + flucloxacillin 500 mg i.v. at induction and every 8 hours for 48 hours.
Hip replacement	Cefuroxime at induction and every 8 hours for 48 hours.

PRACTICAL POINTS IN THE ADMINISTRATION OF ANTIBIOTICS

1. Oral penicillins and tetracyclines should be given 30 minutes before meals to facilitate absorption. Erythromycin, sodium fusidate and metronidazole should be given with or after food to minimize nausea.

2. In general, intravenous antibiotics should be given as a bolus. A few, e.g. piperacillin, are given as short-term infusions. If long-term infusions are used, remember that some antibiotics are unstable in certain solutions and

rapidly lose their potency. Among the most important are:

Ampicillin — Loses activity in dextrose solutions.

Gentamicin — Unstable in solution and inactivated if combined with penicillins.

Do not as a rule mix drugs in an infusion bottle and, if this is necessary, check their compatibilities with the pharmacist.

3. When making up solutions for injection avoid contamination of hands, etc., due to the risk of contact dermatitis. Hands should be washed after as well as before giving injections and in certain circumstances gloves may be worn.

4. When patients are taking antibiotics at home, compliance must be assured by full explanation of its importance.

FURTHER READING

Angel J 1992 The modern management of pulmonary tuberculosis. Prescribers Journal 32: 144

Barry M G et al 1995 Zidovudine in HIV infection. Which patients should be treated and when? British Journal of Clinical Pharmacology 40: 107

Begg E J, Barclay M L 1995 Aminoglycosides – 50 years on. British Journal of Clinical Pharmacology 39: 597

Classen D et al 1992 The timing of the prophylactic administration of antibiotics and the risk of surgical wound infection. New England Journal of Medicine 326: 281

Como J A, Dismukes W E 1994 Oral azole drugs as systemic antifungal therapy. New England Journal of Medicine 330: 263

Editorial 1993 Floroquinolones reviewed. Drug and Therapeutics Bulletin 31: 69

Editorial 1996 Interferon Beta-1B – hope or hype. Drugs and Therapeutics Bulletin 34: 9

Editorial 1997 Major advances in the treatment of HIV-1 infections. Drug and Therapeutics Bulletin 35: 25

Editorial 1997 Postexposure treatment of HIV. Taking the risk for safety's sake. New England Journal of Medicine 337: 1542

Editorial 1999 Tackling antimicrobial resistance. Drug and Therapeutics Bulletin 37: 2: 9

Gerberding J L 1995 Management of occupational exposure to blood-borne viruses. New England Journal of Medicine 332: 444

Gold H S, Moellering R C 1997 Antimicrobial drug resistance. New England Journal of Medicine 335: 1445

Griffith G, Krishna S 1998 Infectious diseases. Journal of the Royal College of Physicians, London 12: 306

Mossad S B 1998 Treatment of the common cold. British Medical Journal 317: 33

Rodvold K A, Danziger L H, Quinn J P 1997 Single daily doses of aminoglycosides. Lancet 350: 1412

Stamm W E, Hooton T M 1993 Management of urinary infection in adults. New England Journal of Medicine 329: 1328

Taylor D, Littlewood S 1998 Pneumonia. Nursing Times 94 (7): 48

Taylor D, Littlewood S 1998 Tuberculosis. Nursing Times 94 (11): 51

Tunkel A R, Scheld W M 1995 Acute bacterial meningitis. Lancet 346: 1675

Walters J 1993 How antibiotics work. Professional Nurse 8(12) 788

17

Immunity, sera and vaccines. Antihistamines. Immunosuppression

SERA AND VACCINES

THE IMMUNE REACTION

The human body is continually subjected to the risk of infection by microorganisms (bacteria, viruses, fungi) or to damage by toxins produced by bacteria. These foreign substances are known collectively as *antigens*.

The cells that recognize and react to antigens are called lymphocytes. They are distributed throughout the body in blood, lymph and lymphoid tissues (spleen, lymph nodes, tonsils and adenoids). All lymphocytes originate in the bone marrow, but there are two main groups, the B and T cells, which mature differently and help to defend the body against foreign antigens in different ways (Fig. 17.1).

Humoral immunity

Humoral immunity is a property of the B lymphocytes which mature in the spleen and lymph nodes after they leave the bone marrow. B lymphocytes are specific for particular antigens and the body can produce hundreds, possibly thousands of types of B lymphocytes, each able to respond to a different microorganism. When an antigen gains access to the tissues the B lymphocytes become activated, dividing many times to form a clone of identical *plasma cells*. The plasma cells release proteins called *immunoglobulins* also known as *antibodies*. Antibodies circulate in the blood and react with antigens to neutralize their effects and destroy them. Once the antigens

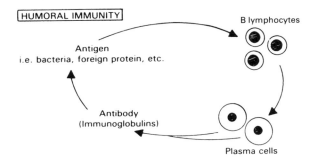

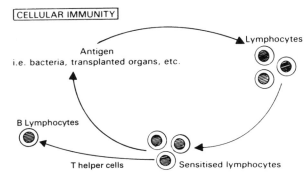

Figure 17.1 The sequence of events in the production of humoral and cellular immunity.

have been removed most of the plasma cells disappear, but a few persist as memory cells. If a second exposure occurs the memory cells multiply rapidly and release antibodies even more swiftly than during the first exposure. This establishment of 'memory' by the B lymphocytes forms the basis of active immunization against bacteria and the harmful toxins they produce (see later).

Cell-mediated immunity

Cell-mediated immunity is a property of the T lymphocytes which mature in the thymus gland before they enter the circulation. T lymphocytes do not produce antibodies, but are an essential component of the immune response as B lymphocytes require them to function properly. Some T lymphocytes (T helper cells) appear to play an important part 'switching on' the immune response when antigens invade, while others 'switch off' the immune response when the body no longer requires it. Cell-mediated immunity is especially important in the rejection of foreign materials such as transplanted organs, and in chronic infections such as tuberculosis. People whose cell-mediated immunity is impaired by HIV infection, which destroys the T helper cells, become very prone to fungal and protozoal infections which T lymphocytes usually keep in check.

ACTIVE IMMUNIZATION

The principle of this method is to promote the production by the patient of antibodies or sensitized lymphocytes to certain bacteria or toxins produced by bacteria before infection occurs. If the patient then becomes infected, the antibodies are quickly produced and are capable of rapidly dealing with the infecting organism or its toxin and thus preventing or minimizing the disease.

Antibodies are usually produced by injecting into the patient killed or modified bacteria which, although harmless, are still capable of producing antibodies. These organisms are known as a *vaccine*. Two good examples of this method are the production of immunity to typhoid by injection of dead typhoid bacilli and the widespread immunization against poliomyelitis by the Sabin vaccine, which is a live virus which has been attenuated (rendered harmless).

Similarly, bacterial toxins may be modified to produce toxoids which are no longer harmful, but capable of acting as antigens. They are then injected and protect against future damage from the particular toxin. Good examples of toxoids are the various diphtheria toxoids which produce immunity to the very dangerous toxin produced by the diphtheria organism (*C. diphtheriae*).

Following injection of the antigen, whether vaccine or toxoid, there is usually an interval of a few days before antibodies appear; these may then persist for varying periods from a few months up to many years. It is often the practice to give two or more injections of the antigen to produce a higher level of immunity.

Active immunization is used in the prevention of the following diseases: measles; mumps;

rubella; diphtheria; whooping cough; tetanus; typhoid; typhus; yellow fever; cholera; tuberculosis; smallpox; poliomyelitis; hepatitis A and B; influenza; meningitis; anthrax; pneumococcal infections; and rabies.

Active immunization may take several weeks before enough antibodies are produced to be effective. This is satisfactory as a prophylactic measure, but is not much good to treat established disease. Under these conditions passive immunization is used.

PASSIVE IMMUNIZATION

In this method of immunization the appropriate antibody against the invading organism or toxin is injected. This antibody is produced on a large scale by injecting an antigen, either vaccine or toxoid, into an animal until a high blood level of antibody is obtained. Some of the animal's blood is then removed and the antibody extracted and stored until it is required. Following injection of antibody, immunity will last about 2 weeks.

This method suffers from the disadvantage that it is not possible to completely purify the antibodies produced and there is therefore a risk of a hypersensitivity reaction. Certain types of antibody can be obtained from human blood, either after the subject has been actively immunized or has suffered a particular infection. These antibodies, usually called *human immunoglobulin*, are safer and rarely produce a serious reaction, although there may be discomfort at the injection site. Common examples are diphtheria antitoxin, which is obtained from horse serum, and antitetanus immunoglobulin injection from human blood.

ADMINISTRATION OF SERUM

Antitoxin raised in animals, often called *antiserum*, carries a real risk of a hypersensitivity reaction. This is particularly liable to occur in patients who have had previous serum injections or who suffer from allergic disorders (e.g. asthma). It is due to the antibody in the serum reacting with antigens already present in the patient, releasing histamine and other substances. If possible, antibodies obtained from the blood of immune humans should be used. They are called immunoglobins and reactions are much less likely to occur. Serum reactions take two forms.

Immediate or anaphylactic reaction (see p. 297). Within a few minutes of injection the patient collapses with difficulty in breathing, low blood pressure and, sometimes, widespread urticaria. Rarely it can be fatal.

Serum sickness occurs about a week after injection of serum. The patient is pyrexial with a rash and arthritis. It clears up in a few days.

Nursing point
Sera and vaccines should be kept in a refrigerator at the correct temperature. Guidelines are given in Immunisation against infectious disease, HMSO (1996).

Precautions when injecting serum

Ask the patient:

- Have you had serum before?
- Have you had asthma or eczema?

If both answers are negative, give a test dose of serum subcutaneously and if there is no reaction in 30 minutes the rest may be given and the patient kept under observation for a further 1 hour.

These precautions may well be unnecessary if human immunoglobin is used, but are mandatory for diphtheria antitoxin which is raised in animals.

The management of anaphylaxis and serum sickness are considered on page 297.

Whenever serum is injected by any route a syringe of 1 : 1000 epinephrine, an antihistamine and hydrocortisone hemisuccinate should be ready at hand in case of immediate reaction.

ANTISERA

Diphtheria antitoxin is an antiserum raised in animals and there is a real risk of a hypersensitivity reaction.

Dose: Prophylactic— Erythromycin + vaccine

Therapeutic — Not less than 10 000 units of antitoxin intramuscularly or intravenously.

Tetanus antitoxin is an immunoglobin prepared from human sources, with little or no risk of a hypersensitivity reaction. Following injury:

Immunized patients require a booster dose of vaccine to stimulate immunity. Extensive and dirty wounds may need, in addition, tetanus immunoglobin plus antibiotic cover.

Non-immunized patients require 250 units of tetanus immunoglobin and a course of tetanus vaccine should be started. These should not be given in the same syringe nor into the same site. This should be combined with antibiotic cover.

VACCINES

Adsorbed diphtheria vaccine for adults and adolescents is prepared by adsorbing toxoid onto aluminium phosphate:

Dose: Adult: Primary   — 0.5 ml, three doses at
     immunization   monthly intervals.
     Reinforcement — 0.5 ml, one dose.
  Child: Dose as instructed.

Adsorbed tetanus vaccine Dose: three doses of 0.5 ml i.m. at intervals of 4 weeks. In addition to single vaccines, combined vaccines stimulating immunity to diphtheria, whooping cough and tetanus are available and are frequently used for immunizing infants.

Hib is a vaccine against *Haemophilus influenzae type b*. Three doses are given at monthly intervals in the first year of life. Immunization is not required after the age of 4 years as infection is much less likely.

Diphtheria, tetanus and pertussis vaccine is given in doses of 0.5 ml i.m. For initial immunization three injections are given at intervals (see Table 17.1).

Whether pertussis vaccine should be given and to whom is outside the scope of this book, but the dilemma serves to underline the fact that no active drug is entirely safe and that possible benefits have to be weighed against risks.

Table 17.1 Immunization of children

Age	Vaccine	Note
During first year of life	Triple (diphtheria tetanus and pertussis) + polio + Hib	First dose at 2 months 3 doses at 4-weekly intervals
During second year of life	MMR Hib	One dose if not previously given
At school entry	Diphtheria, tetanus +polio MMR	
At 10–14 years	BCG	If tuberculin test is negative
On leaving school	Diphtheria, tetanus + polio	

Smallpox vaccination is not now given as a routine unless the subject is going to a country which still requires a certificate of vaccination despite the elimination of the disease! It should also be offered to laboratory workers at special risk.

Nursing point

Children who develop a fever after receiving the MMR vaccine can be given paracetamol (see p. 125) which can be repeated once if necessary, after 4–6 hours.

In the past there have been fears that brain damage might, rarely, follow the use of pertussis vaccine and, although the frequency was difficult to assess, a figure of less than 1:80 000 was given. More recently, even this low risk is considered unlikely. The dangers attached to having whooping cough, especially in infancy, are considerably greater (see Fig. 17.2).

Subjects at risk from tetanus should receive a booster dose of toxoid.

Typhoid. Both oral and injected vaccines are available for those visiting a high-risk area. They are effective for about 3 years.

Bacillus Calmette–Guérin vaccine. A suspension of living bacilli which will produce tuberculosis antibodies. Dose 0.1 ml by intracutaneous injection.

Poliomyelitis vaccine may be either inactivated poliomyelitis viruses type 1, 2 and 3 (Salk vaccine) or attenuated live virus (Sabin vaccine) —the latter is to be preferred as it avoids injections, provides a more prolonged immunity

Pertussis notifications to ONS and vaccine coverage figures for children by their 2nd birthday England and Wales (1940–1995)

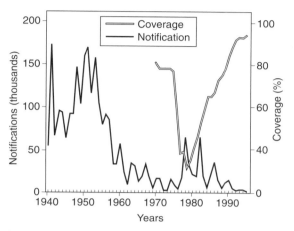

Figure 17.2   The importance of coverage on the incidence of pertussis. (Published by permission of HMSO.)

and by producing antibodies in the intestine it prevents the spread of infection.

The dose is three drops on a lump of sugar.

Rubella vaccine should be offered to sero-negative women of childbearing age. It is important to exclude pregnancy when giving the vaccine and to avoid it for 1 month thereafter. The dose is 0.5 ml by deep subcutaneous injection.

> **Nursing point**
>
> Nurses should ensure that they are immune to rubella, especially if they are working in an obstetric role.

Measles, mumps and rubella vaccine (MMR). This combined vaccine should be given as a single dose of 0.5 ml by intramuscular or deep subcutaneous injection to children aged 12–15 months and 4–5 before starting school. It occasionally produces malaise, fever, a rash and parotid swelling about 1 week after injection. Meningitis due to the mumps component occurs in about 1 in 1 000 000 doses. There is no evidence that MMR vaccine is a cause of autism or bowel disease.

Meningococcal A & C vaccine is used for visits overseas where meningitis is common. The Group C conjugate vaccine which is more effective in infancy, is recommended from 2–4 months to 18 years.

Pneumococcal vaccine is given to people who are at special risk from pneumococcal infection, including those with chronic lung and heart disease, diabetes and patients who have had a splenectomy, are immunosuppressed or have sickle cell disease.

Influenza vaccine. The 'flu' viruses are changing continually so the WHO recommends which strains of virus should be included in the vaccine for a particular year. The vaccine only protects about 70% of subjects for about 1 year and its use is confined to those at special risk, e.g. the elderly, those with heart, lung or renal disease and patients with diabetes. There may be some local discomfort, but systemic reactions are rare.

> **Nursing point**
>
> **Vaccines and safety.** Vaccination is one of the most successful methods of preventing disease. Vaccines should be safe as they are given to large numbers of healthy people and, often, to very young children. They certainly have side-effects but these are usually minor and transient, such as a short bout of fever. From time to time an adverse effect of a serious nature is reported, which ultimately turns out to be very rare or based on insecure evidence. Meanwhile, the public become confused and anxious, the rate of immunization falls and the incidence of the disease in question may rise (Fig. 17.2).
>
> It is therefore very important for nurses, especially those involved in immunization programmes, to be familiar with the adverse effects of vaccines and to distinguish between those caused by the vaccine and those which are coincidental. No vaccine is absolutely safe but the patient (or parent) should consider the risk against the benefit.

Immunization against viral hepatitis

1. *Hepatitis A.* This virus is spread by poor hygiene, and infection is usually due to contaminated food and water. A vaccine is now available and is given as a single injection with a booster dose after 6 months. It appears to be very effective in preventing hepatitis A, but the

---

Nursing point

A doctor may delegate the responsibility of immunization to a nurse provided that:

1. The nurse is willing to be accountable for the work.
2. The nurse has received training in the subject.
3. The nurse has been trained in the diagnosis and treatment of anaphylaxis.

Consent must always be obtained before immunization.

Anaphylaxis is very rare with active immunization but treatment should be immediately available (see above).

Contraindications to immunization

1. Acute illness.
2. Live vaccines should not be given to those who have reduced immunity due to:
   a. High doses of steroids or cytotoxic drugs
   b. Active lymphomas including Hodgkin's disease
   c. Other causes of reduced immunity.
3. Pregnancy. Rarely the risk of infection outweighs this precaution.
4. HIV-positive subjects should not receive BCG, yellow fever or oral typhoid vaccine. Their response to immunization may be reduced.

Immunization programmes are constantly reviewed and altered from time to time. In case of doubt, nurses are referred to *Immunization against infectious disease*, HMSO (1996) or to the current edition of the *British National Formulary.*

---

duration of protection is not yet known. There may be local soreness at the site of injection.

Alternatively, normal human immunoglobin given by intramuscular injection confers passive immunity for up to 2 months.

2. *Hepatitis B.* This viral infection is of particular importance to the health professional as it can be spread by infected body fluids (blood and saliva) and precautions should be enforced when nursing all patients as it is impossible to predict who are carriers from the history alone.

A vaccine prepared from the surface antigen of the virus is available (H-B-Vax). Three injections of 1 ml i.m. are given into the deltoid muscle—the first and second, 1 month apart, and the third after 6 months. Immunity persists for at least 2 years. Passive immunization is also possible using a special serum containing large

amounts of antibody against the hepatitis B virus.

DRUGS WHICH BLOCK THE IMMUNE REACTION

The immune response can be blocked either:

1. By interfering with the effects of immunity or with some aspects of them
   Antihistamines
   Steroids
   Sodium cromoglicate.
2. By suppressing cells involved in cellular or humoral immunity (immunosuppression)
   Azathioprine
   Methotrexate
   Cyclophosphamide
   Corticosteroids

THE ANTIHISTAMINES

The histamine released following an antigen–antibody reaction is responsible, with other factors, for a variety of clinical syndromes. These include anaphylactic shock, serum sickness, hay fever and urticaria. A series of drugs have been produced which block this action of histamine and thus relieve or partially relieve some of these conditions. It is believed that these drugs prevent the stimulation of H_1 receptors by histamine and must be distinguished from H_2 receptor blockers (see p. 95) which interfere with an entirely different action of histamine.

The antihistamine drugs are usually given orally and are well absorbed from the intestinal tract.

In addition to their antihistamine properties, some of these drugs enter the central nervous system and have sedating and anti-emetic effects. Some also have anticholinergic effects such as dry mouth and urinary retention.

Therapeutics

Nonsedating antihistamines are used mainly for hay fever and other allergic reactions.

Terfenadine in doses of 60 mg once or twice daily is useful and is rarely sedating.

It can, rarely, cause dangerous cardiac arrhythmias. Therefore:

1. The recommended dose should not be exceeded
2. It should not be given to patients with liver disease
3. It should not be combined with erythromycin, clarithromycin, and certain antifungals which slow its metabolism and leads to accumulation.

Other non-sedating antihistamines are **cetirizine** and **loratadine** and they are available without prescription.

Sedating antihistamines are used for various allergic reactions but also for non-allergic itching and as anti-emetics and sedatives.

Chlorphenamine (Chlorpheniramine) can be given orally or slowly intravenously, the oral dose being 4.0 mg two or three times daily.

Clemastine, cyproheptadine and **triprolidine** are similar. **Trimeprazine (Alimemazine)** is very sedative and is used for this purpose. **Promethazine** is a useful anti-emetic which can be used in pregnancy.

The wide range of antihistamines is useful as patients vary in their response to treatment and it may be necessary to try several before finding the most suitable one.

Adverse effects. Except for *drowsiness*, already mentioned, toxic effects are rare.

The drugs should be kept out of the reach of children as they may mistake them for sweets and overdosage produces dangerous results.

Antihistamines are also available for local application to bites and stings. This is not recommended as they are not particularly effective and can cause local reactions.

Sodium cromoglicate

This compound prevents the release of substances from mast cells, which constrict the bronchi and produce an attack of asthma. It is given by inhalation in a 'Spincap' capsule, as 20 mg of sodium cromoglicate. Usually one capsule is inhaled night and morning and at 4–6 hourly intervals—this dosage can be reduced.

Sodium cromoglicate is thus used to prevent asthma rather than treat the established attack. It is particularly effective in the allergic type of asthma occurring in young people.

It is available as a 2% solution as eye or nasal drops and as a nasal spray. Drops are instilled four to six times daily. It can also be given orally four times daily before meals for treating various intestinal disorders.

Corticosteroids (see p. 183)

This group of drugs suppress the immune response in several different ways and are widely used to treat disorders of immunity such as autoimmune disease—systemic lupus, polyarteritis, etc.; organ rejection after transplantation; and anaphylactic shock. Corticosteroids are also applied locally in hay fever and various dermatological disorders.

The main problems with their long-term use is the development of adverse reactions and the lowest effective dose must be used.

Epinephrine (Adrenaline)

Although not specifically blocking any of the substances which mediate the immune response, epinephrine is very effective in *acute anaphylaxis* as it reverses bronchospasm and vasodilatation. The usual dose is 0.5 ml of 1 :1000 solution i.m.

Anaphylactic shock: The treatment is considered on p. 297.

Hay fever

This is a common disorder caused by an allergic response to pollen, with the release of histamine in the nose and eyes. It is therefore most severe in late spring and early summer. A similar allergic rhinitis may occur at any time of year or be more or less continuous.

Treatment can be systemic or local. Systemic oral antihistamines are useful and a non-sedative preparation is the first choice. If this fails a nasal spray containing a steroid (beclomethasone or budesonide) can be added to the regime. Alternatively, sodium cromoglicate nasal spray can be used on a regular basis. Local applications have the advantage of avoiding systemic side-effects, but may cause local stinging.

The associated conjunctival inflammation requires eye wash solution or local sodium cromoglicate. In severe intractable cases systemic steroids may be necessary for a short period.

IMMUNOSUPPRESSION

The antibody-producing system may become deranged and produce antibodies against various body tissues. Diseases which arise in this way are called *'autoimmune'* and may include some types of nephritis, systemic lupus erythematosus, polyarteritis nodosa and possibly rheumatoid arthritis. If the antibody system can be suppressed there is reason to hope that the disease process can be controlled. This can be achieved to a certain degree by steroids (see p. 183), but often incompletely and more recently various cytotoxic drugs which are active against antibody-forming cells have proved useful. Those most frequently used are **azathioprine, cyclophosphamide and methotrexate**; the dose has to be carefully adjusted to avoid leucopenia. Such drugs are also used for the same reason to prevent rejection of transplanted organs by sensitized lymphocytes.

Cyclosporin. The greatest problem in organ transplantation is rejection of the graft by the immune system of the recipient. This is largely mediated by the lymphocytes and most drugs which have been used to prevent rejection (see earlier) suppress all aspects of immunity and also interfere with the formation of polymorphs and platelets. Cyclosporin affects the T lymphocytes which are particularly concerned with graft rejection and is thus very useful in transplant surgery and is being tried cautiously in various autoimmune diseases.

It is, however, a difficult drug to use. It can be given orally or intravenously and is used to cover the organ or bone marrow transplant and then continued orally at a lower maintenance dose to prevent rejection. Estimation of blood levels are required to control dosage.

Adverse effects include disturbances of renal and hepatic function, nausea and vomiting and tremor. There is also the possibility of the development of cancer as a delayed complication.

Interactions with other drugs may increase absorption and alter the metabolism of cyclosporin in the liver. Combination with aminoglycosides (e.g. gentamicin) or NSAIDs can be nephrotoxic.

FURTHER READING

Bedford H 2000 Concern about immunisation. British Medical Journal 320: 240

Coppola J, Johnston R 1998 Cold comfort. Nursing Times 94 (11): 72

Cross S 1997 The foundations of allergy. Nursing Standard 12 (7): 94

Cross S 1997 The misery of hay fever. Nursing Standard 11 (37): 26

Editorial 1992 Treating anaphylaxis with sympathomimetic drugs. British Medical Journal 305: 1107

Editorial 1994 Immunosuppressing drugs and their complications. Drug and Therapeutics Bulletin 33: 66

Editorial 1998 MMR vaccination and autism. British Medical Journal 316: 715

Gangarosa E J et al 1998 Impact of anti-vaccine movements on pertussis control: the untold story. Lancet 351: 356

Green T 1997 Anaphylaxis. Nursing Times 93 (42): 60

HMSO 1996 Immunization against infectious disease. HMSO, London

Lockhead Y J 1991 Failure to immunise children under five years. Journal of Advanced Nursing 16: 130

Rankin A C 1997 Non-sedating antihistamines and cardiac arrhythmias. Lancet 350: 1115

Simons F E R, Simons K J 1994 The pharmacology and use of H_1 receptor-antagonist drugs. New England Journal of Medicine 333: 1663

Suthanthiran M, Strom T B 1994 Renal transplantation. New England Journal of Medicine 331: 365

Thakker Y, Woods S 1992 Storage of vaccines in the community. British Medical Journal 304: 756

18

Drugs used to treat tropical and imported diseases. Anthelmintics

Tropical diseases, like their background, are inclined to be dramatic and florid. The majority are infective or due to dietary deficiency and in former times, and even to some degree today, great epidemics have caused widespread disease with a very high death rate. During the last 50 years the causative organisms of nearly all these diseases have been discovered and drugs have been devised which are capable of dealing with them. The problem of treating tropical disease is further complicated by the primitive conditions which prevail in many parts of the tropics and the lack of proper medical and nursing facilities. However, in spite of these difficulties, immense progress has been made in this sphere. In recent years, air travel has brought tropical diseases much nearer home for it is possible to catch malaria in Central Africa and not be taken ill until after arrival in London. Some knowledge of these disorders is therefore necessary even if the nurse does not intend to work in tropical countries.

The consideration of tropical disease will be carried out under headings of the disease rather than the drug.

TRAVELLERS' DIARRHOEA

A holiday in tropical or subtropical countries is often interrupted by an attack of diarrhoea, colic and vomiting, which, although rarely severe, interferes with a few days' pleasure. It is believed that there is usually an infective cause and the organism most often implicated is an unusual variant of *Escherichia coli*. Prevention should include care over drinking water and washing uncooked foods such as fruit and vegetables in chlorinated water. The prophylactic use of antibiotics is not recommended except for those at special risk (e.g. bowel disease) or if for social or business reasons diarrhoea must be avoided. In these cases *trimethoprim* 200 mg daily or *doxycycline* 100 mg daily are satisfactory. For the developed attack, fluid replacement with added glucose and electrolytes (e.g. Dioralyte or a similar preparation) is important. Symptoms can be improved with *loperamide* which should not be given to children under 4 years. In severe cases trimethoprim 200 mg twice daily or ciprofloxacin 500 mg as a single dose is effective.

AMOEBIC DYSENTERY

Amoebic dysentery is an infection of the lower bowel with an organism called *Entamoeba histolytica* and is characterized by chronic diarrhoea. Sometimes the infection spreads outside the bowel, particularly to the liver, where it causes an abscess.

The chief drug used in this infection is:

Metronidazole is now the first choice in treating amoebic infection of the bowel and abscess of the liver. It is given in doses of 800 mg three times daily, and a 5-day course is often sufficient (see also p. 235). At this dose level, vomiting can be troublesome. Metronidazole can be combined with *diloxanide furoate*, which is active against organisms in the bowel lumen, but not in the tissues. The dose is 500 mg three times daily for 10 days and the combination appears to be even more efficient at eradicating the infection.

GIARDIASIS

Giardiasis is due to the organism *Giardia lamblia* which affects the intestine causing distension, gas and frothy stools. Infection can occur in many parts of the world and symptoms often develop on return from a holiday abroad.

Metronidazole 2 g daily for 3 days is an effective treatment.

BACILLARY DYSENTERY

This may be caused by a variety of organisms of the *Shigella* group. In mild cases symptomatic treatment only is required and there is no evidence that antibiotics produce a more rapid cure. In severe cases the organism should be cultured and its sensitivity to antibiotics defined. If there is no time for culture, treatment may be started with trimethoprim 200 mg twice daily. Ciprofloxacin is used if trimethoprim resistance is a problem. Fluid and electrolyte replacement is important.

CHOLERA

Cholera is due to an organism, the *Cholera vibrio*, which invades the intestine, producing severe and copious diarrhoea and vomiting. This leads to intense dehydration and sodium and potassium deficiency and is often fatal. The most important part of treatment is to replace the lost water and salts orally or by intravenous infusion.

The *Cholera vibrio* is sensitive to tetracycline and ciprofloxacin, which can be used to eradicate the infection and shorten the course of the illness.

In developing countries, where this disease reaches epidemic proportions, large-scale intravenous infusion may be difficult. An important advance has been the discovery that if glucose is added to the electrolyte replacement solution and given orally, water and electrolytes are well absorbed and i.v. infusion is less often required. The oral replacement solution contains:

Sodium chloride 3.5 g
Sodium citrate 2.9 g
Potassium chloride 1.5 g
Glucose 20 g
Made up to 1 litre.

The volume given is titrated against the loss in the stools and by vomiting.

A cholera vaccine is available, but is of little use.

LEPROSY

Leprosy is a disease of great antiquity and is

referred to in the Bible. It is caused by the *Myco-bacterium leprae*; these bacteria cause chronic infection of the skin, visceral nerves and other parts of the body. Leprosy has long resisted treatment, but in recent years the introduction of new drugs has made the outlook more hopeful.

The *Mycobacterium leprae* can become resistant to the drugs used in treatment; therefore at least two antibacterial drugs should be given together to prevent this. Three drugs are used in leprosy at present:

Dapsone is widely used. It is given orally, usually over long periods.

Adverse effects are uncommon, but include headaches, cyanosis, anaemia and blood dyscrasias.

Clofazimine is useful in treating leprosy and is combined with other agents. It is given orally over long periods.

Adverse effects are rare, but it may cause pigmentation of the skin.

Rifampicin (see p. 232) is also effective against the *Mycobacterium leprae,* although resistance may develop.

Treatment of leprosy

In patients with florid infection (*multibacillary*) treatment is:

Rifampicin 600 mg once a month
Clofazimine 50 mg daily with a 300 mg dose
  once a month
Dapsone 100 mg daily.

The course should be continued for a minimum of 2 years. With a less florid infection (*paucibacillary*) treatment is:

Rifampicin 600 mg once monthly
Dapsone 100 mg daily.

The course is continued for 6 months.

MALARIA

Malaria has been known for thousands of years and is one of the most widespread diseases which attack humans.

Although it is largely confined to tropical and subtropical zones, air travel has led to its increased frequency in this country. Malaria is caused by a small organism called a plasmodium. There are three varieties of plasmodia which produce the commonly found varieties of human malaria. They are:

- *Plasmodium vivax*—causing benign tertian malaria.
- *Plasmodium malariae*—causing quartan malaria.
- *Plasmodium falciparum*—causing malignant tertian malaria.

These plasmodia are injected into the human victim by the mosquito. They are carried to the liver where they go through a stage of division known as the exo-erythrocyte stage. After a short period some plasmodia enter the red cells of the bloodstream. Here they divide in a simple asexual fashion to form more plasmodia, which rupture the red cells and then re-enter further red cells: the breaking up of the red cells corresponds with the rise of temperature with rigor and later sweating which is so characteristic of the disease.

Other plasmodia which have entered the red cells form male and female gametes. These may be sucked out when a mosquito bite occurs and then continue the cycle in the infected mosquito. The cycle is shown graphically in Figure 18.1. The drugs which are effective in treating malaria may be divided into two groups:

1. Those which act on the asexual stage of the malarial parasite in the blood.

Quinine
Chloroquine
Proguanil
Halofantrine
Mefloquine
Pyrimethamine.

2. Those which act on the exo-erythrocyte stage in the liver and the gametocytes.

Primaquine.

Quinine. Quinine is described first, because it was the first effective remedy.

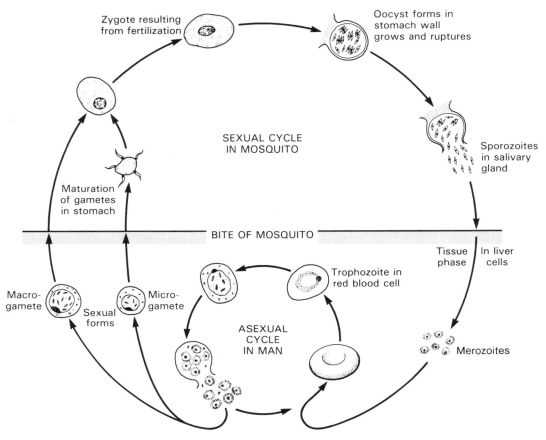

Figure 18.1 The malarial cycle.

It is one of the alkaloids obtained from the bark of the cinchona tree and has been known to be effective against 'fever' for several hundred years.

For some years it was largely replaced by newer antimalarial drugs, but is now proving very useful in *Plasmodium falciparum* infection when it is resistant to other drugs.

Quinine is given either orally or intravenously. It is well absorbed from the intestine.

It suppresses the multiplication of the plasmodia in the bloodstream. It does not, however, have any effect on the gametes or exo-erythrocyte stages of the malarial life cycle and thus symptoms may recur when quinine is stopped.

Quinine has a number of other actions. It has a depressing action to the heart similar to that of quinidine; it is also said to cause contraction of the uterus and should, therefore, be avoided in

pregnancy. It is sometimes used in the treatment of *muscle cramps*.

Adverse effects are common with quinine—the syndrome produced being known as cinchonism. This may occur with large doses—but some people are hypersensitive to the drug and develop toxic effects after small amounts; the chief symptoms are vertigo, tinnitus, deafness and visual disturbances. In addition, it can cause delirium, haemolytic anaemia, thrombocytopenia and renal failure.

Therapeutics. The usual therapeutic dose of quinine sulphate for treating malaria is 600 mg (540 mg base) three times a day for 7 days.

If quinine is given intravenously, which is required in fulminating malignant tertian malaria, it should be given as quinine dihydrochloride.

Chloroquine is a most useful drug to treat

malaria, but resistant strains of *P. falciparum* are common.

It can be given orally, intramuscularly or intravenously. It is rapidly absorbed and is stored in various organs of the body, part being destroyed and part excreted in urine.

It is effective against the asexual forms of the plasmodia in the bloodstream, but has no effect on the gametes or on the exo-erythrocyte stages. Strains of malaria which are resistant to chloroquine have appeared in South-east Asia and South America and Central and East Africa.

Adverse effects are rare, but include nausea and headaches, and as it may cause fetal damage it should not be used during pregnancy.

Therapeutics. In an acute attack of malaria, adults should receive 600 mg of chloroquine base followed by 300 mg after 6 hours, then 300 mg daily for 2 days. Prophylaxis against malaria is obtained by taking 300 mg of chloroquine base weekly.

Mefloquine is effective against chloroquine-resistant *P. falciparum* and is used in parts of the world where this is common. It is excreted very slowly so a single or divided dose of 20 mg/kg is used.

It can also be used prophylactically in doses of 250 mg once weekly, but not for more than one year.

Adverse effects. Nausea and giddiness are fairly common. Psychotic disturbances, including hallucinations, panic attacks and depression, can occur and the patient should be warned of this possibility. Mefloquine should not be used during pregnancy nor in subjects with epilepsy.

Halofantrine can be used to treat resistant infection due to *P. falciparum* but, owing to adverse effects, it has fallen from favour.

Artemisinin and its derivatives are obtained from sweet wormwood—they originated in China. They appear to be rapidly effective in treating severe *P. falciparum* infections, either alone or combined with other antimalarials, and are given by injection, although oral and rectal routes are possible. They are not yet generally available in the UK.

Atovaquone acts against the three types of malaria but, if used alone relapses are common.

However, when combined with **proguanil** (**Malarone**), it is effective both in treating *P. falciparum* malaria and also as a prophylactic.

Proguanil. Proguanil is given by mouth. It is rapidly absorbed, but disappears rapidly from the bloodstream.

It is effective against the bloodstream asexual phase of the plasmodia and also has some action against the gametocytes and against the exo-erythrocyte stage of *P. falciparum*.

It is, however, slower at relieving an acute attack of malaria than chloroquine and, furthermore, resistant strains of plasmodia have been encountered. Toxicity is very low.

Therapeutics. Proguanil is very slow in its antimalarial action and it is therefore largely used as a suppressant. The usual dose for this purpose is 100–200 mg daily.

Doxycycline is effective against resistant *P. falciparum* and has been used with success in the Far East. It should be taken after meals with copious fluids and the dose is 100 mg daily.

Pyrimethamine. Pyrimethamine is effective against the asexual bloodstream phase of the malarial parasite, but it is too slow to be used in treating an acute attack. Owing to the emergence of resistant strains it is now only used in combination, e.g.

Pyrimethamine + dapsone—Maloprim
Pyrimethamine + sulfadoxine—Fansidar.

It can be seen that all the drugs so far described, with the possible partial exception of proguanil, while effectively suppressing the asexual bloodstream phase of the malaria organism and relieving acute symptoms, are ineffective against the exo-erythrocyte stage in the liver and against the gametocytes.

This is particularly important when the malaria is caused by *P. vivax* or *P. malariae* as a relapse may occur on stopping treatment. In these types of malaria the initial treatment should be followed by a drug which acts against the parasites in the exo-erythrocyte stage.

Primaquine. Primaquine is effective against the exo-erythrocyte stage and against the gametocytes. It is not free from toxic effects and may produce nausea and vomiting.

It is not used alone in the treatment of the acute malarial attack, but may follow treatment of *T. vivax* or *ovale* with chloroquine, when it is particularly valuable in eradicating benign tertian malaria. Relapses will not occur unless there is reinfection.

Before starting treatment it is important to test the patient for G6PD deficiency, an inherited disorder of the red blood cells which results in severe haemolysis with primaquine and some other drugs.

The treatment of malaria

It is impossible to give precise instruction as to the best drug or drugs in the treatment of malaria as this is always changing and may also vary with different forms of malaria infection.

It must be realized that there are two possible ways in which malaria may be attacked by drugs.

Suppressive.* Regular administration of a drug to prevent clinical manifestation of the disease.

The best drug for this purpose varies in different parts of the world. This is because the widespread use of antimalarial drugs has led to the development of resistant strains of *P. falciparum*, particularly in South-east Asia, but also South America and parts of Africa. At the time of writing the following may be recommended, but *it is wise to obtain up-to-date advice before travelling.*

North Africa	Chloroquine 300 mg weekly Very low risk Egypt, Turkey, Algeria
Sub-Saharan Africa and South Asia	Mefloquine 250 mg weekly (preferred) or Chloroquine 300 mg weekly + Proguanil 200 mg daily
Oceania	Mefloquine 250 mg weekly or Doxycycline 100 mg daily
South America (depends on area)	Chloroquine 300 mg weekly and/or Proguanil 200 mg daily

> **Nursing point**
>
> Any unexplained fever occurring within 1 year (and especially the first 3 months) of returning from a risk area could be malaria.

The chosen drug must be started 1 week (2 weeks for mefloquine) before entering the malarial area and *continued for 1 month after leaving it.*

In addition, *precautions should be taken against mosquito bites* including the use of nets at night as drug prophylaxis is not totally effective.

Travellers in highly malarious areas who are likely to be remote from medical care should take an emergency treatment kit.

Treatment of established disease. The really dangerous type of malaria is that due to *P. falciparum*, which may prove fatal unless treated rapidly. Strains from many parts of the world are resistant to one or more antimalarial drugs and it is safest to regard all *P. falciparum* infections as chloroquine-resistant.

P. falciparum	Quinine 600 mg 8 hourly for 7 days followed by Fansidar[†], a single dose of 3 tablets. In severely ill patients quinine can be given by i.v. infusion. This is a potentially dangerous procedure. A loading dose of 20 mg/kg of the salt[‡] is infused over 4 hours. After 12 hours a dose of 10 mg/kg is then repeated at 8-hourly intervals. If it is impossible to monitor the infusion, quinine salts can be given, well-diluted, intramuscularly. Oral treatment with quinine is continued when the patient can swallow. This is followed by Fansidar as above.

*Full details are given in the British National Formulary.
†Fansidar is combination of pyrimethamine and sulfadoxine. Its long-term use is not recommended as it can cause a severe and unpleasant rash (Stevens–Johnson syndrome).
‡This dose is correct provided quinine dihydrochloride is used.

An alternative is Malarone (atovaquone + proguanil) 4 tablets, given once daily for 3 days.

Quinine is the preferred drug for treating *P. falciparum* malaria during pregnancy.

P. vivax or *P. malariae* — Chloroquine (see p. 256) followed by primaquine base 15 mg daily orally for 14 days to eliminate exo-erythrocyte forms.

Recommendations for prevention and treatment are always changing and nurses are advised to seek up-to-date advice from the Malaria Reference Laboratory (0171 530 3500). Travellers can telephone 0171 388 9600.

LEISHMANIASIS (KALA-AZAR)

There are several varieties of kala-azar caused by closely related organisms. These organisms may invade the spleen, liver, lymph glands and bone marrow producing a generalized disease with constitutional symptoms or produce a local ulcerative lesion. It may complicate HIV infection.

The most useful drugs for treating leishmaniasis are those which contain antimony. They are believed to interfere with enzymes within the parasite.

Sodium stibogluconate given intravenously for 20 days is usually adequate. Sometimes it may be necessary to repeat courses at intervals of 2 weeks.

Adverse effects include irritation at the site of injection, muscle aches and cardiotoxicity with arrhythmias.

The patient usually responds within 2 weeks and should be restored to full health within 2 months.

Aminosidine, an antibiotic, is also effective, either alone or combined with sodium stibogluconate.

Adverse effects are uncommon but include ototoxicity.

SCHISTOSOMIASIS

This disease is caused by flukes which inhabit the veins of the bladder and the lower bowel, leading to haematuria and rectal bleeding.

Praziquantel has now emerged as the most useful drug in schistosomiasis. It is effective against all types of the disease and, unlike drugs formerly used, it appears free from serious adverse effects. 40 mg/kg in divided doses is adequate for *Schistosoma mansoni* and *S. haematobium* and three doses of 20 mg/kg for *S. japanicum*. The cure rate is around 80%.

ANTHELMINTICS

Anthelmintics are drugs which are used to treat worm infestations. Although such infestations, with the possible exception of threadworms, are not common in this country, they may occur in immigrants, being endemic in some regions of the world, and are of great medical and economic importance.

The anthelmintics are a diverse group of substances with widely differing properties and they will be described under the headings of the type of infestation they are used to treat.

THREADWORMS (*Enterobius vermicularis*)

These worms appear like short lengths of thread. They live in the caecal region and the females migrate to the anus, where they lay eggs and provoke intense itching. The resulting scratching leads to the hands becoming contaminated with eggs which may then be transferred to food and thus further infestation occurs.

General cleanliness and scrubbing of the nails before meals is important in treating this disorder.

It must be remembered that the whole family of an infected patient must be examined for infestation as it is common to find several members of a family harbouring worms and reinfection will occur unless the worms are eradicated from the whole family.

Mebendazole as a single dose of 100 mg is effective. It should not be given to children under 2 years or during pregnancy and, rarely, it causes nausea and diarrhoea. A second dose can be given after 3 weeks as reinfection is common. It is available without prescription.

Piperazine. This is effective in treating thread-worm infections and is not liable to produce side-effects.

It is conveniently prepared as an elixir (750 mg/5 ml). The dose for an adult is 15 ml once daily. This should be given for a week followed by a week's rest and then a further week's treatment if necessary.

Pripsen sachets containing piperazine and sennosides are also available.

Adverse effects are rare, but it should not be used in patients with epilepsy, during pregnancy or in patients with peptic ulcers. It may cause gastrointestinal upsets and rashes.

STRONGYLOIDES STERCORALIS

This worm, which is common in the tropics, lives in the intestines. The larvae of *Strongyloides stercoralis* can penetrate the anal skin and thus reinfect the host, so infection can last for a long time. Usually they only cause mild intestinal symptoms, but if the patient is immuno-suppressed (i.e. given large doses of steroids or has AIDS) widespread penetration of the bowel occurs which may be fatal.

Thiabendazole in doses of 25 mg/kg twice daily for 3 days is effective, but side-effects of nausea and drowsiness are common. It should not be used during pregnancy.

TAPEWORMS

There are two common types of tapeworm. They are *Taenia solium* and *Taenia saginata*. Both these worms inhabit the small intestine of humans where they may reach several feet in length. They consist of a head which is embedded in the wall of the intestine and a body consisting of a large number of segments. These segments containing eggs are shed and pass out in the faeces.

The eggs may then infect the animal host, which is the pig in the case of *Taenia solium* and the bullock in the case of *Taenia saginata*. In the animal's gastrointestinal tract the larval form is released and migrates via the bloodstream

throughout the carcase where it remains until the animal is killed, the meat is eaten by humans and reinfection occurs.

There are several drugs which can be used to treat tapeworms, the most effective being:

Niclosamide. This is effective against tapeworm. No preparation is required. In the morning 1 g of the drug is chewed and swallowed on an empty stomach. After 1 hour the dose is repeated. This is followed 3 hours later by a saline purge. In *Taenia solium* infestation a more powerful purge should be used as it is important to clear all the ova from the gut. Treatment may be preceded by metoclopramide to minimize the risk of vomiting.

The drug appears very free of side-effects and acts by actually killing the worm.

Alternatively, a single dose of **Praziquantel** is effective.

ROUNDWORMS (*Ascaris lumbricoides*)

The roundworm is similar to a pale-coloured earthworm. It lives in the small intestine and its eggs are passed out in the faeces. If reinfection occurs, the larval forms are liberated in the gastrointestinal tract and pass via the bloodstream to the lungs. They then migrate up the trachea to the pharynx and are swallowed, thus completing the cycle.

Piperazine. This is useful in treating round-worms. It paralyses the muscle of the worm which is passed alive via the rectum. A single dose of 30 ml of the elixir, for an adult, is effective and should be repeated after 14 days. Alternatively, one Pripsen sachet (containing piperazine + sennosides) may be used, the purgative helping to clear the bowel of worms.

Mebendazole 100 mg twice daily for 3 days is an alternative.

HOOKWORM

The hookworm, although not seen in this country, is extremely common in tropical and subtropical countries in both the Old and New World.

This worm lives in the small intestine of humans, the fertilized eggs are passed out in the faeces and develop into larvae in the soil. The larvae penetrate the skin and pass via the bloodstream to the lung. Here they enter the bronchial tree and migrate to the intestinal tract via the trachea.

Severe infestation can cause iron deficiency anaemia.

Mebendazole in doses of 100 mg twice daily for 3 days is effective. It should not be used during pregnancy or for children under 2 years old.

FILARIASIS

The parasitic worms *Loa Loa*, which cause subcutaneous swellings, and *Wuchereria bancrofti*, another filarial parasite which causes elephantiasis, may be eradicated by **diethylcarbamazine**.

FURTHER READING

Du Pont H L, Ericsson C D 1993 Prevention and treatment of travellers' diarrhoea. New England Journal of Medicine 388: 1821

Editorial 1988 Imported diseases: a symposium. Prescribers Journal 28: 69

Liu L X, Weller P F 1996 Antiparasitic drugs. New England Journal of Medicine 334: 1178

Lockwood D N J, Pasvol G 1994 Recent advances in tropical medicine. British Medical Journal 308: 1559

Payling K 1994 The prevention and treatment of malaria. Professional Nurse 9: 506

Prophylaxis against malaria for travellers from the UK 1995 British Medical Journal 310: 709

Winstanley P 1998 Malaria treatment. Journal of the Royal College of Physicians, London. 32: 203

The BNF carries a useful section on malaria prophylaxis.

19

Vitamins

Vitamins are substances which are present in certain foods, but which humans cannot manufacture for themselves and are necessary for the proper functioning of animal tissues. Deficiency of vitamins in the diet leads to a number of diseases which are specific for each particular vitamin. Many of the vitamins exert their action by taking part in the complex chemical reactions which occur within the cell.

It is important to realize that provided a sufficiency of vitamins is taken, which should be provided by a good mixed diet, there is no advantage to be gained by taking further large doses of the various vitamins unless there is some form of malabsorption. In fact, the taking of excessive amounts of certain vitamins can even be harmful. At present there is no firm evidence that extra vitamins protect against cancer and heart disease to any appreciable extent and reports that supplementary vitamins given to children increase their IQ should be treated with scepticism until confirmed.

The vitamins may now be considered in detail.

Vitamin A (retinol)

Retinol is a fat-soluble, oily liquid. It is present in dairy products such as milk, butter and cream and in fish liver oils.

Betacarotene, a substance which is closely allied to retinol and can be converted to retinol by the body, is found in carrots, green vegetables and liver.

The absorption of retinol is helped by the presence of fat and bile salts in the intestine. Retinol is concerned with maintaining the health of the epithelium. Deficiency leads to keratinization of the epithelium of the nose and respiratory passage and to changes in the conjunctiva and in the cornea which may lead to blindness.

Retinol is also concerned with the mechanism of dark adaptation by the retina and deficiency leads to night blindness.

Therapeutics. Retinol should be given in cases of deficiency causing night blindness or epithelial changes.

Minimum human requirements. Adult 2250 IU daily.

Therapeutic dose. 50 000 IU.

Toxicity. Overdosage with retinol can produce liver damage, headache and vomiting.

Pregnant women are advised to avoid vitamin A supplements or liver products as there is some evidence that excessive intake is associated with fetal defects.

Retinoids

These substances are related to vitamin A, but are used for their effect on the skin.

Acitretin causes desquamation of the skin and is very effective in the treatment of psoriasis.

Isotretinoin can be applied locally and taken systemically in the treatment of acne where it reduces the secretion of sebum.

Both drugs are *teratogenic* and should not be taken during pregnancy or for a period afterwards. Their use requires expert supervision.

Vitamin B1 (thiamine)

Vitamin B1 is a white crystalline solid, soluble in water. It is obtained from wheat germ, yeast, egg yolk, liver and some vegetables.

Vitamin B1 is essential for certain stages in carbohydrate metabolism. Deficiency of this vitamin leads to a disorder known as **beri beri**. This deficiency may not only result from an inadequate intake of vitamin B1, but may also occur in disturbances of metabolism in which requirements of vitamin B1 are higher than normal, a good example being chronic alcoholism. Beri beri is characterized by heart failure and polyneuritis.

Therapeutics. Beri beri responds rapidly to vitamin B1. Severe cases will require up to 100 mg daily by i.m. injection; in milder cases oral administration is satisfactory.

Vitamin B1 is also used in high doses in the polyneuritis of chronic alcoholism and in Wernicke's encephalopathy, which is also usually due to excess alcohol.

Minimum human requirements. Adult 2 mg daily.

Therapeutic dose. 50 mg orally or i.v. daily. For severe deficiency, 200 mg daily.

Vitamin B2 (riboflavin)

This vitamin is found in vegetables, yeast and liver. It is concerned in intracellular metabolism. Deficiency in humans causes cracking and fissures at the corner of the mouth and a sore tongue. Vitamin B2 may be given in doses of 2 mg daily.

Nicotinic acid

Nicotinic acid is found in yeast, dairy products and liver. Deficiency of nicotinic acid leads to a disorder known as **pellagra** which may occur in alcoholism and renal failure as well as with deficient diets. This disease is characterized by the 3 Ds, diarrhoea, dermatitis and dementia. It may be relieved by nicotinic acid. It is worthwhile remembering that nicotinic acid is also a vasodilator. If it is taken in large doses flushing and tingling of the face may occur.

Although the deficiency of vitamins in the B group have been discussed separately, it is common to find that deficiencies are often mixed and in treating patients who show evidence of vitamin B deficiencies it is worth giving all the vitamins of the group.

Pyridoxine is concerned with protein metabolism. It is sometimes used in the treatment of vomiting of pregnancy or following radiation. It can be used to prevent the polyneuritis which rarely complicates the use of high-dose isoniazid in doses of 10–20 mg daily (p. 232) and it has been tried with varying success in the treatment of premenstrual syndrome.

There is some evidence that high doses of pyridoxine can damage peripheral nerves and such doses should be avoided, particularly when pyridoxine is being used as a food supplement and not for a specific medical purpose.

Vitamin B12 (cyanocobalamin)
(see p. 271)

Vitamin C (ascorbic acid)

Vitamin C is a crystalline solid, soluble in water. It is found in fresh fruits, particularly citrus fruit, blackcurrants, tomatoes and green vegetables. It is important to remember that vitamin C is relatively unstable and it is destroyed by boiling, especially in an alkaline solution. Thus green vegetables should be eaten raw if required for their vitamin C content.

Vitamin C is necessary for the formation and maintenance of a cement-like substance between cells and deficiency leads to a disorder known as scurvy. Requirements are increased with prolonged exercise and illness.

Scurvy has been recognized for hundreds of years. It was particularly liable to attack mariners who in the days of sailing ships were away from land for long periods and were thus deprived of fresh food and vegetables. Infants and children are also susceptible, for although breast milk contains about 6 mg of vitamin C per 100 ml, cow's milk contains considerably less.

Scurvy is rarely seen in England at the present time, although it is occasionally found in people who for medical reasons, or more often supposed medical reasons, have been living on a very restricted diet such as bread and weak tea.

Scurvy is characterized by a tendency to bleed due to increased capillary fragility. Haemorrhages occur into the skin and mucous membranes; sponginess and haemorrhage around the gums may be found in those with teeth. Bleeding also occurs under the periosteum of bones and into joints producing great pain and tenderness; the patient is anaemic. If vitamin C is not given the disease will prove fatal.

Therapeutics. Scurvy is cured by giving vitamin C, the dose for adults being 500 mg daily. The bleeding is arrested and the anaemia, which is not entirely secondary to haemorrhage, is relieved. Vitamin C is also used in a number of other disorders where it is of doubtful value; it does appear, however, to be useful in promoting the healing of wounds in those who, although showing no evidence of scurvy, have a mild degree of deficiency.

Very high doses of vitamin C are sometimes taken to prevent colds and other forms of ill health. The efficacy of this medication is not proven, but it does not seem to do any harm.

Minimum human requirements:

- Children 100 mg daily
- Adults 50 mg daily
- Pregnancy 200 mg daily
- Lactation 150 mg daily.

Therapeutic dose. 500 mg daily.

Pabrinex contains high doses of B and C vitamins and is given intravenously or intramuscularly. Rarely, it can cause a severe allergic reaction and infusion should be over at least 10 minutes and facilities should be available for treating an acute allergic reaction.

Vitamin D (cholecalciferol) (Fig. 19.1)

This fat-soluble vitamin is found in fish liver oils and dairy produce and is also formed in the skin on exposure to sunlight. It is essentially concerned with calcium metabolism and bone formation. After absorption it is modified in the liver to form *25-hydroxycholecalciferol*, and undergoes further change in the kidney to form *1,25-dihydroxycholecalciferol*. This substance is highly active in facilitating calcium absorption from the gut and the laying down of calcium and phosphate during bone formation. A deficiency in vitamin D leads to inadequate calcification of the bones, resulting in their becoming soft and easily deformed. This disorder when it occurs in children is known as **rickets** and these children with their bowed legs and deformed chests were a familiar sight in former times; with the arrival of cheap milk, cod liver oil and Infant Welfare

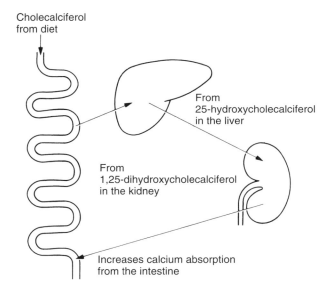

Cholecalciferol from diet

From 25-hydroxycholecalciferol in the liver

From 1,25-dihydroxycholecalciferol in the kidney

Increases calcium absorption from the intestine

Figure 19.1 The changes undergone by cholecalciferol (vitamin D) in the body.

Centres it has now become rare, although there has been a reappearance of the disease in coloured immigrants to this country. In adults, prolonged deprivation of vitamin D gives rise to a disorder similar to rickets, but it is very rarely seen in this country, although certain groups, e.g. the elderly, Asians and vegetarians, are at some risk.

Vitamin D deficiency can also result from poor absorption from the intestine, as in coeliac disease, and from resistance to the action of vitamin D which is found in renal failure leading to stunting in children (*renal rickets*).

Therapeutics. Patients at risk of deficiency can be given one calcium and ergocalciferol tablet daily (400 units of vitamin D per tablet),* which should be crushed or chewed before swallowing. 5000 IU of vitamin D daily is adequate for the treatment of established rickets. In coeliac disease doses of vitamin D up to 50 000 units daily may be required at first, but these requirements diminish as the disease is controlled by diet. In chronic renal failure large doses of vitamin D or alfacalcidol are used.

---

*400 units of vitamin D ≡ 10 micrograms of ergocalciferol.

Overdose with vitamin D is dangerous and leads to deposition of calcium in the kidneys and other organs.

Patients receiving high doses should have their plasma calcium measured regularly.

Minimum human requirements:

- Young children 600 IU daily.*
- Adults 400 IU daily.
- Pregnancy and lactation 1000 IU daily.

Alfacalcidol (1-alpha-hydroxycholecalciferol) is closely related to vitamin D and is used in treating various disorders in which there is a resistance to the action of vitamin D.

Vitamin E (tocopherol)

Vitamin E is found in nuts and wheat germ and deficiency produces no clear clinical syndrome. It is, however, an antioxidant and it is believed that by this action it may reduce the incidence of cancer and vascular disease, although at present there is little hard evidence to support this view.

Vitamin K (phytomenadione)

Vitamin K is a precursor of prothrombin, which is essential for the coagulation of blood.

Vitamin K is fat soluble and requires bile salts for proper absorption from the intestine. It is also synthesized in the gut by bacteria. After absorption it is used by the liver for the synthesis of prothrombin.

Deficiency in vitamin K will lead to bleeding and may result from insufficient uptake due to various intestinal diseases or to deficient utilization following liver disease or anti-coagulant drugs.

In the newborn there is a lack of vitamin K because it has not been synthesized by the gut bacteria and this may lead to bleeding (*haemorrhagic disease of the newborn*). It occurs at birth and, more seriously, about a week later when it is often intracranial. It can be prevented by giving vitamin K. There has been some anxiety that injected, but not oral, vitamin K may be associated with childhood cancers, but this fear appears to be unfounded.

The *options* at present are to give:

1. 2.0 mg of Konakion MM Paediatric orally at birth and repeat the dose 4–7 days later. Breast-fed infants should be given a further dose at one month.
2. 1.0 mg of vitamin K by injection at birth.

Konakion MM Paediatric, unlike previous preparations of vitamin K, is quite well-absorbed orally and thus avoids the need for injections.

Trace elements

Certain elements, including zinc, manganese, boron, cobalt and copper, exist in very small amounts in the body. They are essential for some important metabolic processes and deficiency can cause or contribute to several disorders. Adequate amounts are present in a full, normal diet but insufficiency can arise in those whose diet is severely restricted, or with malabsorption. Patients who are on total parenteral nutrition are especially at risk of deficiency and trace elements may be added to their intravenous infusion.

Patients who are poorly nourished and are about to undergo surgery may be given dietary supplements before operation. Zinc and vitamin C are thought to be of particular importance in aiding wound healing and improving immunity to infection.

Antioxidants (see also page 88)

Antioxidants include some vitamins and other compounds which are not usually classified as vitamins but are considered to be important constituents of the diet.

Oxidation is a metabolic activity occurring in nearly all tissues and is necessary for life. It can however, produce substances called *free radicals* which are chemically very active and can damage constituents of cells. They are believed to play a part in the development of vascular diseases, cancer and possibly, some other diseases. Antioxidants suppress the formation of free radicals and might therefore, be expected to protect against these conditions.

Although it has been shown that there is a relationship between the dietary intake of antioxidants and the development of certain diseases, there is, at present, little evidence that adding them to the diet has a prophylactic effect, other than a possible reduction of coronary artery disease by vitamin E. Among those being used are vitamins C and E, betacarotene and selenium. In addition, antioxidants are present in fruit and vegetables which should form part of a healthy diet.

FURTHER READING

Bates C J 1995 Vitamin A. Lancet 345: 31
Editorial 1995 Vitamin A and birth defects. New England Journal of Medicine 333: 1414
Editorial 1996 Dietary habits and mortality in 11 000 vegetarians and health-conscious people, results of a 17 year follow-up. British Medical Journal 313: 775
Editorial 1998 Which vitamin K preparation for the newborn? Drug & Therapeutics Bulletin 36: 317
Fraser D R 1995 Vitamin D. Lancet 345: 104
Gregory J et al 1990 Dietary and nutritional survey of British adults. HMSO, London
Ministry of Agriculture, Fisheries and Food 1991 Dietary supplements and health foods. Report of the Working Group. MAFF Publications, London

20

Drugs used in the treatment of anaemia

IRON DEFICIENCY ANAEMIA

Iron is an essential constituent of haemoglobin, which is contained in the erythrocytes (red cells) of the blood. Haemoglobin is concerned with the transport of oxygen from the lungs to the tissues. When the red cells break down, the iron is retained by the body and built up again into further haemoglobin molecules. There is very little iron held in storage depots, the major portion being constantly in use (Fig. 20.1). A little iron, probably about 2 mg a day or less, is lost by desquamation of cells by the skin and gut, but the chief drain of iron from the body occurs in the various forms of blood loss, either menstruation or parturition or due to chronic bleeding, usually from the gastrointestinal tract. In pregnancy the growing fetus requires a certain amount of iron and during lactation iron is lost in the mother's milk.

It can be seen, therefore, that although the average diet which supplies about 25 mg of iron a day is sufficient for most people, if there is any prolonged iron loss, a deficiency will occur. This leads to failure to produce enough haemoglobin with resulting anaemia.

Iron, when taken by mouth, is converted into the ferrous form in the stomach. It is absorbed from the upper part of the small intestine, forming a loose compound with a protein in the intestinal wall which is called *transferrin*; in this form it is transported across to the bloodstream where it is carried to the bone marrow for the synthesis of haemoglobin. The absorption of

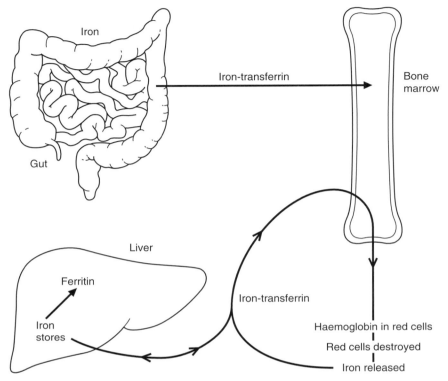

Figure 20.1 Metabolism of iron.

iron is carefully regulated so that just enough is absorbed to make good any deficiency. Iron is also stored in the liver in the form of *ferritin*.

Iron deficiency anaemia is sometimes associated with deficient secretion of hydrochloric acid by the stomach and this leads to a failure of release of ferrous iron from the diet. It can occur as a result of diseases of the intestine which interfere with iron absorption.

If a deficiency of iron occurs, less haemoglobin is synthesized and the amount of haemoglobin in the erythrocytes decreases.

Iron is given to correct a deficiency. It is usually given orally. The rise in blood haemoglobin level should be at least 0.7 g/dl per week and *treatment should be continued for 4 months after the blood haemoglobin level has returned to normal to replace depleted iron stores.*

It is also given during pregnancy when the iron requirements increase (see under folic acid, p. 271).

Ferrous sulphate

Ferrous salts are rapidly changed to ferric salts in the air and thus ferrous salts are given as coated tablets. Ferrous sulphate tablets are a satisfactory way of giving iron to most people. The therapeutic dose is 200 mg, three times a day. In sensitive subjects ferrous sulphate may cause gastric discomfort and nausea or diarrhoea or sometimes constipation.

Ferrous sulphate tablets are usually coated with sugar; *children are therefore very liable to take them and fatal poisoning by ferrous sulphate is not uncommon.* Like all drugs they should therefore always be kept in a position of safety.

Ferrous gluconate is another ferrous salt. It is less irritating to the stomach than most ferrous salts.

Ferrous glycine sulphate is a complex of ferrous sulphate and the amino acid glycine. It is perhaps less liable to cause gastrointestinal disturbances and is useful in sensitive subjects.

Liquid preparations are also available. **Sodium ironedetate (Sytron)** and a **polysaccharide–iron complex (Niferex)** are satisfactory and do not stain the teeth. Although slow-release iron preparations are used they may be less effective as iron absorption takes place in the upper small intestine, but these preparations release it lower down the gut.

Iron can also be given by intramuscular injection in those who are not absorbing iron satisfactorily. *Before injecting iron, oral iron should be stopped for at least 72 hours as this appears to reduce the chances of a reaction after injection.*

Iron-sorbitol citrate is an iron preparation for intramuscular injection. It is rapidly absorbed from the injection site. It contains 50 mg of iron per ml of solution. Side-effects appear slight but shock-like reactions can occur and care must be taken when giving the injection to prevent leakage along the needle track and subsequent staining of the skin.

DRUGS USED IN TREATING OTHER ANAEMIAS

Cobalamins (vitamin B12). There are several factors required for the proper maturation of the red cells. The best known of these is vitamin B12. A deficiency of this vitamin leads to a failure in production of erythrocytes. There is, therefore, a decrease in the number of circulating erythrocytes and those which do manage to mature appear abnormal, being large and irregular in shape and size. Primitive red cells may also appear in the blood.

In addition to the change in the blood, deficiency in cobalamin leads to glossitis and degenerative changes in the nervous system. The syndrome produced by cyanocobalamin deficiency is known as *pernicious* or *Addison's anaemia*. This deficiency is believed to be due to a failure to absorb cobalamin from the intestine. In the normal person, a factor (*the intrinsic factor*) is produced by the stomach and is necessary for the absorption of cobalamin in the intestine. In patients with pernicious anaemia there is a lack

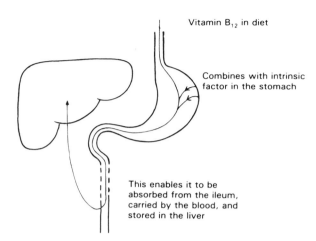

Vitamin B$_{12}$ in diet

Combines with intrinsic factor in the stomach

This enables it to be absorbed from the ileum, carried by the blood, and stored in the liver

Figure 20.2   Absorption of vitamin B12.

of this gastric factor and cobalamin cannot therefore be absorbed (Fig. 20.2). Failure to absorb cobalamin can also result from diseases of the intestine.

Treatment is to give cobalamin by injection. There are two cobalamins available, **hydroxocobalamin**, which is stable and which is highly bound by the plasma proteins so that it is excreted slowly and thus its action is prolonged, and **cyanocobalamin**, which is effective but more rapidly excreted.

Therapeutics. Treatment is started with hydroxocobalamin 1 mg three times weekly and then reduced to 1 mg every 6–8 weeks when a satisfactory remission has been produced. Maintenance doses of cyanocobalamin, however, should be given every 3–4 weeks.

The lesions in the nervous system also respond to cobalamin, but it may be many months before the full effect of treatment is seen.

Occasionally, vegans may develop vitamin B12 deficiency due to a shortage in the diet. To prevent this 1 mg of *hydroxocobalamin* can be added weekly to their food.

Folic acid. Folic acid is obtained from animal and vegetable sources and is also synthesized by bacteria. It is necessary for the maturation of red cells, and deficiency will produce changes in the blood similar to those found in pernicious anaemia.

The common causes of deficiency in this country are:

1. Malabsorption syndromes such as coeliac disease.
2. Pregnancy. Some women do not absorb folic acid in the later months of pregnancy and thus become anaemic. In addition, folic acid taken early in pregnancy reduces the incidence of *neural tube defects*. Iron deficiency is also common in pregnancy and it is usual to give both folic acid and iron supplements which are taken throughout pregnancy.

Therapeutics. Folic acid can be given orally in doses of 15 mg daily. Larger doses may be required in malabsorption states. Tablets containing both iron and folic acid are available for use in pregnancy. 'Pregaday' contains ferrous fumarate equivalent to 100 mg of ferrous iron plus folic acid 350 micrograms, the dose being one tablet daily. If possible, a woman considering pregnancy should start taking folic acid (400 micrograms daily) before conception and for the first 3 months of pregnancy, to minimize the risk of neural tube defects which occur very early in pregnancy. To prevent recurrence of a defect, a dose of 5.0 mg of folic acid daily should be used and continued for the first 3 months of pregnancy. There is also some evidence that the addition of folic acid to the diet reduces the incidence of cardiovascular disease. *It is important not to treat pernicious anaemia with folic acid for, although it will improve the anaemia, it will worsen the neurological complications of pernicious anaemia.*

Erythropoietin deficiency

Erythropoietin is a hormone manufactured by the kidney, which is necessary for erythrocyte formation. If the kidneys fail, the level of erythropoietin in the blood falls with resulting anaemia.

Patient education

Severe hypertension requires immediate treatment. Patients or relatives should be told to report headaches or confusion at once.

Epoetin is a genetically engineered analogue of erythropoietin and two forms, alpha and beta, are available commercially. They are essentially the same. In patients with renal failure and anaemia epoetin is given three times weekly by subcutaneous or intravenous injection until a satisfactory haemoglobin level is produced. Treatment then continues with maintenance doses.

Adverse effects. Hypertension is fairly common and may be severe. The blood pressure should be measured every week in the initial stages of treatment and then at 6-weekly intervals. Thrombosis and 'flu'-like symptoms occasionally occur.

Blood growth factors

Factors which stimulate the growth of white blood cells are now available and are especially useful in patients whose white cells have been depressed by cancer chemotherapy, immunosuppression or treatments associated with the AIDS virus.

Human granulocyte-colony stimulating factor (filgrastim and **lenograstim)**, given by subcutaneous or intravenous injection, increases the production of neutrophils.

Human granulocyte macrophage-colony stimulating factor (molgramostim) also increases the white cells in the blood.

The use of these factors has considerably improved the treatment of a wide range of serious disease in which it is necessary to suppress temporarily the white count to achieve a satisfactory therapeutic effect. They accelerate the recovery of the bone marrow and thereby decrease the risk of serious infection which accompanies leucopenia.

FURTHER READING

Editorial 1993 Filgras H M – human granulocyte colony stimulation factor. Drug and Therapeutics Bulletin 31: 33

Editorial 1998 Eat right and take a multivitamin. New England Journal of Medicine 338: 1060

Hibbard B M, Horn E 1988 Iron and folate supplements during pregnancy. British Medical Journal 297: 1324

Kong C H, Brown S M 1991 Recombinant human erythropoietin in the management of anaemia. Professional Nurse 6(11): 650

21

Drugs used in the treatment of malignant disease

Although a great deal has been discovered about normal cell function and cell division, after many years of research it is still not known exactly why malignant cells behave as they do. The pattern of their behaviour is familiar. Instead of differentiating in an orderly fashion to take their place in the formation of some organ, they multiply in a haphazard way showing little, if any, attempt at differentiation and, further, instead of remaining in their organ of origin they invade neighbouring structures. Cell emboli from new growths are swept in the blood or lymphatic circulation to distant parts of the body, take root and set up further tumours knows as secondary deposits or metastases.

CELL DIVISION AND CYTOTOXIC DRUGS

The cells of the body vary enormously in appearance and function but all share some common characteristics. With very few exceptions (e.g. erythrocytes), cells consist of a nucleus surrounded by cytoplasm. The most vital component of the nucleus is deoxyribonucleic acid (DNA), which consists of two chains of molecules arranged into a double helix. DNA contains the code which determines the types of protein that are made by the cell and thus ultimately how the cell functions.

One of the important components of the cell cytoplasm is ribonucleic acid (RNA). This substance receives instructions from the DNA in the cell nucleus and is actually responsible for the manufacture of protein.

Most cytotoxic drugs interfere with DNA or RNA and thus they have a profound effect on cells and their functions. Unfortunately, these actions are not confined to the malignant cells, but affect normal cells as well.

Some cells in the body divide frequently to replace those which have become worn out, particularly the cells of the bone marrow, the lymphatic system and the lining of the intestinal tract, and these are particularly sensitive to the action of cytotoxic drugs.

During its life the cell passes through a series of changes, and cell division itself is a complicated process. The newly formed cell enters the G_1 stage, which is a period of protein synthesis and intense metabolic activity. This may last for a variable time, from a few hours to many years. Many cells remain in this phase throughout the

life of the organism, but some undergo division and enter the S phase. This phase is short and is concerned with DNA and RNA synthesis so that the DNA strands may split when cell division occurs. It is a period of great metabolic activity. The G_2 phase which follows is a short period of consolidation before cell division occurs. In the mitotic phase the DNA spiral splits longitudinally so that each daughter cell has its full complement of DNA, which is exactly the same as that in the parent cell (Fig. 21.1).

Some cytotoxic drugs will affect cells at any phase in their life cycle; others will only act at a single phase of the cell cycle, usually when the cell is dividing, and are called *phase specific*. It follows therefore that when using phase specific drugs repeated dosage is necessary if the maximum effect is to be achieved.

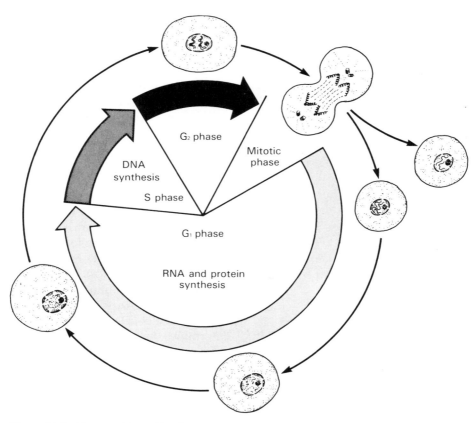

Figure 21.1 Phases of the cell cycle.

A proportion of the cells in a cancer are in a resting phase, sometimes called the G_0 phase, when they are not dividing. This is important because in this stage they are very resistant to chemotherapy.

The aim of treating neoplastic disease with drugs is to find a drug which will kill the neoplastic cells while leaving the normal cells of the body unharmed. However, the metabolic process of the neoplastic cells is so very similar or perhaps even the same as that of normal cells that so far it has been impossible to reach this ideal. Nearly all drugs which have so far been discovered, although having a marked toxic effect on neoplastic cells, have some adverse effect on the normal cells of the body, especially those of the bone marrow. The best that can be done is to give the cytotoxic drug or drugs at repeated intervals so arranged that the recovery of normal cells can occur, but little recovery of cancer cells is possible. It *may* then be possible to progressively reduce the number of malignant cells without unduly reducing the normal cells until ultimately all the malignant cells are eradicated (Fig. 21.2).

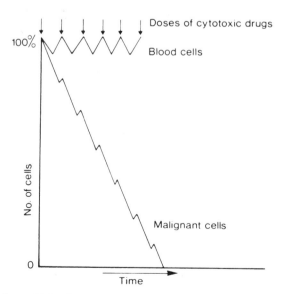

Figure 21.2 Progressive reduction in the number of malignant cells produced by repeated doses of a cytotoxic drug, with recovery of the normal blood cells. An ideal therapeutic response.

The natural history of cancer

The growth rate of tumours varies considerably and the development of clinical symptoms and signs occurs at a late stage in the disease process (Fig. 21.3). Note particularly the long subclinical period and that after chemotherapy, although the patient is apparently in full clinical remission, a small amount of tumour may remain.

As a result of these considerations and a large amount of work on animal models of cancer, certain principles of treatment have emerged.

1. Cytotoxic drugs are usually given in intermittent high-dose treatments over long periods.

2. The smaller the mass of tumour treated, the better the result because small tumours have less resting cells which are insensitive to chemotherapy.

3. Suppression of the bone marrow is very common as cytotoxic drugs have to be given at the maximum tolerated dose.

ALKYLATING AGENTS

These are chemically very active substances which combine with the DNA in the cell nucleus and thus damage or kill the cell. Unfortunately, although these substances have a marked effect on certain types of malignant cells, they also damage normal cells, particularly those of the bone marrow and gastrointestinal tract which have a high rate of division.

There are a number of alkylating agents now available.

Chlormethine (mustine) is related to mustard gas and is used in the treatment of neoplastic diseases of the lympho-reticular system such as Hodgkin's disease, and with less success in certain carcinomas such as those of the ovary and bronchus. Because of toxicity its use is decreasing.

Therapeutics. Chlormethine is given by intravenous injection and as it is very irritant it is common practice to set up an intravenous drip of saline and inject the chlormethine into the drip tubing and flush it through the vein with saline.

Adverse effects. Most patients experience nausea and vomiting for some hours after treatment.

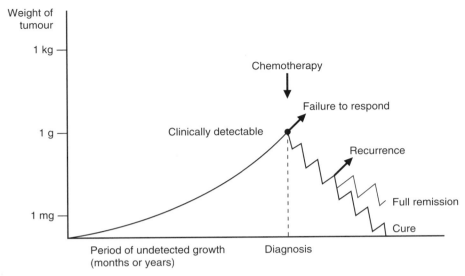

Figure 21.3 Tumour growth and possible responses to chemotherapy. Modified from Ritter, Lewis and Mant, A textbook of clinical pharmacology, 3rd edn, Edward Arnold, London.

Bone marrow suppression is an ever-present risk, usually affecting the white cells and platelets.

Chlormethine may also be injected into malignant effusions and may either slow down or prevent their formation.

Cyclophosphamide was developed in an attempt to improve the therapeutic effectiveness of this type of drug. Cyclophosphamide itself is non-toxic, but in the liver it is split by enzymes which release cytotoxic metabolites. It can be given orally or intravenously, either daily or weekly and is frequently combined with other cytotoxic agents. The therapeutic effect is usually delayed for a week or more.

Adverse effects include depression of the bone marrow and loss of hair. A metabolite is excreted in the urine which can cause severe cystitis. This may be avoided by giving a high fluid intake (4 litres a day) or combining it with mesna (see later).

Ifosfamide is closely related to cyclophosphamide, from which it differs slightly in efficacy. It is less likely to depress the blood count than cyclophosphamide, but is more likely to damage the kidneys and bladder. To prevent this adverse effect it is combined with a drug called **mesna** which neutralizes ifosfamide in the kidneys and bladder and thus prevents toxicity.

Chlorambucil is a useful drug of the chlormethine group. It is effective by mouth and although depression of the bone marrow can occur, vomiting is unusual.

Therapeutics. Chlorambucil is given orally over long periods. It is one of the few cytotoxic drugs which is used continuously rather than as high-dose intermittent treatment. It can be used on an outpatient basis, but the patient should attend regularly for blood counts and if severe bone marrow suppression occurs recovery may be slow. It is effective against various forms of Hodgkin's disease and non-Hodgkin lymphoma and is probably the drug of choice in chronic lymphatic leukaemia.

Busulphan is particularly used in chronic myeloid leukaemia where it has a selective depressing action on the abnormal white cells. Excessive dosage will produce dangerous depression of normal white cells and platelets.

Therapeutics. Busulphan is given orally. Treatment is continued over weeks or months and is modified by the response of the patient.

Adverse effects. In addition to bone marrow depression it can cause pigmentation and fibrosis of the lungs.

Melphalan is used particularly in multiple myelomatosis. It is usually given daily for a week, and may be repeated if the blood count is satisfactory. Melphalan is a powerful depressant of white cells and platelets.

Lomustine (CCNU) is similar in many ways to the alkylating agents and, though its mode of action is different, it is effective against the same types of cancer. It is given orally as a single dose and should not be repeated for 4 or preferably 6 weeks as depression of white cells and platelets may be delayed. Nausea and sometimes vomiting is common for about 12 hours after dosage.

ANTIMETABOLITES

These agents resemble substances used by the cells for their metabolic processes. They thus become incorporated in the cells and because they cannot be metabolized they normally cause the cell to die.

Malignant cells often have a very rapid metabolic turnover and thus incorporate antimetabolites more rapidly than normal cells. It is thus possible to kill the majority of malignant cells without interfering too drastically with normal cells. Excessive dosage will inhibit normal cell production, particularly in the bone marrow.

Methotrexate. This is similar in structure to folic acid and it blocks one of the chemical processes necessary for the production of cell nuclear material from folic acid. Methotrexate can be given orally, intravenously or intrathecally, but large doses are not well absorbed from the intestine and must be given by injection. Dosage schedules depend on the type of cancer being treated. It is excreted via the kidney and it is essential that renal function is measured before starting treatment. With impaired function the dose is reduced.

In certain types of malignant disease, a very large and potentially lethal dose of methotrexate is given; then, after 24 hours, the action of the drug is reversed by giving folinic acid. It is extremely important that this is carried out precisely.

This method is known as *folinic acid rescue.*

Methotrexate in low doses is also used as an immunosuppressant in rheumatoid arthritis and psoriasis.

Adverse effects. In addition to bone marrow suppression methotrexate can cause liver damage and mouth ulceration.

Mercaptopurine is closely related chemically to adenine and hypoxanthine, two substances used in the formation of the cell nucleus.

It is believed that mercaptopurine replaces these substances in the nucleus of cells and thereby prevents their further division. It is used in combination with other drugs in the treatment of acute leukaemia, a disease where the bone marrow is rapidly overgrown by very malignant white cells.

Mercaptopurine can also be used in chronic myeloid leukaemia.

Therapeutics. Mercaptopurine is given daily, by mouth, and the course of treatment is determined by the response of the patient. Excessive or prolonged treatment will produce depression of normal white cells.

Fluorouracil is another antimetabolite which is used with some benefit in a wide variety of tumours, including those of the gastrointestinal tract. It is given by intravenous infusion or as a bolus; the dose varies with circumstances. It can also be applied locally to certain skin cancers. It produces leucopenia and in particular ulceration of the mouth.

Cytarabine is a drug which interferes with the nuclear function in the malignant cell and is used in acute leukaemia. It can cause bone marrow depression.

VINCA ALKALOIDS

Vinblastine is an extract of periwinkle. It is believed to act at the stage of cell division (mitosis) and is therefore phase specific. Vinblastine is useful as part of a cytotoxic drug regime in treating certain lymphomas and is given in a single weekly injection. It can cause a leucopenia which is, however, usually short-lived.

Vincristine, which is related to vinblastine, is also given intravenously, at intervals. It is used

---

Nursing point

Vinca alkaloids should be given intravenously and, under no circumstances, intrathecally.

---

as an initial drug in acute leukaemia to induce a remission and is also useful in treating lymphomas and other cancers. It is less likely to cause leucopenia, but may also damage peripheral and autonomic nerves, producing constipation with abdominal distension and tingling and numbness in the limbs.

MISCELLANEOUS DRUGS

Doxorubicin (adriamycin). This cytotoxic drug is an antibiotic; it has a fairly wide antitumour range. It is given by intravenous injection, every 3 weeks, usually in combination with other cytotoxic drugs. It is believed to interfere with DNA and RNA function.

Adverse effects. It can depress bone marrow and this occurs about 2 weeks after treatment, rather later than with most cytotoxic drugs. It is toxic to heart muscle and this requires regular ECG monitoring. Toxicity is dose related and the total cumulative dose of the drug should not exceed $450\,\text{mg/m}^2$. Other effects are nausea, vomiting and hair loss.

Etoposide is related to podophyllin, an extract of mandrake which can be applied locally in the treatment of warts. Its action is to prevent cell division.

Etoposide can be given orally or intravenously and is usually used in combination in the treatment of a wide range of malignancies.

Adverse effects include bone marrow depression and vomiting in a small number of patients.

Procarbazine is also used in the treatment of lymphomas. Nausea is less likely if the drug is given after meals and it may have to be combined with an anti-emetic. If alcohol is taken at the same time as the drug it may produce a reddish flush.

Dacarbazine is largely used in treating Hodgkin's disease and melanomas. It has to be given intravenously and is highly irritant so it must be injected *very* slowly into a fast running drip. It also causes considerable vomiting and severe myelodepression.

Bleomycin, another antibiotic with relatively weak anticancer effects, is used in combination to treat lymphomas and testicular cancers. However, unlike all the drugs already discussed, it does not depress the bone marrow. It is usually injected at weekly intervals, and injection may be followed by a spike of fever. Prolonged use (usually more than a total cumulative dose of 300 000 units) leads to lung fibrosis.

Cisplatin is based on the metal platinum. It is effective in a number of cancers, but has found a particular use in regimes designed to treat cancer of the testicle and ovary and has proved very successful.

Therapeutics. Cisplatin is given intravenously and usually in combination with other anticancer agents at 3–4 week intervals. Certain precautions must be observed:

1. A diuresis is essential when the drug is given or it will damage the kidneys.
2. Hearing should be tested regularly as it damages the inner ear.
3. Vomiting is usually very troublesome.

It follows, therefore, that this drug should only be given by those who are aware of the complications which can occur.

Carboplatin is similar and is used in ovarian carcinoma. It is not, however, so nephrotoxic as cisplatin.

Mitoxantrone (mitozantrone) is given as a single injection at 3-weekly intervals. It is used in a variety of cancers. The incidence of adverse effects is relatively low and it is useful in controlling the disease, particularly on an outpatient basis.

Taxanes: paclitaxel, docetaxel

These drugs are obtained from yew. They inhibit cell division in the G_2 and M phase (see Fig. 21.1) and are used to treat ovarian and breast cancer when other regimes have failed. They are given by intravenous infusion. They both depress the blood count and there is a risk of hypersensitivity reactions with flushing, rashes, dyspnoea and collapse. To prevent this, patients are given a steroid and an antihistamine before infusion.

HORMONES IN MALIGNANT DISEASE

Various hormones will produce a temporary remission in malignant disease. Their mode of action is not clear, but it is believed that certain malignant tumours are in part dependent on hormones. By removing these hormones (i.e. by removing the endocrine glands where they originate) or by suppressing them by giving other hormones, the stimulus to growth is removed from the malignant cells and they regress.

Examples of such forms of treatment are the orchidectomy or the administration of *estrogen* or androgen blockade by drugs in patients with carcinoma of the prostate (see p. 210) and adrenalectomy or the administration of estrogen or testosterone to patients with carcinoma of the breast.

Tamoxifen competes with estrogens for receptors in the malignant cells. In some way which is not understood this causes regression of the tumour in carcinoma of the breast. It is given in doses of 20 mg orally daily for metastatic disease in both pre- and postmenopausal women and is also used in the adjuvant treatment of postmenopausal women.

Trials are being undertaken to determine whether it could prevent breast cancer in normal women at high risk. This project is subject to some debate as it means giving the drug to apparently fit women. The initial results in the USA suggest that there is a reduction in the incidence of breast cancer in those treated, but further results are required to show the effects of long-term treatment and to see whether it also affects mortality. An additional advantage of its long-term use may be to prevent osteoporosis and decrease the incidence of heart disease.

Adverse effects are mild and include occasional nausea, oedema, flushing and bone pain and a slightly increased risk of endometrial cancer.

Interactions. Tamoxifen increases the anticoagulant effect of warfarin.

Aminoglutethimide inhibits steroid synthesis in the adrenals and also suppresses estrogen and androgen production in the peripheral tissues. For this reason it is used in the treatment of advanced breast cancer. It can also be used to control the overproduction of adrenal steroid hormones in Cushing's disease.

A number of estrogen antagonists including **anastrozole** and **letrozole** inhibit the enzyme aromatose and thus prevent the production of estrogen. They are used in the treatment of advanced breast cancer in postmenopausal women.

Adverse effects are usually minimal but they can cause thrombotic episodes.

Corticosteroids not only have a general tonic effect in malignant disease, but have a specific cytotoxic action in lymphomas and some leukaemias and are included in several multidrug regimes.

IMMUNOTHERAPY

Repeated attempts are being made to induce specific antibodies against cancer cells. Although some results are promising, as yet there has been no substantial therapeutic advance. However, two types of immunotherapy are in use.

Interferons are produced by cells in response to viral infection and have some antitumour activity. They are being tried for a variety of cancers and have proved very effective in the rare hairy-celled leukaemia.

Levamisole is an immunostimulant and is being used in carcinoma of the colon.

COMBINATION TREATMENT

In most forms of malignant disease which can be treated successfully by drugs, better results with less toxicity are achieved if several cytotoxic agents are combined in the course of treatment. Most regimes consist of repeated courses given at intervals of 1–2 weeks and extending over 6–12 months or even longer. This enables the malignant cells to be attacked at different stages in their cell cycle; also careful timing enables the normal cells of the body to recover while the malignant cells remain suppressed. Treatment can often be carried out on an outpatient basis, or with patients remaining in hospital overnight when they receive the drugs. As an example of a treatment which has been used for widespread lymphomas, the CHOP regime, is shown below:

Cyclophosphamide days 1 and 8
Doxorubicin (adriamycin) day 1
Vincristine days 1 and 8
Prednisolone daily for 5 days.

The course is given in cycles of 3–4 weeks and repeated about six times.

Many combination regimes are being used in the treatment of various types of cancer. Among the malignant diseases which can nearly always be improved and quite often cured by chemotherapy are:

- Various leukaemias, particularly acute lymphoblastic in children
- Hodgkin's disease
- Non-Hodgkin's lymphomas (some types)
- Testicular cancer
- Ovarian cancer
- Retinoblastoma
- Chorioncarcinoma.

Other types of cancer can often be improved without effecting a cure—these include carcinoma of the breast and prostate and myeloma.

Chemotherapy may be combined with surgery or radiotherapy and the management of a patient is often an integral operation.

Although much cancer is still treated in general hospitals, it is preferable for this to be carried out in special units experienced in this type of work and such units are being widely established.

In terms of nursing organization it requires frequent short-term admissions or special outpatient facilities and careful checks on the general health of the patient and the blood count.

Special training is now available for nurses who wish to work in the field of cancer treatment.

ADJUVANT TREATMENT

It is common experience that, although a malignant growth appears to have been totally removed, a recurrence may occur somewhere else in the body at a later date. This must mean that at the time of operation there was already a seedling deposit, and the object of adjuvant treatment is to give cytotoxic drugs *after* operation even if there is no evidence of spread to eradicate hidden small deposits which are particularly susceptible to drug treatment. For example, over half the women who have operative treatment for *carcinoma of the breast* will ultimately die from metastases, although these were not apparent at the time of operation. Results of trials in this condition have made it clear that adjuvant treatment improves the long-term prognosis in all age groups. The type of chemotherapy is determined by the age of the patient, the nature of the cancer cells and whether the axillary nodes are involved. It varies from tamoxifen, given alone to postmenopausal low-risk patients, to polychemotherapy, perhaps combined with ovarian ablation, for high-risk younger patients. It must be remembered, however, that adjuvant treatment results in some patients receiving chemotherapy who in fact have no metastases and which is therefore unnecessary. This presents a difficult ethical problem.

A similar strategy, which is being investigated, is to give chemotherapy *before* operation (primary treatment).

PALLIATIVE CHEMOTHERAPY

In some types of advanced cancer, chemotherapy can relieve symptoms and prolong life, but is not curative. Most regimes have some side-effects and before embarking on palliative chemotherapy it is very important to weigh possible benefits against disadvantages. This will require a compassionate discussion with the patient and ascertaining the views of relatives, nursing staff and others who are involved. As with all chronic diseases much supportive care will be necessary, and, generally, such treatment should be given in specialist oncology units.

It is impossible to discuss the palliation of all the cancers in which this treatment is an option, but the group includes:

- Carcinoma of the breast
- Small cell carcinoma of the lung
- Carcinoma of the ovary and cervix
- Colorectal carcinoma
- Carcinoma of the bladder
- Head and neck cancer
- Various lymphomas
- Malignant melanoma.

SOME PRACTICAL POINTS

Storage of drugs and preparation of solutions

Oncology units should have a pharmacist with special experience and expertise in handling cytotoxic drugs to advise and supervise others. Solutions for injection should be prepared in a designated area by:

- Nurses who have received special training
- Pharmacists
- Medical staff.

Nursing point

Although some cytotoxic drugs can be used for some time after the solutions have been prepared, it is usually best to discard all unused remnants at the end of a treatment session.

Some of these substances are very irritant and, in addition, can be highly dangerous if absorbed. The following precautions should be observed:

1. Wear plastic gloves and a plastic apron when making up solutions or crushing tablets. If any of the drug splashes onto the skin it should be washed off immediately. Some of the drugs are irritant and there is always the risk of an allergic reaction.

2. Wear protective spectacles to protect the eyes. If the drug comes into contact with the eyes, they should be washed out with water and further advice should be sought.

3. Care should be taken to avoid absorbing the drug either systemically or by inhalation. Hands should be washed after preparing a drug (even when gloves are worn). Although at present there

is no evidence that those who handle cytotoxic drugs are more liable to suffer long-term ill-effects, there are certainly no grounds for complacency and every care must be taken.

4. Pregnant staff should not prepare cytotoxic solutions.

5. If spillage occurs, it should be mopped up with absorbent paper which must be disposed of properly and the whole area washed down thoroughly.

6. Waste material should be disposed of safely.

Administration of cytotoxic drugs

In view of the possible danger when giving cytotoxic drugs, the following authorization should be applied:

1. Oral—no special restriction.
2. i.m. or i.v. infusion, which may be by a pump—nurses with special training.
3. Intravenous bolus—nurse with special training or medical staff.
4. Intrathecal or intra-arterial—medical staff.

Never use the brachial vein for vesicant drugs.

Use a No. 23 butterfly or a cannula (22–24) for intravenous administration.

Vesicant drugs should be given into a fast running infusion over at least 5 minutes. For patients with difficult veins or when frequent injections are given, a Hickman catheter/Portacath may be used.

Extravasation of cytotoxic drugs on injection

Even if great care is taken, some leaking of the injected drug may occur around the vein and this can cause problems.

Vesicant drugs carry a high risk of severe tissue necrosis if they extravasate.

Vesicant drugs:

Chlormethine	Melphalan
Dactinomycin	Mitomycin
Daunorubicin	Vinblastine
Doxorubicin	Vincristine
Epirubicin	Vindesine

Bleomycin and ifosfamide are irritant drugs which cause pains but do not lead to tissue damage. For vesicants the following full extravasation procedure should be carried out.

1. The needle should be left *in situ*, the infusion stopped and as much as possible of the extravasated fluid removed.
2. The needle can now be removed.
3. Ice packs should be applied to the area.
4. The area should be kept cool for the next 24 hours and 1% hydrocortisone cream applied twice daily.
5. The episode and subsequent progress should be recorded in the patient's notes.
6. An expert should be consulted.
7. The area should be inspected after 24 hours and as often as necessary thereafter.

Policies may vary in different units and local policies and procedures should be available and strictly followed.

Occasionally, necrosis occurs despite all the measures and skin grafting may be required.

Vomiting with cytotoxic drugs

Many cytotoxic drugs cause the patient to vomit a few hours after administration.

Severe	*Moderate*	*Mild*
Cisplatin	Cytarabine	Bleomycin
Cyclophos-	Etoposide	Busulphan
phamide	Procarbazine	Chlorambucil
(high dose)	Vinblastine	Fluorouracil
Dacarbazine		Melphalan
Daunorubicin		Mercaptopurine
Doxorubicin		Methorexate
Lomustine		Vincristine
Chlormethine		
Plicamycin		

There is as yet no complete remedy for this troublesome side-effect. A variety of regimes may be tried in an attempt to mitigate the symptoms and patients vary in their preference. It is usual to give cytotoxic drugs in the late evening so that the patient may sleep as much as possible through the period of nausea.

For mildly or moderately emetic cytotoxic drugs, dexamethasone, prochlorperazine, domperidone or low-dose metoclopramide can be used.

Combinations are often more effective and intravenous dexamethasone and metoclopramide initially, followed by both orally, is useful.

It is believed that the most severely emetic drugs (e.g. cisplatin) stimulate the 5-HT_3 receptors in the gastrointestinal tract and brain stem. *Ondansetron*, a 5-HT_3 antagonist, combined with dexamethasone given intravenously, immediately before treatment and followed by further doses of ondansetron, either orally or intravenously, or by dexamethasone with domperidone is the most effective anti-emetic for this type of cytotoxic drug.

Some patients, particularly towards the end of their course of treatment, become anxious and tense before treatment and may indeed vomit before receiving their drugs. This is a difficult problem. Lorazepam an hour before coming to hospital may be tried and sometimes psychiatric support with a desensitization programme helps.

Care of the mouth

Mouth ulceration may occur with many cytotoxic regimes. This is partially due to the direct effect of the drugs on the mucous membrane of the mouth and also the general suppression of immunity, particularly of the leucocytes, encourages infection. This unpleasant complication can be minimized.

1. Before starting treatment, the patient should be seen by a dentist or dental hygienist and have any infections treated.
2. If the white blood cell count drops or the mouth becomes sore, the patient should have nystatin pastilles (for candida) every 6 hours and Corsodyl mouth washes twice daily. Some units use fluconazole systemically.
3. If ulceration develops, the pain can be relieved by Difflam Oral Rinse which contains benzydamine, a local anaesthetic. The mouth is rinsed out every 3 hours with the undiluted solution. Lidocaine gel can also be applied to the painful area.

Alopecia

Hair loss may occur with many cytotoxic drugs (particularly doxorubicin, etoposide and ifosfamide). It will recover, but causes embarrassment to patients. With doxorubicin ice-cold water caps applied to the scalp during treatment may decrease the loss, otherwise wigs may help, while other patients will prefer to just put up with it. It is important to warn the patient of this problem *before* treatment is started.

Bone marrow suppression and infection

Cytotoxic drugs (except bleomycin and vincristine) depress bone marrow function. This leads to a low white blood cell count and, sometimes, to low platelet and red blood cell counts usually after 7–10 days As a result, immunity is suppressed and the patient is liable to develop an infection or to bleed. In addition to those caused by the usual bacteria, infections may be due to fungi, viruses and even organisms which do not normally cause disease in healthy people. Attempts have been made to diminish the risk of infection by isolating the patients, but this is difficult and, if strictly implemented, very expensive. In most cases it appears to be sufficient to avoid obvious sources of infection. Those caring for these people should always watch for signs of infection and the patients should be told to report any suspicious symptoms. Immunosuppressed patients often respond poorly to antibacterial treatment and the infecting organism may be obscure, so a combination of antibiotics is often used.

The extent and duration of the low blood count can be minimized by giving *haemopoietic growth factor* (see p. 272) and this has proved a useful adjunct to the more intense courses of chemotherapy.

Sometimes very large doses of cytotoxic drugs are given in an attempt to eradicate a tumour which is poorly sensitive to chemotherapy and this will destroy the blood-forming cells in the bone marrow. In these circumstances, bone marrow is removed from the patient before starting treatment or stem cells, which can form bone marrow, are harvested from the patient's peripheral blood and stored. After the chemotherapy is finished the stored cells are injected back into the patient to multiply and restock the bone marrow. This is rather a high-risk procedure with an appreciable morbidity and mortality, but potentially will extend the range of cancers which can be controlled or cured.

Long-term risks of the use of cytotoxic drugs

Most cytotoxic drugs interfere in some way or other with the structure of the cell nucleus and this can have serious long-term implications.

1. Second malignancy. These drugs may induce changes in normal cells so that they ultimately become malignant. This means that although the original cancer is eradicated, a different malignancy may develop at a later date. Second malignancies are more common after certain cytotoxic drugs and if drugs are combined with radiotherapy. It is necessary to put this risk in perspective as the chance of dying from the initial cancer, if untreated, is much greater than that of developing a further cancer. Some information is now available as to the risk of second malignancies with various cytotoxic drugs and the situation is becoming increasingly well defined. This risk will be one factor to be considered when choosing a suitable regime.

2. Many cytotoxic drugs damage the gonads. In men permanent sterility may result; in women amenorrhoea is common but periods usually return after stopping treatment. It is possible to store a man's sperm before treatment in case gonadal function is permanently suppressed.

3. Most cytotoxic drugs are potentially teratogenic, especially in early pregnancy. If pregnancy is avoided during and for 6 months from the end of treatment, there does not seem to be an increased risk of an abnormal infant being born.

The role of the nurse in cancer chemotherapy

The establishment of units specializing in oncology has enabled nurses to receive advanced training which is of direct benefit to patients and their families. A multidisciplinary approach is important in the treatment of cancer and the team will consist of nurses, doctors, pharmacists and social workers. In most centres part of the work will be concerned with therapeutic trials and this will require ancillary staff.

The management of malignant disease may be by chemotherapy alone or may involve surgery or radiotherapy. In this book only the problems of chemotherapy are considered. In addition to technical knowledge the nurse will have a most important role in patient support. The distress and fear of having cancer is enough to shake the stoutest heart and, indeed, chemotherapy is usually prolonged and often unpleasant.

In the initial assessment nurses should try to establish what patients know about malignant disease and their beliefs, if any, about treatment. They will appeal to the nurses for information and this provides an opportunity to dispel myths and at the same time explain what treatment will entail. Patient education is multipronged and can take the form of booklets, videos, question and answer sessions and group discussions so that sufferers can gain support from others in similar circumstances. Patients usually attend oncology units at regular intervals for treatment and follow-up so it is possible for the nursing staff to build up a supportive relationship with those who know and trust them.

A good deal of research is in progress by oncology units to mitigate the unpleasantness of chemotherapy and one of the key areas being examined is the use of self-help measures at home.

FURTHER READING

Banks C 1991 Alleviating anticipatory vomiting. Nursing Times 87 (16): 42

Byrne J et al 1987 Effects of treatment on fertility in longterm survivors of childhood or adolescent cancer. New England Journal of Medicine 317: 1315

Dodds L et al 1993 Case-control study of congenital abnormalities in children of cancer patients. British Medical Journal 307: 164

Editorial 1998 Tamoxifen in the prevention of breast cancer. British Medical Journal 316: 1181

Freeman E 1990 Making sense of cancer chemotherapy. Nursing Times 86 (31): 45

Gelmon K 1994 The taxoids. Lancet 344: 1267

Gibbs J 1991 Handling cytotoxic drugs. Nursing Times 87 (11): 54

Goodkin D E 1994 Interferon beta 1b. Lancet 344: 1057

Hawthorn J 1995 Understanding and management of nausea and vomiting. Blackwell Scientific, Oxford

Holmes S 1990 Cancer chemotherapy. Lisa Sainsbury Foundation, Austin Cornish, London

Hortobaggi G N 1998 Treatment of breast cancer. New England Journal of Medicine 339: 974.

Kaye S B 1998 Prevention of vomiting due to cytotoxic drugs. Prescribers Journal 28: 144

Luther J M, Robinson L 1993 The Royal Marsden Hospital standards of care. Blackwell Scientific, Oxford

Molassiotis A 1998 Cancer, chemotherapy and pregnancy. Nursing Times 94 (9): 48

Richards M A, Smith J E, Dixon A M 1994 The role of systemic treatment for primary operable breast cancer. British Medical Journal 309: 1363

Richardson A 1992 The Royal Marsden Hospital manual of core care plans for cancer nursing. Scutari Press, London

Robinson S 1993 Principles of chemotherapy. European Journal of Cancer Care 2: 55

Stuard N S A, Blackledge G R P 1989 Side effects of cytotoxic chemotherapy. Prescribers Journal 28: 155

Swerdlow A J et al 1992 Risk of primary cancer after Hodgkin's disease. British Medical Journal 304: 1137

Traynor B 1991 Haemopoietic growth factors. Nursing Standard 23 (18): 32

22

Drugs in pregnancy and at the extremes of age

Most facts about drugs are obtained from observations on adults. However, age may modify the way drugs are handled by the body and also the way the body reacts to the actions of drugs. In recent years, increasing interest has led to studies of drugs given at the extremes of age and in pregnancy.

DRUGS IN PREGNANCY

Drugs can affect the fetus either by interfering with some important function in the mother which indirectly damages the fetus or by passing across the placenta and acting directly on it. *Most drugs cross the placenta.*

The fetus may be damaged at three stages of pregnancy.

1. Implantation (5–15 days). Drug toxicity at this stage usually results in abortion.

2. Embryo stage (15–55 days). During this period the embryo is changing from a group of cells into a recognizable human being. The embryo is particularly susceptible to drug toxicity at this time, which leads to fetal malformation (teratogenesis) such as occurs with thalidomide.

3. Fetogenic stage (55 days–birth). As the fetus continues to grow and develop, drug damage becomes less likely, but it is still possible.

4. Delivery. Drugs at this stage may interfere with labour and modify the behaviour of the neonate immediately after birth.

In this country about 30% of women take some drug during pregnancy, though only 10% take one in the first trimester when the fetus is most vulnerable to damage. Those most commonly taken are mild analgesics and antibiotics.

It is important to discover which drugs can produce fetal damage and which are safe to use. This is difficult for two reasons:

1. Fetal abnormalities can occur for various reasons even when no drugs are taken. About 2% of babies have some abnormality at birth, but only about 5% of these are believed to be drug-related.

2. If the drug only rarely causes an abnormality, thousands of pregnant women need to be studied before a connection between a certain drug and fetal damage can be confirmed. Experiments with pregnant animals have only a limited value.

At present drugs can be divided into three groups:

A. Drugs known to produce fetal abnormalities

Thalidomide
Folic acid antagonists
Tetracyclines
Androgens
Danazol
Warfarin (during the first 4 months of pregnancy)
Diethylstilbestrol
Etretinate
Lithium
Some anticonvulsants

B. Drugs suspected of producing fetal abnormalities

Oral hypoglycaemic agents cause neonatal hypoglycaemia
Various cytotoxic drugs
Anorexics (amphetamines)
ACE inhibitors and thiazides should not be used for hypertension in pregnancy

There are a number of other drugs which are under suspicion or for which information is not available.

C. Drugs which probably do not harm the fetus (see also British National Formulary, Appendix 4)

Simple analgesics	— Paracetamol for minor pain.
	— NSAIDs can be used if really necessary and ibuprofen, being mild and short-acting is preferred.
Cough	— Codeine
Powerful analgesics	— Opioids can be used (but see below).
Diabetes	— Insulin
Drugs for dyspepsia	— Antacids, advice on diet.
Drugs for constipation	— Bulk purges, lactulose
Drugs for nausea	— Avoid if possible and treat by modifying diet.
	— Promethazine if necessary.
Antibacterial drugs	— Penicillins, cephalosporins, erythromycin.
	— Trimethoprim should be avoided in the first 3 months of pregnancy if possible.
Hypotensive agents	— Methyldopa
	— Hydralazine for rapid lowering of blood pressure.
	— β blockers can be used, but retard fetal growth.
Antimalarial drugs	— Chloroquine (low dose) proguanil.
Antiasthmatic drugs	— β_2 agonists, inhaled steroids, short courses of systemic steroids if really necessary.
Centrally acting drugs	— Benzodiazepines (but see below).
	— Neuroleptics and tricyclic antidepressants probably safe.
	— Antiepileptics—see page 171.

Hay fever   — Topical preparations.
— Antihistamines (chlorphenamine, terfenadine).

Further information can be obtained from: The *British National Formulary, Appendix 4*, The *National Teratology Information Service* (tel. 0191 232 1525 or from a drug information unit.

When treating pregnant women some general rules should be observed:

1. Avoid giving drugs if possible, especially in the first 3 months of pregnancy.
2. Give drugs at the lowest effective dose for as short a time as possible.
3. Avoid recently introduced drugs if possible.
4. Drugs on lists A and B should be avoided if possible. The problem arises when there is no satisfactory substitute and treatment is vital. This is a matter of risk to the fetus against risk to the mother (and often therefore, the fetus as well).
5. *Ethanol and street drugs.* Alcohol taken by the mother during pregnancy can damage the fetus, resulting in an infant with a small head, facial abnormalities and of low intelligence. Although it may well be better to avoid alcohol altogether in pregnancy, there is no evidence that one glass of wine, or its equivalent, daily causes any harm. If the mother is dependent on opioids, the newborn infant may suffer acute withdrawal symptoms. Regular use of cocaine is associated with an increased risk of fetal abnormality.

Pregnancy and dosage

Pregnancy causes a number of changes in the way the drug is handled by the body. The volume of water in the body is increased so that the concentration of a given dose will be decreased, though this may be offset by a fall in protein binding which leaves more free active drug in the blood.

Liver enzymes increase so that some drugs are broken down more rapidly and renal excretion may also be enhanced. Where dosage is not critical this does not matter, but for a few drugs

(e.g. anticonvulsants and theophylline) adjustment of the dose may be necessary.

DRUGS IN NEWBORN INFANTS

During the hours of labour drugs may be given to the mother and some of these can pass via the placenta to the neonate. Among those which are important are:

Analgesics and hypnotics. Morphine and similar drugs affect the fetus and may lead to difficulties in starting breathing immediately after birth.

Excessive dosing of the mother with barbiturates and benzodiazepines leads to accumulation of these drugs in the fetus and after birth the infant will be floppy with depressed breathing and failure to suck.

β blockers pass to the fetus and produce a slow pulse rate.

Kernicterus and drugs. Certain drugs given to the mother late in pregnancy or to the infant in the first few days of life bind onto the plasma protein and displace bilirubin from the binding sites. This can be dangerous because too much uncombined bilirubin in the blood causes brain damage. Drugs that have been implicated are:

Sulfonamides
Tolbutamide
Aspirin.

Chloramphenicol. Newborn infants are not able to break down drugs as effectively as older children or adults, thus accumulation may occur after repeated dosing. With chloramphenicol this can be dangerous as accumulation of the drug produces the '*grey syndrome*' which is due to collapse of the circulation.

Oxygen. Treating a newborn infant with a high concentration of oxygen is known to cause blindness due to *retrolental fibroplasia*.

BREAST FEEDING AND DRUGS

Most drugs will pass into the breast milk, but usually at very low and innocuous concentrations. However, this is not inevitable and a few drugs being taken by the mother can be a hazard to the baby. Generally, drugs should be avoided by nursing mothers, but if a drug is essential the baby should feed just before the mother takes her dose when blood levels will be low.

Certain drugs should not be used by nursing mothers and, if unavoidable, will require transfer to bottle feeding.

For further information there is a comprehensive list of safe and unsafe drugs in the *British National Formulary, Appendix 5.*

DOSAGE OF DRUGS IN CHILDREN

Children should not be regarded as small adults when prescribing for them, particularly in the first few months of life. They differ in:

1. Body composition
2. Elimination of drugs.

In the first few weeks of life the breakdown of drugs by the liver is reduced, but thereafter, because of the relatively large size of a child's liver, the rate of breakdown is greater, weight for weight, than in adults. This discrepancy progressively disappears until adulthood.

Renal excretion is similarly reduced in the first few weeks of life, but reaches normal levels by about 6 weeks. It follows therefore that except for the first few weeks of life, weight-related doses of most drugs are higher in children than in adults.

This means that dosage has to be carefully considered for each individual drug. Young children find it difficult to swallow tablets, so liquid preparations are preferable. However, they should not be mixed in the feeding bottle as milk may interfere with drug absorption. Older children respond to drugs more like adults but, even here, there may be differences.

There is no completely satisfactory way of calculating the correct dose of a drug for children. In practice three methods may be used:

1. Dose = Adult dose $\times \dfrac{\text{Patient's weight in kg}}{70}$

2. Dose = Adult dose $\times \dfrac{\text{Patient's body surface area (metres}^2)}{1.8}$

3.
Age	Wt in kg	% of adult dose
Newborn	3.5	12.5
4 months	6.5	20
1 year	10	25
3 years	15	33
7 years	23	50

Note: This assumes that the child is 'average'.

The first is most satisfactory in deciding the initial loading dose but the second, which takes into account the rate of breakdown of the drug, is to be preferred for maintenance dosage. These methods are only approximate and with certain drugs the dose in adults and children differs considerably.

Administration of drugs to children may present difficulties (see p. 21). Children under 5 years of age cannot usually swallow tablets and will require liquid preparations. Volumes of less than 5.0 ml should be given via an oral syringe. These should be free of sucrose, which causes dental damage. For certain drugs (e.g. diazepam) the rectal route is useful.

Further information can be found in the *British National Formulary* or in various paediatric formularies. The Guy's, St. Thomas's and Lewisham Paediatric Formulary is particularly useful.

DRUGS IN ELDERLY PATIENTS

Elderly people are responsible for about one-third of the expenditure on drugs by the National Health Service and a high proportion of them are receiving regular drug treatment. It is therefore important to know whether the action of drugs is modified by old age and how advancing years may alter the handling of drugs by the body.

1. Drug absorption. At present there is little evidence that the absorption of drugs after oral administration changes with age, provided there is no disease of the gastrointestinal tract.

2. Drug distribution. After absorption drugs are carried round the body in the blood. They are to a greater or lesser extent bound to the plasma proteins, particularly albumin. Elderly people have less albumin in the blood so, of certain drugs less is protein-bound and more is free in the blood and tissue fluids and can therefore produce a greater pharmacological effect.

3. Drug metabolism (breakdown). Many drugs are broken down by enzymes in the liver, but with advancing age these enzymes become less active and, in addition, the blood supply to the liver decreases. Some drugs may be more slowly broken down with a tendency for accumulation to occur and signs of overdosage to develop. Those implicated include:

Lidocaine	Tricyclic antidepressants
Propranolol	Caffeine
Benzodiazepines	

4. Drug excretion. Drugs are also excreted via the kidney. Old age, sometimes associated with kidney disease, leads to a decline in renal function, so that by the age of 80 years renal function is only half that at age 40. This again may cause drug accumulation and among the most important drugs in this case are:

Digoxin	Aminoglycosides
Propranolol	

5. Organ sensitivity. This is more difficult to assess, but there is evidence that certain systems become more sensitive to drug action with advancing years. Brain function is easily disturbed in elderly people so that hypnotic and other centrally acting drugs can easily produce confusion and excessive drowsiness. The control of blood pressure is more easily disturbed, causing fainting, not only with hypotensive drugs but with tricyclic antidepressants and levodopa.

6. Compliance. Complicated drug regimes may be impossible for elderly people to follow so they either give up taking their drugs or take the wrong doses at the wrong times, sometimes with disastrous results.

7. Adverse reactions to a drug are two or three times more common in the elderly than in younger adults and there are several reasons for this:

1. Elderly patients often need several drugs at the same time and there is a close relationship between the number of drugs taken and the incidence of adverse reactions.

2. For reasons given above, the elimination of drugs may be impaired in elderly patients so that they are exposed to higher concentrations unless the dose is suitably adjusted.

3. Elderly patients are often severely ill and this may interfere with elimination.

4. Drugs which are associated with adverse reactions such as digoxin, diuretics, NSAIDs, hypotensives and various centrally acting agents are often prescribed for elderly patients.

This does not mean that diseases should not be treated in elderly people, but drugs must be prescribed with care.

All these considerations have made it necessary to observe certain general principles when using drugs for elderly patients:

1. A full **drug history** is important as the patient may have experienced an adverse effect from a drug in the past. Medication already being taken (including over-the-counter preparations) may raise the possibility of an interaction. It will also enable the nurse to assess the patient's ability to manage the regime alone or whether help may be needed from relatives.

2. Keep the regime simple and use as few drugs as possible.

3. Prescribe the smallest effective dose and if possible, use drugs which are short-acting.

4. Do not continue to use a drug for longer than necessary.

5. If an elderly person's condition deteriorates, remember that a drug may be responsible.

6. Certain formulations such as elixirs may be easier than tablets for an elderly person to take, particularly if the tablets are very large or very small.

7. Clear and simple instructions should be given to the patient and the container must be clearly labelled. Various types of calendar packs are available, but it is important to ensure that the patient can use them.

Specific therapeutic problems

Sleep. Elderly people generally require less sleep than younger adults and broken sleep during the night is common. They do not usually require a hypnotic, but should avoid sleeping in the day and take more exercise. Alcohol, taken in the evening, may induce sleep, but often leads to waking in the night because its hypnotic effect wears off rapidly. If, however, the patient is used to a little alcohol before sleep it is usually best not to interfere. Various disorders can cause sleeplessness and they should be sought and treated if possible:

Pain	Depression
Urinary frequency	Heart failure
Constipation	Dementia
Caffeine taken in the evening	

The main dangers of hypnotic drugs for elderly people are:

1. They may cause mental confusion during the night.
2. They may have hangover effects into the next day.

Elderly people appear to be very sensitive to most centrally acting drugs. Those most commonly used for insomnia are the *benzodiazepines*. *Temazepam* 5–10 mg is short-acting and is preferred.

Despite their relative safety, these drugs can produce excessive drowsiness, confusion and ataxia and the smallest possible dose must be used. If possible, they should only be given for short periods and a careful watch kept for adverse effects and falls.

Tranquillizers. Agitation with restlessness is common in elderly people, especially if they are demented. This can be controlled by phenothiazines, such as *thioridazine* 25–50 mg, but with all phenothiazines remember postural hypotension, Parkinson-like symptoms and akathisia (restlessness and anxiety).

Depression. Tricyclic antidepressants are useful, but postural hypotension, urinary retention, dry mouth, exacerbation of glaucoma and a liability to fall can all be troublesome. The 5-HT re-uptake inhibitors are a considerable improvement as far as most adverse effects are concerned and are equally effective. However, they are much more expensive.

Parkinson's disease. (See p. 171) Small doses of *levodopa*, combined with a dopa decarboxylase inhibitor, are useful. In the elderly postural hypotension can be a problem. Anticholinergic drugs often cause troublesome side-effects, i.e. urinary retention and glaucoma and constipation should be avoided.

Hypertension. There is now considerable evidence that treating hypertension in older subjects is worthwhile and it is possible to reduce cardiovascular complications in this group. The cardiovascular systems of elderly people do not adapt to change so well as in younger patients, therefore a gentle approach is needed. A low-dose thiazide diuretic (bendroflumethiazide 2.5 mg daily) is often adequate. Calcium-channel blockers can be used, but must be avoided in heart failure. ACE inhibitors are also effective and well tolerated, but renal function must be monitored. β blockers are rather less effective in elderly patients. The blood pressure should be taken standing and lying as elderly patients may have a large postural fall.

Chronic heart failure is increasingly common and is usually, but not always, due to coronary artery disease. Treatment is along the same lines as in younger patients (see p. 58), but certain problems are more liable to arise in older people:

Diuretics	— Sodium deficiency may develop causing postural hypotension and fainting on standing.
	— With loop diuretics, the rapid diuresis can cause acute retention in men with enlarged prostates.
	— With large doses, potassium deficiency occasionally occurs, requiring potassium supplements or the addition of a potassium-sparing diuretic.
ACE inhibitors	— Hypotension, particularly with the first dose and in those already receiving diuretics.
	— Developing renal failure. Renal function should be monitored.
Digoxin	— Toxicity due to reduced renal

Nursing point

It is important not to confuse ankle oedema due to long periods of sitting with that due to heart failure.

elimination. Low doses should be given.

Oral hypoglycaemic agents. Diabetes in elderly people can be treated with these drugs. Tolbutamide or glipizide are to be preferred as they are rather short-acting and the risks of hypoglycaemia are less.

Epilepsy due to cerebrovascular disease is not uncommon in elderly patients. The most useful drugs are carbamazepine, sodium valproate and phenytoin. The same problems arise as in younger patients (see p. 168). The initial dose should be small and adverse effects are more easily pro-

voked, mainly because of slower elimination. It is also important to remember that interference with cognitive function, which occurs with many centrally acting drugs, is more marked in elderly people.

Antibiotics. There is no particular contra-indication to antibiotics in elderly patients as long as care is taken with aminoglycosides, as reduced renal function can lead to high blood levels and toxic effects.

Analgesics. Elderly patients are more sensitive to opioids and particular care is necessary if the patient has chronic obstructive airways disease. Co-codamol (codeine + paracetamol) can be used, but the resulting constipation may require a laxative. Paracetamol is preferred for minor pains because NSAIDs are especially liable to cause gastric bleeding in older people. If an NSAID is really necessary ibuprofen is the safest.

FURTHER READING

Cargill J 1992 Medication compliance in elderly people: interfering variables and interventions. Journal of Advanced Nursing 17: 422
Conn V C 1991 Older adults: factors that predict the use of over-the-counter medication. Journal of Advanced Nursing 16: 1190
Editorial 1996 Preconception, pregnancy and prescribing. Drug and Therapeutics Bulletin 34: 25
Glasper A, Oliver R W 1984 A simple guide to infant drug calculations. Nursing 2nd Series 22: 649
Grant E, Golightly P 1992 Drugs in breast feeding. Prescribers Journal 32: 90

Guy's, St. Thomas's and Lewisham Hospitals Paediatric Formulary (1999)
Iro S 2000 Drug treatment in breast-feeding women. New England Journal of Medicine 343: 118
Koren G, Partuszak A, Ito S 1998 Drugs in pregnancy. New England Journal of Medicine 338: 1128
Rajaen-Dehkordi Z, Macpherson G 1997 Drug-related problems in older people. Nursing Times 93 (28): 54
Rubin P 1998 Drug treatment during pregnancy. British Medical Journal 317: 1503
Rylance G 1998 Prescribing for infants and children. British Medical Journal 296: 984
Swift C G, Shapiro C M 1993 Sleep and sleep problems in elderly people. British Medical Journal 306: 1468

23

Adverse reactions to drugs. Testing of drugs. Pharmacovigilance

TYPES OF ADVERSE REACTIONS

During the last few years, adverse reactions to drugs have become increasingly common. They are responsible for about 5% of admissions to hospital and occur in 10–20% of hospital inpatients. This is probably due to the enormous increase in the range and number of drugs now in use. It is particularly important for nurses to be aware of the possibility of drug reactions as they may be the first to realize that something is wrong, and so the drug can be stopped before too much damage is done.

Drugs most commonly causing adverse reactions are:

Warfarin	Diuretics
Digoxin	Tranquillizers
Antibacterials	Steroids
Potassium	Antihypertensives

The classification of adverse reactions to drugs has been simplified by Professors Rawlins and Thompson of the University of Newcastle. They have suggested that reactions can be divided into:

Type A reactions are more common and are due to the normal pharmacological actions of the drug which for various reasons are greater than would normally be expected. They are therefore predictable.

Type B reactions (idiosyncratic) are considerably less common and are unrelated to the drug's normal pharmacological action. They are therefore unpredictable and not related to the dose of the drug.

Type A reactions

They can be due to:

1. Incorrect dose

Excessive absorption. This is uncommon.

2. Decreased elimination

This is due to slower breakdown or poor excretion by the kidneys. This in turn leads to accumulation of the drug in the body and adverse effects.

Examples:

- Slow breaking down of morphine by the liver in patients with liver damage, causing undue sedation and even coma.
- Poor elimination of gentamicin by the kidneys in renal failure, causing accumulation of the antibiotic and damage to the ears.

3. Undue sensitivity of organs

Undue sensitivity to the action of a drug.

Examples:

- The increased sensitivity of the heart to digoxin, leading to toxicity in patients with potassium deficiency.
- The respiratory centre of patients with chronic lung disease may be unduly sensitive to opioids, so that normal therapeutic doses cause symptoms of overdose.

This type of reaction is usually related to the dose of the drug and can be relieved if a lower dose is given or the drug is stopped for a time.

Type B reactions

These are bizarre and unexpected reactions and are not dose-related. In many cases the reason for and mechanism of this type of adverse reaction is not known—for example, chloramphenicol causes severe depression of the bone marrow in about 1 : 30 000 treatment courses. It is therefore very difficult to relate the adverse effect to the drug when it occurs in such a small proportion of patients.

Among the known causes of type B reactions are:

1. Genetic factors

A tendency to certain reactions of this type is related to the genetic make-up of the individual.

Example:

- Subjects of tissues type HL-A D3 are more likely to suffer from gold toxicity.

Genetic factors may make the drug act in a completely abnormal way.

Example:

- Primaquine, an antimalarial agent, causes breakdown of red cells in a number of people of African and Indian descent. This has been shown to be due to an enzyme deficiency in the red cell (glucose-6-phosphate dehydrogenase deficiency).

A similar deficiency is responsible for favism, in which red cells break down as a result of eating certain beans.

2. Host factors

Host disease may predispose to a certain adverse reaction.

Example:

- Patients with infectious mononucleosis (glandular fever) are liable to get a rash if given ampicillin.

3. Environmental factors

These have been little studied, but it is possible that in certain individuals diet, tobacco or alcohol consumption and other, as yet unknown, factors may influence the response to a drug.

4. Allergic reactions

Allergy plays an important part in unexpected

drug reactions, although here the mechanism is partially understood.

This type of reaction implies that the patient has been exposed to the drug on some previous occasion. This exposure has resulted in the production of an antibody against the drug. Antibodies are proteins which are formed in the body as the result of the introduction of some foreign substance (antigen). They often serve a useful purpose—for example, antibodies formed against bacteria combine with and destroy the bacteria. Several different types of antibodies are produced in response to drugs. Sometimes these antibodies combine with a drug in such a way as to cause damage to tissue and so produce the symptoms of an allergic reaction. Four types are described:

Type I—The antibody (produced in response to a drug) may become attached to the surface of certain cells called *mast cells* which are scattered throughout the body. If the drug is given on a second occasion the drug (antigen) and antibody combine on the surface of the mast cells which are destroyed, liberating substances such as histamine which cause an acute anaphylactic reaction (see later).

Type II—The antibody may become attached to the surface of red cells. On second exposure to the drug, the combination occurs on the surface of the red cells which are destroyed, producing a haemolytic anaemia.

Type III—Antigens and antibodies may combine in the bloodstream to form immune complexes. They may penetrate various organs where they are deposited, together with a further substance called complement which is present in the blood. The antigen/antibody/complement combination stimulates inflammation which may affect the skin, kidneys and other organs.

Type IV—Drugs acting as antigens may sensitize lymphocytes which, on further contact with the antigen, will cause tissue damage. This type of reaction usually causes rashes.

Although the exact mechanism of all allergic reactions is not understood, some form of drug/antibody combination is always involved.

Allergic reactions cause a number of clinical disorders:

Acute anaphylaxis may be caused by certain foods (especially nuts and fish), by drugs (notably penicillin), by wasp and bee stings, by injection of foreign serum and by contact with latex rubber. The onset is usually rapid.

Mild cases show urticaria, nausea and coughing. More severe attacks include bronchospasm, facial oedema, hypotension, substernal pain and collapse. Severe anaphylaxis can be fatal.

Treatment. Acute anaphylaxis should be avoided if possible. *Patients must always be questioned about previous reactions before they are given a drug and particular care is required with sufferers from certain allergic disorders (asthma, hay fever and infantile eczema)* as they are more prone to analphylactic reactions.

The treatment depends on the severity of the reaction; if severe it consists of:

1. The patient should be recumbent.
2. Ensure a clear airway and give 100% oxygen.
3. Give epinephrine (adrenaline) 1: 1000 solution 0.6 ml (600 micrograms) *intramuscularly* and repeat as required at 10-minute intervals.
4. Give hydrocortisone hemisuccinate 100 mg intravenously, and repeat as required, although its effect may be delayed.
5. Give chlorphenamine (chlorphenizamine) 10 mg intravenously or intramuscularly.
6. Give an intravenous infusion of 500–1000 ml of colloid, if circulatory collapse occurs.
7. Use a nebulized bronchodilator if bronchospasm is marked.
8. Nurses should never leave the patient alone.
9. Follow up to determine the cause of the reaction and to prevent a recurrence.

Serum sickness develops about a week after the serum or drug has been administered. There is usually an urticarial rash with stiffness and swelling of joints, sometimes a mild nephritis and lymph node enlargement. Spontaneous recovery is usual, but calamine lotion applied to the rash and oral chlorphenamine together with prednisolone for a few days in more severe cases will relieve the symptoms and speed recovery.

Rashes may occur as a result of drugs allergy, but not all rashes which occur when drugs are given are due to allergy. A good example of a non-allergic drug rash is the typical erythematous rash which often occurs when ampicillin is taken.

Renal disorders. Damage to the glomerulus by several drugs including penicillamine and gold can cause gross proteinurea. NSAIDs and ACE inhibitors can cause renal failure and there are a number of other types of drug-induced renal disease.

Other allergies have been implicated as the cause of various other disorders, including depression of the bone marrow leading to leucopenia, thrombocytopenia and anaemia, haemolysis (breakdown) of red cells, jaundice and renal damage. These drug reactions are not always caused by allergic mechanisms and in many cases the exact way in which a drug damages the tissues and organs is not known.

Nursing point

Adverse reactions cannot be eliminated entirely, but they can be minimized by:

1. Taking a *drug history* to discover whether patients are already taking medicines and whether they have had adverse effects from a drug or drugs in the past.
2. Reducing prescribing to a reasonable minimum.
3. Remembering that certain patients (i.e. the elderly, those with liver or renal disease) may not handle drugs in the usual way and dose modifications may be required.
4. Always remembering that some unexpected change in a patient's condition may be due to an adverse drug reaction.

The Committee on Safety of Medicines and the Medicines Control Agency publish, at regular intervals, Current Problems in Pharmacovigilance, which provides up-to-date reports of adverse drug reactions.

DRUG INTERACTIONS

If the prescription sheet of a patient in hospital is examined it will probably show that he or she is receiving at least half a dozen separate drugs. This treatment with multiple drugs which has become a feature of medical practice has brought with it the danger that certain drugs may interact, occasionally with disastrous consequences. Dangerous interactions are particularly liable to occur:

1. In seriously ill patients because they will probably be taking several drugs at the same time.
2. In elderly patients because they may be very sensitive to relatively small changes in the blood concentration of certain drugs.
3. When there is only a small difference between the toxic and therapeutic dose of the drug.

Interaction may occur before the drugs enter the body. Intravenous infusions are commonly used, particularly in very ill patients, and a veritable cocktail of drugs may be mixed in the infusion bottle. Some of these drugs may be incompatible in solution, and precipitation or modification may occur. It is therefore very important that when drugs are given via a drip infusion, they should wherever possible be given as a bolus injected into the plastic tubing and flushed into the patient. If drugs have to be mixed in the infusion bottle, the advice of the pharmacist or doctor should be sought.

After administration of drugs, interactions can occur at numerous sites (Fig. 23.1):

1. In the intestine
2. In the blood
3. At the site of action of the drug
4. At the sites of elimination of the drugs
   a. Liver
   b. Kidney.

The intestine

Most drugs are absorbed by diffusion through the gut wall. If a drug which is well absorbed becomes attached to a drug which is poorly absorbed, the well-absorbed drug will be held in the intestine and absorption will be decreased. For example, if tetracycline and iron are given together, the tetracycline is held in the intestine by the iron which is poorly absorbed.

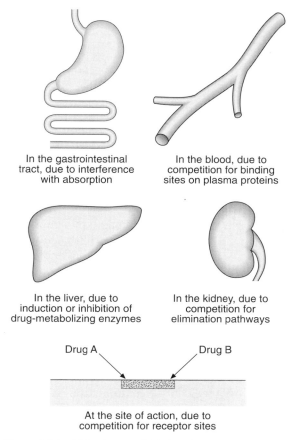

In the gastrointestinal tract, due to interference with absorption

In the blood, due to competition for binding sites on plasma proteins

In the liver, due to induction or inhibition of drug-metabolizing enzymes

In the kidney, due to competition for elimination pathways

Drug A   Drug B

At the site of action, due to competition for receptor sites

Figure 23.1   Main sites at which drug interactions can occur.

The blood

Many drugs are transported partially attached to the plasma proteins and partially free in the blood. Only the free drugs have any pharmacological action. If two drugs (A and B) of this type are given together they may compete for sites of attachment to the carrier plasma protein. Drug A may be displaced from the carrier sites by drug B so that there is more drug A free, and thus drug A has an increased pharmacological action. For example, the anticoagulant warfarin is largely carried by the plasma proteins. If chloral hydrate is given to a patient taking warfarin, the warfarin is pushed off the carrier protein and more free warfarin becomes available, resulting in increased pharmacological action and bleeding.

Drugs which will displace others from the plasma protein include NSAIDs, sulfonamides and tolbutamide.

At site of action

Drugs may antagonize or augment each other at their site of action—for example, the effect of a drug depressing the nervous system (e.g. a benzodiazepine) will be enhanced by another depressant (e.g. alcohol).

There may be antagonism at the receptors—for example, β agonists (e.g. salbutamol) and β blockers (e.g. propranolol) compete for receptors in the walls of the bronchi and thus produce bronchodilatation or bronchoconstriction depending on their relative concentrations.

At sites of elimination

Many drugs are broken down in the liver where enzymes can be modified by drugs in two ways:

1. They can be made more active (*enzyme induction*) so that other drugs are broken down more rapidly and their effect decreased. Phenytion, rifampicin and erythromycin are powerful enzyme inducers.
2. They can suppress enzyme activity. The antibiotic chloramphenicol is an enzyme suppressor.

One of the most important enzymes which breaks down drugs, and also some naturally occurring substances such as epinephrine and norepinephrine, is monoamine oxidase. It is possible to inhibit this enzyme with drugs called monoamine oxidase (MOA) inhibitors which are used in treating depression (see p. 163). If patients receiving MOA inhibitors are given certain drugs or even foods containing amines, these substances will accumulate in the body and cause an abrupt and serious rise in blood pressure.

Such drugs are:	*Such foods are:*
Epinephrine	Cheese
Norepinephrine	Broad beans
Amfetamine	Marmite and Bovril

In addition, the effects of some drugs are potentiated, particularly those of:

Meperidine
Barbiturates
Anaesthetics.

Drugs may also be excreted via the kidney and in many cases they are passed through the renal tubular cell into the urine. At this site competition can occur. Perhaps the best known examples are probenecid and penicillin, both of which are excreted via the renal tubular cells. Probenecid blocks the excretion of penicillin and this fact is used when very high levels of penicillin are required. Similarly, thiazide diuretics block the renal excretion of lithium and small increases in blood levels of lithium lead to severe and dangerous toxicity.

Important interactions

The number of drug reactions which have been described is now very large and many of them are of little or no clinical importance. In general those interactions which are important occur when the dose of a drug is critical and a small change in the blood concentration or the patient's sensitivity to the drug results in toxicity or, conversely, a lack of therapeutic effect. It is impossible for the nurse or doctor to remember them all, but most of the important ones concern:

ACE inhibitors	Lithium
Anticoagulants	Oral contraceptives
β blockers	Phenytoin
Cimetidine	Rifampicin
Digoxin	Theophylline
Erythromycin	Warfarin
Hypoglycaemic agents.	

When these drugs are being given to a patient the possibility of interactions must be remembered if further drugs are added to the treatment regime. In outpatient prescribing it should be remembered that the patient may be taking over-the-counter drugs.

Many patients would not consider alcohol as a drug, but nevertheless it can cause serious interactions and should therefore be avoided when certain drugs are taken.

> **Nursing point**
>
> Charts are available which show the more important interactions and it would be sensible to display such a chart in every ward and outpatients' department.

Disulfiram Griseofulvin Procarbazine Metronidazole Chloropropamide Hypnotics and sedatives	These drugs interfere with the metabolism of alcohol causing flushing, headaches, sweating and nausea. Potentiated by alcohol.
Warfarin	Anticoagulant action enhanced with acute overdose of alcohol. Chronic overdose may reduce effect by increasing the rate of breakdown.
MOA inhibitors Metformin Aspirin and other NSAIDS	Hypertensive crisis, particularly with Chianti. Risk of lactic acidosis. Increased risk of gastric bleeding. This risk is small and in fact many people take alcohol and aspirin without disaster.

Beneficial interactions

Not all interactions are harmful and some are used deliberately to enhance a therapeutic effect. For example, antibiotics may be combined to increase their efficacy and/or prevent the emergence of bacterial resistance, as in the combination of drugs used to treat tuberculosis. In hypertension, two agents acting in different ways (β blockers and diuretics) help to reduce blood pressure.

THE INTRODUCTION AND TESTING OF NEW DRUGS

There are two ways in which newly introduced drugs can be licensed for use in the UK (Fig.

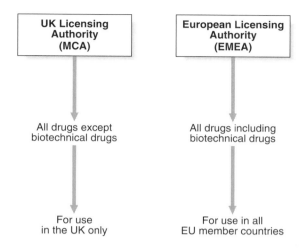

UK Licensing Authority (MCA)	European Licensing Authority (EMEA)
All drugs except biotechnical drugs	All drugs including biotechnical drugs
For use in the UK only	For use in all EU member countries

Many countries have their own licensing authorities and there may be mutual recognition of some licensing procedures between them.

Figure 23.2   Procedures currently available for licensing drugs in the UK.

23.2). The EMEA, which is based in London, covers all member states in the European Union, and is the only agency which can approve biotechnical products as well as other drugs.

Most countries also have their own licensing bodies. In the UK this is the Medicines Control Agency (MCA) and is a division of the Department of Health.

The Committee on Safety of Medicines (CSM) is an independent body, composed of experts in relevant fields who advise the licensing authority on the safety and efficacy of drugs. The CSM is also responsible for monitoring adverse reactions.

The introduction of a new drug is a costly and protracted affair. It takes about 10–12 years from the time a chemical entity is discovered until its release for general use as a therapeutic agent and the process costs about £300 million.

In the past many substances were screened for an action which could be useful in treating disease. With greater understanding of the nature of drug action, it is now possible to design drugs which might be expected to have the desired effect. These are then synthesized in the laboratory. Certain proteins are very complex and difficult to synthesize, but this can be achieved by *biotechnology*. Genes which are responsible in human or animal cells for the manufacture of specific substances, such as hormones, can be introduced into bacteria or yeasts which then produce these substances in large quantities. When harvested, they can be used therapeutically. Human insulin and growth hormone are produced in this way. The drugs are then tested in animals to ensure that they have the required pharmacological action.

A few drugs may appear promising and these have to be thoroughly tested for toxic effects. This is done in two stages. First, large doses of the drug are given to animals over a short period and their actions and toxicity determined. The drug is then given in smaller doses to animals over long periods to see whether there are any toxic effects from prolonged administration or histological changes are found after the animals are killed. At this stage the drug is also tested to see if it produces any fetal abnormalities in pregnant animals or cancer after long-term use. Only if this testing shows satisfactory results is the drug given to humans. Animal toxicology has a limited predictive value and even if a drug appears to be non-toxic in animals it may well cause an adverse reaction in humans.

Phase 1. The first time a new drug is used in humans it is given to normal volunteers. Small doses are used at first and then increased. The subjects are kept under close observation either in hospital or in a special unit. Safety is evaluated and measurements are made of the various actions of the drug and estimation of blood levels will determine the rate and degree of absorption and elimination.

Phase 2. If the preliminary studies are satisfactory permission must be obtained from the licensing authority for limited clinical trials of the new drug to find out whether, in fact, it is useful in treating disease (Fig. 23.3). About 250 patients are involved.

Phase 3. This is a larger trial involving about 2000 patients to confirm the safety and efficacy of the drug.

Only after this process will a *product licence* be given which allows the drug to be released for general use, though the licensing authority may

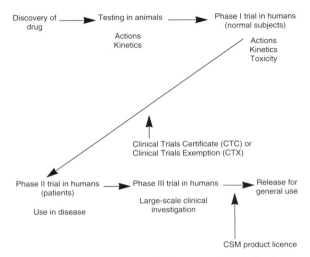

Figure 23.3 Stages in introducing a new drug, indicating when licences are required. A CTC requires full information about a drug.

still stipulate a limited period during which further information as to its effectiveness and possible dangers can be obtained.

This type of preliminary screening will usually discover serious and frequently occurring side-effects, but is of little use in picking up rare and unexpected adverse reactions. Other methods are being used to detect this type of adverse effect.

POST-MARKETING SURVEILLANCE AND PHARMACOVIGILANCE

1. Voluntary adverse reaction reporting

Practising doctors and dentists are asked to fill in a *yellow card* and send it to the CSM if they suspect an adverse reaction to a drug. For older drugs only severe or unusual reactions should be reported, but for recently introduced drugs designated by a black triangle in the *British National Formulary* doctors should report any unusual effect. This method is limited by under-reporting and probably only 5–10% of these untoward reactions are recorded on the yellow cards. At present, nurses cannot report adverse reactions via the yellow card, but they should report any such reactions to the relevant doctor or pharmacist.

2. A study of the national statistics

Statistics such as causes of death may, rarely, give a clue to some adverse reactions—an example being the rise in sudden deaths in young people suffering from asthma which was probably due to overuse of pressurized inhalers. This method usually requires an unacceptable increase in morbidity or mortality before the adverse effect becomes apparent.

3. Hospital-based systems

In a group of hospital patients all drugs given and their effects are carefully monitored—examples being the Medicine Monitoring Unit, Dundee and the Boston Collective Drug Surveillance Scheme. Such schemes provide valuable information, but are limited by the number of patients under surveillance. Nevertheless, large collaborative studies provide a great deal of useful information, not only about drug side-effects, but also about other aspects of the use of drugs.

4. Monitored release and prescription event monitoring

When a new drug is released for the first time for general use it may be limited to certain doctors who are asked to report any untoward reactions. Alternatively, the names of doctors who are using a certain drug can be obtained from prescription returns and they may be asked specifically whether they have noticed any untoward event which has happened to the patient. This method may become popular as a means of following up a newly introduced drug when it is released. It does depend on the collaboration of the doctors concerned, who must be willing to fill in the appropriate reports.

5. Cohort studies

This method involves a large number of patients who are divided (randomly, if possible) into a group taking the drug and a control group. They are then monitored for a long period and the frequency of adverse effects compared between the two groups. Although the results can be useful, it is very expensive and laborious.

6. Case control studies

With this method the problem is approached in a different way. A watch is kept for a cluster of patients with similar symptoms which have occurred for no obvious reason; then the possible causes can be investigated. One problem with this technique is that even if taking a certain drug is a common factor, it does not prove that the drug actually caused the symptoms.

7. Record linkage

This method involves studying the medical records of groups of patients over very long periods to ascertain whether delayed adverse effects emerge.

None of these methods is by any means perfect and, in spite of much effort, adverse effects still pose a difficult problem. One of the most important factors in their early detection is that those who look after patients, especially nurses and doctors, are always on the look-out for something unexpected happening to a patient.

THERAPEUTIC TRIALS

In former times opinion as to the usefulness of a drug depended on impression and anecdote. As a result many drugs in common use were worthless, some of them having no therapeutic effect at all. One important advance in recent years has been the introduction of the *clinical trial* as a means of assessing the true value of a drug.

First of all the question to be answered by the trial should be defined. For example, it may be a simple one such as the prolongation of life or the cure of a disease, or it may be a more difficult question such as the relief of anxiety or improved quality of life.

It is not always easy to assess the efficacy of a drug in practice and its trial requires careful planning. The usual way is to randomize patients into two groups which are as nearly as possible similar. One group receives the drug under trial and the other group—the control group—receives a *placebo* (a placebo being an inert substance which must be similar in appearance to the drug which is being tested) or possibly another active drug against which the trial drug is being compared. This is necessary because suggestion plays a considerable part in the relief of certain symptoms and may be responsible for some apparent therapeutic action of a drug. The usefulness of the active drug is then compared with the placebo by noting the beneficial effect in both groups. It is also important that the nurses and doctors who are looking after the patients during the trial do not know who is receiving the active drug and who the placebo, as even they may bias the result by unconsciously communicating their hopes and fears to the patients. This is known as a *double-blind trial*. The trial is designed so that the number of subjects involved is sufficient to give a clear answer as to the drug's efficacy. When completed the results are subjected to statistical analysis which will allow an estimation of the drug's therapeutic value.

The placebo response

A placebo drug may be defined as a substance which has no pharmacological action but which, when used, produces a therapeutic effect.

There is now good evidence that in a wide variety of symptoms including pain, cough, headache, etc., the administration of an inert substance will produce marked improvement in about 30% of subjects. It is important to realize that this does not mean that the patients's symptoms were imaginary. The mechanism whereby this improvement is produced is not known, but is obviously connected with the powers of suggestion.

The placebo effect has a number of important implications:

1. It is possible in some patients to control symptoms without using active drugs.

2. In assessing the effectiveness of new drugs, the placebo response must be remembered and as far as possible excluded.

3. Further study of the placebo response might be useful in opening up new methods of treatment of symptoms by suggestion, thus making it possible to relieve symptoms without resorting to pharmacologically active drugs.

Meta-analysis

Even with a well-designed controlled trial it is not always certain whether a particular new drug is more effective than those in current use. This is usually because the difference between the treated and control groups is small and the number of patients involved not large enough to give a clear result. To get round this difficulty the technique of meta-analysis has been introduced. This takes an overview of all properly controlled randomized trials of a particular drug or treatment. This technique has become very sophisticated and is giving useful information and guidance as to the best treatment in certain clinical circumstances. For example, meta-analysis of the trials in the use of streptokinase in coronary thrombosis has firmly established that it reduces mortality and it is now standard treatment.

Risk:benefit analysis

When a drug is licensed by the CSM or when it is used to treat a patient, it is important to consider the benefits which will result from its use and the possible risks involved.

When granting a product licence, the CSM needs to be convinced that the new drug is not only effective, but that the risks entailed in its use are acceptable in the context of the disease being treated (for example, greater risks are reasonable for an anticancer drug than for a hypnotic).

It is essential that prescribers explain clearly to the patient the benefits and possible adverse effects of the drugs to be used.

It may not be easy for nurses to obtain up-to-date information about drugs, but prescribers should have a current edition of the *British*

National Formulary available and should use (if possible) drugs with which they are familiar.

ETHICS COMMITTEES

Experiments on human subjects, whether they be normal volunteers or patients, should be approved by an independent ethics committee before being started. This review is not statutory, but any investigator would be most unwise to proceed without it and many journals will not accept articles if the work has not been approved by an ethics committee.

These committees have now been set up by most major medical institutions such as medical schools, research bodies and pharmaceutical companies. They have no approved constitution but should contain a wide medical representation and, in addition, nursing and lay members. Their main task is to protect the subject of an experiment from unnecessary risk and to ensure every safeguard is provided. They should also see that the subject will receive proper compensation if something goes wrong and some ethics committees take upon themselves the duty of criticizing, if necessary, the design of the experiment and ascertaining that the work is worth doing.

GENERIC PRESCRIBING

When a new drug is introduced it is given two names—a generic (approved) name and a brand name applied by the pharmaceutical manufacturer. If a drug is prescribed by its brand name the pharmacist must dispense that brand.

On introduction there is usually only a single brand of a drug so that the generic and brand names apply to the same product. However, when the patent expires (after 20 years) several manufacturers may produce a particular drug, each giving it a different brand name.

For many years there has been a move to use generic names only and to abolish brand names. This would eliminate the confusion due to a drug having several different names and would reduce the cost, particularly after the patent has expired. Against this it is argued that different brands may differ in quality and the doctor should know which brand is being dispensed. Also, it would reduce the profitability of the drug to the company which had introduced it and had spent many millions of pounds on its development.

FORMULARIES

Formularies and pharmacopoeias were originally introduced as reference books and were mainly concerned with the preparation and composition of drugs in an attempt to achieve some uniformity of composition. The first formulary in England was published by the Royal College of Physicians in 1618 (Fig. 23.4). Since then, formularies have become more concerned with which drugs are available or approved and with their actions and uses.

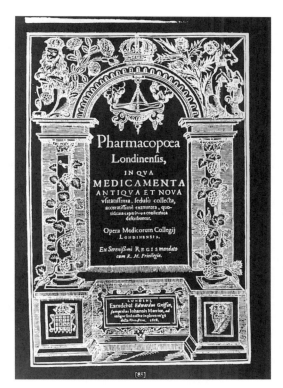

Figure 23.4 Cover of the first formulary in England published by the Royal College of Physicians in 1618.

The *British National Formulary* (BNF) lists the drugs and pharmacological preparations available in the UK together with indications for their use, dosage, adverse effects and cost. It also includes notes on the treatment of many conditions and useful guidance on a variety of problems encountered when using drugs. A copy should be available in every ward, outpatient department and doctor's surgery. It is updated twice a year. The BNF, however, is not selective—for example, the current edition lists 15 β blockers and it is obviously wasteful and extravagant for a hospital pharmacy to stock all of these. A number of hospitals or districts and a few general practices have constructed their own formularies which list the drugs available in the pharmacy and chosen on the basis of efficacy and cost; these may also contain background information. Local formularies do seem to have reduced prescribing costs and have had some educational benefits by stimulating interest in rational and sensible prescribing.

PHARMACOECONOMICS

In recent years there has been concern over the rising cost of health care. This has to some extent been caused by an increase in the number of elderly people, the introduction of new and more costly methods of treatment and the increased expectations from medical care.

In the UK the drug bill, at approximately 10% of the NHS budget, is the third largest area of NHS expenditure. The available resources are insufficient to meet all needs and so various attempts are being made to control this expenditure. Methods used include increasing the patient's contribution to the drug costs (i.e. raising prescription charges); introducing restrictive formularies which evaluate drugs and indicate which are considered most useful in patient care, i.e. 'best value for money'; limiting the drugs prescribable on the NHS; and appointing pharmaceutical advisers who help general practitioners to prescribe in a cost-effective manner.

Pharmacoeconomics has emerged as a branch of health economics relating specifically to the area of drug usage. It is a tool which allows the comparative assessment of the costs and consequences of various uses for the available resources. Choices have to be made as resources used for one treatment cannot be used for another; pharmacoeconomics provides a framework to aid the decision-making process. Resource allocation does not only limit costs, but should maximize the benefit received from the use of these resources.

All health care workers, administrators and the pharmaceutical industry will increasingly need to participate in the practical application of pharmacoeconomics. This will be important as audit and the development of treatment protocols begin to define what should be used, how it should be used and who should receive it. This will move the emphasis of drug decision-making away from acquisition costs and therapeutic efficacy towards the total effect of drug treatment on the life of the patient. Nurses by virtue of a special relationship with patients, both in and out of hospital, are in an ideal position to be involved in this process.

The four main types of pharmacoeconomic evaluation, differing in how the consequences (outcomes) are measured, are cost-minimization, cost-effectiveness, cost-utility and cost-benefit analysis (Table 23.1). Each of these methods involves the systematic identification, measurement and, where appropriate, valuation of all relevant costs and consequences of the treatment options under review. The costs and benefits will vary according to the viewpoint used in the analysis; for example, the patient or the hospital, the broadest viewpoint is that of 'society in general'.

Table 23.1 Four types of pharmacoeconomic evaluation

Type of analysis	Definition
Cost-minimization	Determines the least costly of two interventions that produce clinically identical outcomes
Cost-effectiveness	Costs* are compared with outcomes measured in natural units; for example, per life saved, per symptom-free day
Cost-utility	Costs* are compared with outcomes measured in 'utility based' units — that is, quality adjusted life years
Cost-benefit	Places monetary values on both costs and outcomes

*All relevant costs are measured in monetary terms.

FURTHER READING

Brodie M J, Feely J 1988 Therapeutic drug monitoring and clinical trials. British Medical Journal 296: 1110

Brodie M J, Feely J 1988 Adverse drug interactions. British Medical Journal 296: 845

Davies D M, Ferner R E, de Glanville H 1998 Textbook of adverse drug reactions, 5th edn. Chapman and Hall Medical, London

Editorial 1992 Clinical trials and meta-analysis. New England Journal of Medicine 327: 273

Editorial 1994 European Medicine Evaluation Agency and the new licensing arrangement. Drug and Therapeutics Bulletin 32: 89

Editorial 1995 Risk/benefit analysis of drugs in practice. Drug and Therapeutics Bulletin 33: 33

Ewing D W 1998 Anaphylaxis. British Medical Journal 316: 1442

Morrison-Griffiths et al 1998 Reporting adverse drug reactions: practice in the UK. Nursing Times 94 (10): 52

Naylor C P 1997 Meta-analysis and the meta-epidemiology of clinical research. British Medical Journal 315: 617

Pirmohamed M et al 1998 Adverse drug reactions. British Medical Journal 316: 1295

Rawlings M D 1995 Pharmacovigilance. Journal of the Royal College of Physicians 29: 41

Robinson R 1993 Economic evaluation of health care: what does it mean? British Medical Journal 307: 670

Systemic analysis of controlled trials (meta-analysis) 1992 Drug and Therapeutics Bulletin 30: 25

Symposium 1991 Drug development and clinical trials. Prescribers Journal 32: 219

Walley T, Davey P 1995 Pharmacoeconomics: a challenge for clinical pharmacologists. British Journal of Clinical Pharmacology 40: 199

24

Drug dependence (drug addiction)

Drug dependence may be defined as a state resulting from the interaction of a person and a drug in which the person has a compulsion to continue taking the drug to experience pleasurable psychic effects and sometimes avoid discomfort due to its withdrawal.

Drug abuse is the use of a drug for recreational rather than medical reasons, often in excessive quantities.

There are several groups of drugs of dependence:

1. Opioids
2. Cocaine
3. Amfetamines
4. Alcohol
5. Barbiturates
6. Cannabis
7. Hallucinogens (LSD, etc.)
8. Volatile solvents (glue sniffing).

It is usual to divide dependence into:

1. *Psychic dependence* where the drug produces a pleasant feeling, often relaxation, freedom from worry, or heightened awareness and increased energy and sexual drive. The patient suffers mental anguish when it is withdrawn.

2. *Physical dependence* where repeated administration produces biochemical changes in the subject taking the drug. If the drug is withdrawn, unpleasant symptoms and signs of a physical nature develop which may last for a varying period, but will finally disappear. During this period there is an intense craving for the drug which, if given, will temporarily relieve the

unpleasant symptoms. *Tolerance*, in which increasing doses are required to produce the same effect, often develops with drugs causing dependence.

Drugs may be used intermittently for social or emotional reasons – for example, to relieve a stressful situation. Subjects who are truly dependent take drugs continually and may reach a state in which their whole life centres round obtaining and using drugs.

Dependence may not be confined to one drug or group of drugs. It is common to find dependent subjects who have escalated from minor drugs (for example, cannabis) to hard drugs (for example, heroin) and some subjects may alternate or combine drugs; for example, cocaine and morphine would produce alternating stimulation and relaxation.

Why do people become dependent?

This is a very difficult question and the answer is still incomplete. It appears that there is no single cause for drug dependence, no single set of circumstances or special type of personality which becomes dependent. Among the motives which may be important are:

1. *Curiosity and wanting to belong*. Many young people start taking drugs because they want to know what it feels like. Pressure from peer groups may also play a part, particularly with drugs such as alcohol and cannabis, which are to some degree socially acceptable. This in turn may be tied up with the wish to belong to a group who have a common interest in drug taking and there may be an element of rebellion against accepted values. This need to achieve social acceptance may well be symptomatic of an underlying character disorder so that there are both social and psychological factors at work.

2. Some people take drugs to *relieve mental tension and worries* or to *give themselves more energy and confidence*. Most people have to face difficulties from time to time and look for a prop to help them. This may include advice from a friend, religion, a holiday, or the development of a psychiatric illness. The dependent person has taken what may be termed the 'chemical way out' and by altering his or her psychic state with drugs partially escaped from reality. Unfortunately, this method brings only temporary relief as it does not solve anything and brings in its train further problems which are both physical and psychological.

3. It has long been suggested that people who become drug dependent differ in their genetic or biochemical make-up from those who show no interest in drugs. This has been particularly suggested in alcoholism, which might be regarded as a disease of metabolism, one facet of which is craving for alcohol. This is an attractive hypothesis because it takes the 'sin' out of dependence and puts it in a medical setting, but so far there is little evidence to support it.

4. *Availability*. There is little doubt that the availability and price of drugs of dependence influence both the amount and pattern of dependence. For example, countries where alcohol is cheap, such as France and South Africa, have a high incidence of alcoholism, cirrhosis of the liver, etc.

Opioids and their derivatives

There are probably more than 100 000 people dependent on opioids in this country at present and the number is increasing. Most members of the opium group of drugs are to a greater or lesser extent drugs of dependence. The most frequently used is heroin, which is extremely potent. It may be injected intravenously, taken orally or smoked and produces a feeling of euphoria and relaxation. Dependence is both psychic and physical, and a few hours after withdrawal of the drug the person develops a craving for a further dose, combined with increasing restlessness, anxiety and distress. After 48 hours physical symptoms such as nausea, vomiting and muscle cramps become prominent. Gooseflesh may develop ('cold turkey') and the patient may be pyrexial with a raised pulse rate and blood pressure. The withdrawal symptoms last for about a week.

In addition to the hazards of withdrawal the patient runs further risks:

1. The possibility of overdosage. The drug is often adulterated with other powders and preparations may vary considerably in potency. In addition, the development of tolerance will increase the dose required for the desired effect.

2. The frequent occurrence of sepsis due to injection under nonsterile conditions. This may take the form of septicaemia or endocarditis. In addition, the sharing of injection needles greatly increase the risk of being infected with the virus of hepatitis B or C or the HIV causing AIDS. Between 15 and 60% of intravenous drug users are carrying the HIV and will eventually develop AIDS.

3. Babies born to an addict may have a low birthweight and, in addition, will suffer acute withdrawal symptoms after birth with a mortality of 50%.

4. An addict will go to any length, even serious crime, to obtain further supplies of the drug.

Management. Addicts must be registered and may then receive a supply of their drug from approved doctors. Sometimes patients present to the A and E Department with opioid withdrawal symptoms. Hospitals vary in their approach to this problem, but the main points are:

1. Confirm that the patient is dependent and is genuinely experiencing withdrawal symptoms (e.g. by getting in touch with the patient's doctor and looking for needle marks: a urine sample is useful for screening).

2. Minor withdrawal symptoms can be managed symptomatically with anti-emetics, antidiarrhoeals and minor tranquillizers.

3. Severe withdrawal symptoms are treated with oral methadone mixture (1 mg/ml), the usual dose being 10 mg. If after 6 hours the symptoms are not relieved, the dose should be repeated. It is rare for more than 40 mg/24 hours to be required.

4. Liaison with a specialist unit is essential.

5. In the long term methadone should only be given once or twice daily as it has a long half-life.

6. The Home Office must be informed of subjects who are believed to be opioid or cocaine addicts.

Alternatively, **clonidine** can be used. This drug which lowers blood pressure prevents the rise of norepinephrine in the brain which occurs when opioids are withdrawn and is responsible for many of the unpleasant withdrawal symptoms. Its use in these circumstances requires careful monitoring combined with full support. It is important to tell the patient that the relief of symptoms may be delayed for 12–24 hours.

Lofexidine is similar, but does not lower blood pressure. Whichever method of opioid withdrawal is used, the main problem is to prevent relapse and a great deal of support is needed.

After opioid withdrawal, **naltrexone** can be prescribed. It blocks the action of opioids on the brain receptors and thus prevents the euphoric effect which is linked to addiction.

Nursing point

Nurses should always be on the lookout for patients who are dependent on opioids, but are admitted to hospital for medical or surgical disorders. Multiple needle puncture marks should immediately arouse suspicion.

Cocaine

Cocaine dependence is again on the increase. The drug produces a feeling of elation and appears to temporarily increase physical capacity. In South America the leaves of the coca tree which contain cocaine are chewed for this purpose. Cocaine can be given orally; also it is absorbed through mucous membranes and may be sniffed, which can produce ulceration of the nasal septum. More rapid effects are obtained by giving cocaine intravenously, when it may be mixed with heroin. *Crack* is the free 'base' of cocaine. If this is vaporized and the fumes inhaled the drug is absorbed through the lungs, producing a rapid and intense effect. Because the action of cocaine is short-lived it may be taken in repeated doses every 30 minutes or so and there is risk of dangerous overdose. Dependence is largely psychic and withdrawal symptoms are depression, sleepiness and increased appetite.

Amfetamines

For many years amfetamines were used as appetite suppressors and to treat mild depression, and many people, mainly middle-aged women, became mildly dependent on them. In large doses amfetamines are powerful stimulants producing feelings of confidence, but also, sometimes, hallucinations and other mental disturbances. There is considerable psychic dependence, but the withdrawal symptoms are not severe. Except for special circumstances (p. 46) amfetamines are now rarely used in medical practice.

Ecstasy (MDMA) is an amfetamine derivative which produces a feeling of elation, 'togetherness' and boundless energy. In the UK it is used largely as a dance drug at 'rave' parties. It is manufactured illegally and the strength of tablets is variable. The lethal dose also varies considerably, depending on the individual. The danger is that with vigorous dancing hyperpyrexia, dehydration and electrolyte disturbances can develop with fits, collapse, renal failure and death. In addition, it can cause nausea and bruxism (spasm of the jaw muscles). It appears to have a low addictive potential, but long-term use may cause some cerebral damage. It is a far from safe drug.

Barbiturates

Until some time after the Second World War barbiturates were the most commonly used hypnotic and sedative drugs. It is now realized that prolonged use, particularly in large doses, can lead to dependence. The addict is drowsy, ataxic and examination frequently shows nystagmus. Sudden withdrawal produces well-marked symptoms with anxiety, vomiting and epileptic fits.

Benzodiazepines (see p. 158)

Cannabis (marihuana, hemp)

Cannabis is a resin obtained from a plant which is widely grown in America, Africa and Asia. It is usually smoked but can be taken by mouth. It produces mild excitement combined with a feeling of relaxation and peace. Perception of time is distorted and the passage of time is slowed ('spaced-out') and the subjects may be hungry ('the munchies'). The conjunctivae appear red due to vasodilatation.

Substances related to cannabis (cannabinoids) have been used as anti-emetics for patients who are being treated with cytotoxic drugs.

Cannabis is illegal in the UK, but whether it is more addictive and socially more undesirable than alcohol is a matter of debate.

The main arguments against its legalization are:

1. Repeated use, particularly in high doses, can reduce motivation and interfere with the subject's life. Rarely, it can cause a psychotic state with hallucinations and disorientation.

2. The use of cannabis may lead a person on to take more seriously addictive drugs such as heroin. Although this happens infrequently, most heroin addicts have passed through a phase of using cannabis.

3. Cannabis is a drug of dependence in that there are withdrawal symptoms (anxiety and sleeplessness) and tolerance develops.

Volatile solvents

Various substances contain organic solvents which are volatile and highly fat soluble and therefore easily penetrate the brain causing depression of the cerebral function with euphoria and occasional hallucination.

The problem of 'glue sniffing' has become serious among teenagers and may prove difficult to control as the use of these solvents is widespread.

Hallucinogens

Some drugs cause severe disturbances of cerebral function. The best known of these is **lysergic acid diethylamide (LSD)**. This drug causes hallucinations combined with a variety of mental abnormalities. A return to normal mental function usually occurs, although in some subjects the symptoms persist and others do themselves serious damage while under the influence of the drug. It is doubtful whether such substances have any place in medical treatment.

Mescaline and **psilocybin (magic mushroom)** are similar.

Alcohol

Alcohol presents a special problem as moderate amounts are taken for social reasons by many people and may, in fact, even be beneficial. Dependence on alcohol is very common and its management is a difficult medical and social problem. It occurs most often in those countries where alcoholic drinks are cheap, for instance the United States and France. Not only does it frequently lead to moral and financial breakdown for the patient, but it is a tragedy for his/her family.

Alcohol causes both acute and chronic disorders. Acute consumption of excessive amounts of alcohol produces a deterioration of brain function with changes in behaviour progressing through slurred speech and unsteady gait to unconsciousness.

The relationship between blood concentration and effect is given below:

Blood level	Effect
20 mg/100 ml	Relaxed
30 mg/100 ml	Talkative
50 mg/100 ml	A little uncoordinated (knocks over glass)
100 mg/100 ml	Fall about, vomiting
300 mg/100 ml	Stupor

There is considerable interperson variation.

One half-pint of beer or one glass of wine or one single of spirits raises the blood alcohol level to about 10–20 mg/100 ml. Normally alcohol is rapidly absorbed from the gastrointestinal tract, though food may slow absorption. Peak blood levels are reached in about 1 hour. It is largely metabolized in the liver, though small amounts are excreted in the urine and breath.

Given the same dose of alcohol, women have a higher blood level and appear more prone to develop alcohol-related diseases. This is partly because they are generally smaller than men so the volume of distribution is less, but also because, in women, less alcohol is broken down as it passes from the gastrointestinal tract via the liver to the circulation (greater bioavailability).

Hangovers follow excessive intake of alcohol, although there is considerable interperson variation in their severity. The symptoms of headache, thirst, anxiety and nausea are familiar. To some degree they depend on the type of alcoholic beverage consumed. Brandy is the worst culprit and vodka, the least likely to provoke symptoms. This is because brandy contains substances, other than alcohol, which are toxic. Other factors involved are dehydration, hypoglycaemia, tachycardia, gastric irritability, excessive smoking and lack of sleep.

Chronic alcoholism damages several organs. In the *nervous system* abuse leads to tremor, failure of memory, confusion with ultimate dementia and peripheral neuritis. Some of these changes are linked to vitamin B1 deficiency.

The *liver* may be damaged, leading ultimately to cirrhosis, the *stomach* may develop gastritis and alcohol can affect the *heart muscle* resulting in atrial fibrillation and cardiomyopathy. In addition, high alcohol consumption raises blood pressure and may be a factor in precipitating strokes. Chronic alcoholics are specially prone to *infection* and have a high incidence of tuberculosis.

It is now recognized that excessive consumption of alcohol during pregnancy causes the *fetal alcohol syndrome* with mild mental retardation, small head, turned-up nose and other facial abnormalities.

Alcohol intake. The intake of alcohol is usually measured in terms of units per day or per week.

One unit = Half pint of beer
One glass of wine
One glass of sherry or port
One measure of spirits

Each of these contains about 8 g (10 ml) of alcohol.

A 'safe' level of daily alcohol consumption is very difficult to establish, but a frequently quoted figure is three units per day for a man and two units per day for a woman* and there is now

---

*The Department of Health has recommended four units daily for men and three units for women. Some experts consider this to be too high.

considerable evidence that moderate consumption of alcohol protects against coronary artery disease. It should however be remembered that even if the average intake of alcohol is within the safe range, a bout of high intake is associated with an increased risk of accident and injury.

Treatment. Withdrawal of alcohol from a dependent person leads to tremor, anxiety tachycardia, and vomiting.

Sedation is best achieved with diazepam, starting with 30–50 mg daily and reducing the dose stepwise over 10 days. Clormethiazole is excellent at relieving symptoms, but has its own dependence risk. It is common practice to give large doses of vitamins in the early stages of treatment as deficiency of the vitamin B group may play a part in producing symptoms.

Delirium tremens is a more serious withdrawal disorder with hallucination and disorientation and the patient may be violent. The mortality is around 5%. In these circumstances diazepam (in the form of Diazemuls) may have to be given in 10 mg doses i.v. and repeated as required. Alternately, chlormethiazole can be given by infusion (see p. 134). Because it is normally broken down in the liver, reduced dosage may be required in alcoholics. Vitamins should be given as above and fluid and electrolytes corrected as necessary.

Most alcoholics should give up drinking completely and this requires considerable supportive treatment. Occasionally they may be helped by giving *disulfiram*. This drug inhibits the breakdown of alcohol, producing toxic substances which cause flushing, nausea and headaches and thus the patient is discouraged from further drinking. Alternatively, **acamprosate**, a centrally acting drug which modifies the GABA system, can be used. It reduces the risk of relapse and is started immediately after withdrawal and continued for 1 year.

Alcohol and driving

Increasing doses of alcohol produce a progressive deterioration in physical and mental performance. This is particularly important as it may cause road traffic accidents. Drunk in charge of a car is a serious offence, but the definition of drunkenness is difficult. In the UK it is an offence to have more than 80 mg of alcohol per 100 ml of blood while in charge of a car.

Nicotine

Nicotine is a constituent of tobacco smoke. It stimulates the autonomic nervous system (raised blood pressure and pulse rate) and has a mild cocaine-like stimulant action on the brain. It causes both psychic and physical dependence. Unfortunately, its use is associated with an increased incidence of several diseases, most notably:

- Cancer of the lung, lip and tongue
- Chronic bronchitis and emphysema
- Coronary artery disease
- Peripheral vascular disease.

The death rate among smokers is about twice that of non-smokers and the figure is higher for heavy smokers, whose life expectancy is reduced by about 5 years. Stopping smoking results in a progressive improvement in prognosis.

Withdrawal symptoms include craving for nicotine, constipation and increased appetite.

Nursing point

Compared with other women nurses have a particularly high smoking rate, probably due to the stresses of their job. They should remember that, in addition to the risks outlined above, heavy smoking causes:

- Some reduction in fertility
- Raised perinatal mortality
- Increased risk of thrombosis in those taking oral contraceptives.

Treatment is difficult and requires high motivation on the part of the patient. Subjects vary in their method of withdrawal, some preferring to stop suddenly, others to slowly reduce the number of cigarettes smoked. Various aids such as nicotine chewing gum (Nicorette), skin patches or hypnosis may be used. The success rate at 1 year is about 25%.

Caffeine

Although caffeine is not a serious drug of addiction, transient symptoms of headaches, sleepiness and general depression occur when it is withdrawn from the diet. It is perhaps not generally realized that most people are taking caffeine regularly because, not only is it found in coffee, but also in other dietary components such as tea, chocolate, cocoa and Coca-Cola.

Occasionally, exclusion of caffeine from the diet will cure sleeplessness, anxiety and palpitations.

FURTHER READING

Benowitz N L 1997 Treating tobacco addiction; nicotine or no nicotine. New England Journal of Medicine 337: 1230

Ecstacy (MDMA) 1995 Alerting users to the dangers. Nursing Times 91:30

Editorial 1989 Cocaine and crack. British Medical Journal 299: 338

Farrell M et al 1994 Methadone maintenance treatment in opiate dependence. British Medical Journal 309: 997

Friedman G D, Khatsky A L 1993 Is alcohol good for your health? New England Journal of Medicine 329: 1882

Hall W, Zador D 1997 The alcohol withdrawal syndrome. Lancet 349: 1897

Hall W, Solowij N 1998 Adverse effects of cannabis. Lancet 352: 1611

Henningfield J E 1995 Drug therapy: nicotine medications for smoking cessation. New England Journal of Medicine 333: 1196

Interdepartmental Working Group 1995 Sensible Drinking. London Department of Health

O'Connor P G, Schottenfield R S 1998 Patients with alcohol problems. New England Journal of Medicine 338: 592

Preston A 1992 Substance abuse: pointing the risk. Nursing Times 88 (13): 24

Sievewright N A, Greenwood J 1996 What is important in drug misuse treatment? Lancet 347: 373

Swift R M 1999 Drug therapy for alcohol dependence. New England Journal of Medicine 340: 1482

White I R 1996 The cardioprotective effects of moderate alcohol consumption. British Medical Journal 312: 1179

Woodrow P 1998 The effects of 'ecstasy'. Nursing Standard 12: 39

25

Drugs and the eye

The structure of the eye and orbit is shown in Figure 25.1.

The following types of drug are in frequent use in the treatment of eye disorders:

1. Antibiotics
2. Steroids and other anti-inflammatory drugs
3. Those which affect pupil size
4. Those used in the treatment of glaucoma
5. Local anaesthetics
6. Stains
7. Miscellaneous preparations.

Drugs can be administered to the eye either by local or systemic routes.

LOCAL USE OF DRUGS ON THE EYE

The following preparations are used in the local treatment of eye diseases: eye lotions, eye drops, eye ointments, subconjunctival injections or ampoules for injection into the anterior chamber at operation.

Whenever administering local preparations to the eye it is of paramount importance to ensure that the eye to receive treatment is clearly designated. Often only one eye is to be treated or the two eyes are to be treated differently. For example, after an operation for angle closure glaucoma in one eye it may be necessary to dilate the pupil with drugs called mydriatics. Such treatment given to the other eye could be disastrous.

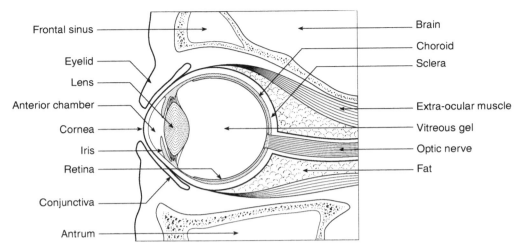

Figure 25.1 Cross-section anatomy of eye and orbit.

Eye lotions prescribed as collyrium

These are used to wash foreign material from the eye and some have a mild antiseptic action. They are applied from an *undine*, which is a small glass container with a fine spout and which resembles a miniature chemistry retort. In an emergency, however, if a little jug is at hand it will serve as well and may save vital minutes in treating a contaminated eye. The patient should lie back or sit in a chair with the head extended. The lotion should be warmed to 35°C (95°F) and before washing the eye it should be run up the cheek into the medial canthus, the lids being firmly separated by the fingers and a small basin held by the patient close to his or her face to catch the effluent. This is less unpleasant than pouring the lotion directly onto the cornea. The lotion should be steadily poured from the undine, the patient being instructed to move their eyes in all directions. There are many types of lotion, but simple normal saline is satisfactory for the removal of foreign material or dirt from the eye. In emergency cases, however, as in chemical contamination, it is better to use plain cold tap water than to lose time in starting the treatment.

In cases of contamination by lime or cement an irrigation with *dihydrogen sodium versenate* is recommended. This substance is a chelating agent and has the action of converting an insoluble heavy metal salt, such as calcium hydroxide, into a soluble complex anion which can be removed in solution.

Eye drops prescribed as guttae

A number of drugs can be applied to the eyes by means of drops which should be instilled into the lower conjunctival sac. The patient is told to look upwards away from the dropper and the lower lid is held down with the finger. One drop only is instilled into the lower fornix and the patient is then told to close their eye for a short while and the excess is wiped away.

All drops and ointment should be sterile when supplied and once opened can no longer be considered so. There is an increasing tendency for them to be dispensed in single dose containers which can be discarded after use. This is particularly useful for patients who require medication over long periods and who may develop

---

Nursing point

Drugs or preservatives in eye drops may become absorbed into hydrophilic contact lenses and cause irritation. Therefore, lenses should be removed before eye drops are instilled and not worn again until treatment is finished. Similarly, contact lenses should not be used with eye ointments.

sensitivity to benzalkonium chloride, the preservative present in most eye drops.

Eye ointments prescribed as oculentum

These can be applied similarly either on a glass rod or from a single dose container; the lower lid is pulled down and the ointment is placed in the lower fornix. About half an inch of ointment as squeezed from the tube should be used at each application. This should be delivered onto the end of a sterile glass rod or a prepacked plastic spatula. A separate applicator should be used for each eye if both are to be treated.

Subconjunctival injections

This method of application is used to obtain immediately a high concentration of a drug in the anterior chamber. This would be appropriate in the treatment of an acute intra-ocular infection.

This treatment is painful and the eye must first be thoroughly anaesthetized by the instillation of several drops of local anaesthetic. Injection is made with a hypodermic syringe and a fine needle.

Some drugs are manufactured in a depot form and are bound to a base substance from which they are released slowly. For example *Depo-Medrone* can be used as a steroid preparation for the local treatment of iridocyclitis. It is given as a subconjunctival injection and its action is continuous over a period of 3–4 days.

Intracameral administration

In certain disorders, it may be desirable to achieve high therapeutic concentrations of antibiotic drugs with a minimum of delay. This calls for delivery of the drug directly into the globe of the eye, either into the anterior chamber or the vitreous cavity.

Anterior chamber administration is frequently used during cataract operations when, to constrict the pupil, the iris is irrigated directly with Miochol, which is an acetylcholine preparation.

In severe intra-ocular infections—for example,

postoperative endophthalmitis—it may be necessary to remove a sample of the vitreous for bacteriological examination. It is then expeditious to inject the vitreous cavity with broad spectrum antibiotics. Several modern antibiotics can be used in this way, although care is needed to avoid any toxic effects on the delicate intra-ocular structures such as the retina. Consequently, the injections need to be carefully prepared and used only in the recommended dosage, and administration should generally be under sterile theatre conditions.

ANTIBIOTICS

Antibiotics are used to treat a wide range of eye infections and they may be administered in three ways:

1. Drops are satisfactory for superficial inflammation such as conjunctivitis, but rapid dilution occurs because of the tears. The drops should be instilled at 2-hourly intervals at least if a reasonable concentration of antibiotic is to be maintained.

2. Ointments release the antibiotic more slowly and their action is helped by the eye being covered.

3. Subconjunctival injection is the best way of ensuring a rapid and high concentration of antibiotic within the anterior ocular segment. The maximum volume which can be injected at one time is 1.0–1.5 ml.

Although, owing to the accessibility of the eye, diseases of the anterior segment can usually be effectively treated by means of the local administration of drugs, for those diseases which affect the posterior part, or the deeper intra-ocular structures, systemic administration is generally necessary.

Eye infections may be due to a variety of agents, both bacterial and viral. The correct antibiotic can be selected as a result of clinical observation and bacterial or viral studies.

The aminoglycosides and chloramphenicol are widely used in the treatment of superficial eye infections. They are active against a broad spectrum of bacteria and are particularly suitable for local administration as this avoids systemic toxicity. They include:

- Chloramphenicol 0.5% drops or 1.0% ointment
- Fusidic acid eye drops 1% in gel base
- Neomycin 0.5% drops and ointment
- Gentamicin 0.3% drops
- Ampoules of gentamicin sulphate 40 mg/ml for subconjunctival injection.

These drugs are active against both Gram-positive and Gram-negative organisms.

The use of *chloramphenicol* has been questioned on account of its tendency to cause blood dyscrasias when given systemically. The evidence that these can arise as a result of local administration to the eye is still far from conclusive. Chloramphenicol remains in general use as it is by far the most effective drug for short-term use in bacterial infections of the eye and for prophylaxis. Fusidic acid, which is used as a substitute, can be effective, especially against straphylococci.

Ofloxacin, a member of the quinolone group, has a broader spectrum of antibacterial action than chloramphenicol and other commonly used antibiotics. It has fewer local side-effects than gentamicin and appears to have a similar spectrum of activity. It rivals chloramphenicol as a general prophylactic antibiotic.

The tetracyclines are wide spectrum antibiotics against bacteria which also show activity against certain viruses and *Rickettsia*, particularly those causing trachoma. Tetracycline is available as a 1% ointment and its use together with systemic administration has helped to bring this widespread and blinding condition under control.

Two ocular disorders which respond well to prolonged administration of systemic tetracycline in low dosage are chronic staphylococal blepharitis (inflammation of the eyelid margins) and ocular involvement in cutaneous acne rosacea. Here the usual dose is 250 mg daily for a period of up to 6 months.

Tetracyclines are contraindicated in young patients before eruption of the second dentition as the permanent teeth can be discoloured. The same caution must apply in administration during pregnancy.

Antibiotics of the penicillin group are rarely, if ever, used as local eye applications as they have a marked tendency to cause allergic reactions. However, they have an important place in the treatment of spreading infections of the eyelids, which are commonly of staphylococcal origin. In such cases the infection is deep in the tissues requiring systemic rather than local administration. In general, a broad spectrum penicillin is best, but if the infection is acquired in hospital one of the penicillinase-resistant type is preferable.

Sodium fusidate is particularly active against penicillin-resistant staphylococci. It has the property of being concentrated in bone and other connective tissues, including the sclera of the eye and the vitreous, and is therefore useful in treating intra-ocular infections, especially those acquired in the operating theatre which can often be due to resistant organisms. Dosage is 500 mg 8 hourly for 5 days. Fusidic acid is also used as eye drops in gel which liquefies on contact with the conjunctiva for a variety of superficial infections.

Frequently after *major intra-ocular operations*, antibiotics are injected subconjunctivally. Prophylaxis against postoperative infection is gaining importance in the face of a growing trend for major surgery, in particular for cataract, to be performed on an outpatient basis. For this purpose gentamicin is often used. This drug, however, causes a degree of toxic damage to the periocular tissues. **Cefuroxime** has recently proved less troublesome in this respect.

Bacterial conjunctivitis

Conjunctivitis is a common complaint with various causes. The bacterial infection is usually by *S. pneumonii* or, more rarely, staphylococci.

Treatment is with chloramphenicol eye drops, every 4 hours, but more florid infections may require more frequent application. Chloramphenicol ointment may be used at night. The alternative is fusidic acid eye drops twice daily.

Acute intra-ocular infections

In acute bacterial infection of the eye much of the damage occurs as a result of the inflammatory response rather than the direct activity of the bacteria. Consequently, it is important to use steroids at the same time as effective antibiotics.

A particular problem exists in severe intraocular infections such as those following eye surgery. It is essential that vigorous antibiotic and anti-inflammatory treatment is started without delay. Otherwise, if the eye is not completely destroyed, it may well lose all useful vision. As time cannot be allowed to obtain the results of bacterial investigations before commencing treatment, a combination of broad spectrum antibiotics and steroids can be used by both subconjunctival and systemic routes and even by direct intravitreal injection, together with a mydriatic.

A combination of antibiotics, steroids and mydriatics which has for many years achieved great success and is still widely used, can be given as follows:

Locally: Framycetin 0.8 ml
(equivalent to
500 mg   by
Cefuroxime 100 mg   subconjunctival
Gentamicin 20 mg   injection
Betnesol 4 mg
Mydricaine 0.3 ml
Orally: Fucidin 500 mg b.d.
Prednisolone 15 mg
q.i.d.

Systemic administration of antibiotics can be either orally or by injection. Their use may be indicated in spreading infections involving the eye, the eyelids and ocular adnexa such as the lacrimal sac. Sepsis around the eye, in particular in the vicinity of the internal angular vein, is of particular clinical importance as it may lead to a septic cavernous sinus thrombosis.

Other antibiotics*

In certain severe cases of intra-ocular infection the following antibiotics have been used success-

*Some of these antibiotic preparations are only available in specialist units and hospitals.

fully when injected directly into the vitreous. Preparations of a suitable strength for intraocular injection are not available yet and the following method of dilution has been devised at Moorfields Eye Hospital.

Vancomycin is effective against Gram-positive bacteria. The injection should contain 1.0 mg dissolved in 0.05 ml of injectable saline and should be prepared as follows. A vial containing 500 mg vancomycin is reconstituted in 8 ml normal saline. The entire contents are then withdrawn and made up to 10 ml, giving a concentration of 50 mg/ml. A volume of 2 ml of this solution is returned to the vial and is further diluted by the addition of 3 ml of normal saline, resulting in a concentration of 20 mg/ml. The therapeutic volume of 0.05 ml, containing 1 mg, is withdrawn into an insulin syringe for intravitreal injection.

Ceftazidime is active against Gram-negative organisms and can be used simultaneously with vancomycin. The therapeutic dose is 2 mg in 0.1 ml, which is the same concentration as for vancomycin and the injection is prepared similarly.

Amikacin treats infections from a wide spectrum of Gram-negative organisms, but its toxicity to the intra-ocular tissues precludes more than one injection. The dose is 0.4 mg in 0.1 ml and is prepared as follows. A vial of non-preserved amikacin with a concentration of 250 mg/ml is required and 2.0 ml is withdrawn. This is diluted up to 10 ml with normal saline, giving a concentration of 50 mg/ml. A 9.0 ml volume is discarded and the remaining 1.0 ml is made up with saline to 12.5 ml to a concentration of 4 mg/ml. The injection of 0.1 ml, containing 0.4 mg of amikacin, is drawn into an insulin syringe.

Amphotericin is used to treat fungal infections such as candida. The therapeutic dose is 0.005 mg in 0.1 ml, and is prepared as follows. A vial containing 50 mg is reconstituted using 10 ml of water for injection (WFI). A 1.0 ml volume is withdrawn and further diluted with WFI up to 10 ml. All but 1.0 ml is discarded and this is made up to 10 ml, using 5% dextrose, giving a concentration of 0.05 mg/ml. The injection of

0.1 ml containing 0.005 mg of amphotericin, is withdrawn into an insulin syringe.

Several more recently developed antibiotics have been used systemically to supplement the effect of those given by intravitreal injection, chief among which are:

Cefazolin which, with few exceptions, is effective against Gram-positive organisms which are sensitive to methicillin. The therapeutic dose is 1 g four times daily, as an intravenous injection, and it may take from 36 to 48 hours to achieve a satisfactory concentration in the vitreous.

Ciprofloxacin is used to treat a wide range of Gram-negative organisms and is similarly effective against many Gram-positive types.

ANTIVIRAL AGENTS

Many eye infections are due to a virus. To mention some of the more common ones, herpes simplex, adenovirus and herpes zoster are all infections that are frequently seen clinically. **Idoxuridine** (*IDU*) was the first generally available antiviral agent and it was and still is effective against the herpes simplex virus that causes dendritic ulceration of the cornea. This drug was available for ocular application under the name of *Kerecid* but is now withdrawn.

A similar preparation called *Herpid* is available for general cutaneous treatment, for example in herpes zoster (shingles). *One warning*, however—Herpid also contains dimethyl sulphoxide which aids cutaneous absorption, but which causes cataracts if applied in the region of the eye. It must therefore *never* be used to treat the eyes or eyelids.

Idoxuridine acts as a competitive inhibitor in that it competes for DNA, an essential component of the virus. For this reason to be effective the concentration in the conjunctival sac had to be maintained at a high level. Prolonged use of IDU led to unwanted toxic effects on the corneal epithelial cells and is no longer available.

As a treatment for ocular herpes simplex infections, the more recently developed *aciclovir* has become the drug of choice. It is highly effective when applied in the form of a 3% ointment five times daily and has minimal, if any, toxic effects. Its action can be supplemented by oral administration and this may well be helpful in cases of herpes simplex keratitis which have been previously treated in error with preparations containing steroids, which greatly reduce the rate of healing. The initial dose is 200 mg five times daily for five days, but owing to the variable absorption from the gastro-intestinal tract, the course may need to be repeated at higher doses.

Herpes zoster may affect the eye, especially when it involves the naso-ciliary branch of the ophthalmic division of the trigeminal nerve. Provided that treatment is commenced at the first appearance of the vesicular rash, aciclovir can significantly reduce the severity of this distressing disorder. For this purpose, however, higher doses are required and 800 mg is given orally, five times daily for five days. When successful, it shortens the time before cutaneous healing occurs and materially reduces the pain in the acute stage and also the post-herpetic pain which often lasts for many years after healing has taken place.

As an antiviral drug **trifluorothymidine (F3T)** shows good activity against herpes simplex. Its main use, however, is against the adenovirus which causes an unpleasant and prolonged acute conjunctivitis, often with corneal involvement which to some extent affects vision, albeit temporarily. In these cases it is the drug of choice as none of the other antiviral drugs has an effect on this virus. It is not readily available, but can often be obtained from the pharmacy of specialist eye hospitals. It is not a particularly stable preparation and must be freshly prepared and kept refrigerated.

ANTIPROTOZOAN DRUGS

Onchocerciasis is a protozoan infection of the eye which is not uncommon in some tropical countries in Africa and South America. This disease is spread by flies which transfer the microfilariae from one human host, who harbours the adult worms in cutaneous nodules, to another individual in whom they spread throughout the body. In the eye they set up inflammation in both the superficial and deeper tissues. Typically they can be seen with a microscope, swimming in the aqueous humour. The drug of choice for treating this disorder is *ivermectin*, which is a semi-synthetic macrocyclic lactone. This is given as a single dose of 150 micrograms/kg and can be repeated after 6–12 months. At the time of writing it is available only from the manufacturer on a named-patient basis.

Since the generalized use of hydrophilic (soft) contact lenses, especially those of the non-sterilizable or disposable type, infections of the cornea with *acanthamoeba* have occurred more often. Diagnosis is made by microscopic examination of deep corneal scrapings and treatment is with the drug *cosmocil*. This is a sterilizing agent with the chemical name polyhexamethylene-biguanide. It is chemically related to chlorhexidine, which has also been used to treat acanthamoeba. Both drugs are made up in 0.02% strength and are applied as eye drops. Neither preparation is generally available and can only be obtained from the pharmacy of certain specialized eye units, such as Moorfields Eye Hospital, at present.

STEROIDS AND OTHER ANTI-INFLAMMATORY DRUGS

The most commonly used steroid for local ophthalmic application is **betamethasone disodium phosphate (Betnesol)**. This can be used in 0.1% drops or ointment. In some preparations the steroid is combined with an antibiotic, for example—*Betnesol-N* contains neomycin. Application can be as frequent as hourly and drugs of this type are used to suppress a wide variety of inflammatory processes within the eye. Steroids should not be used indiscriminately as their improper use may be followed by serious complications. This is particularly so for infective processes which may spread rapidly if steroids are given without a suitable antibacterial agent.

For similar reasons they are rarely applied to virus infections of the eye and never in the presence of active *herpes simplex* (dendritic ulcer).

Administration of *dilute* steroid eye drops is, on the contrary, often beneficial in the treatment of herpetic corneal infection. This, however, is when corneal stromal opacification threatens and *when the viral activity has already been contained*. For this purpose prednisolone eye drops of 0.1% administered two or three times daily can, by suppressing the antibody–antigen reaction in the deeper layers of the cornea, prevent serious loss of vision. For local administration in the form of eye drops, **dexamethasone (Maxidex)** is often used. This drug has good penetration into the eye and is useful in the routine treatment of inflammatory disorders such as iritis. It is available in 1% solution and may be combined with neomycin; it is marketed as 'Maxitrol'.

In severe ocular inflammation a subconjunctival injection of **methylprednisolone acetate (Depomedrone)** produces a continuous level of steroids in the anterior chamber for several days.

In inflammation of the posterior uvea (choroiditis) it is necessary to administer steroids systemically as local applications do not readily reach the site of the disease. Here prednisolone may be used and is generally given in a very high dosage for a short period, followed by a rapid reduction at first which is tailed off more slowly. A usual starting dose may be prednisolone 60 mg a day in divided doses, but on occasions as much as 80–100 mg may be given for a few days.

All steroid drugs, whether administered locally or systemically, can result in a rise in intra-ocular pressure. A steroid more recently developed and named **fluoromethalone** can be used for local administration. It has been shown to be relatively free of the unwanted side-effects that are characteristic of other steroid drugs. It has proved particularly useful in the management of chronic allergic conjunctival inflammations.

For superficial inflammation of allergic origin such as vernal conjunctivitis, a histamine antagonist such as **sodium cromoglicate** is often useful. To be effective the concentration in the conjunctival sac must be maintained at a high level necessitating frequent or continuous administration. This must be done over the entire period of exposure to the antigen, i.e. throughout the pollen season.

NSAIDs. The value of NSAIDs for ocular use lies in their anti-prostaglandin effect. In cataract surgery, prostaglandins are liberated as a response to tissue trauma. These mediators of inflammation can cause constriction of the pupil with consequent surgical difficulties. **Diclofenac sodium**, as a preservative-free 0.1% solution marketed as *Voltarol Ophtha*, seems to protect against this effect.

There is also evidence that patients who receive NSAIDs preoperatively show a lower incidence of macular oedema following cataract removal.

DRUGS WHICH AFFECT PUPIL SIZE

These can be divided into those which enlarge the pupil (*mydriatics*) and those which constrict it (*miotics*).

Mydriatics

Mydriatics are of two sorts:

1. Those which cause paralysis of the muscular sphincter of the iris. The sphincter muscle is innervated by the parasympathetic nervous system and drugs which inhibit it are called parasympatholytic drugs (see p. 35).
2. Those which stimulate contraction of the radial dilator pupillae muscle which is sympathetically innervated. Such drugs are called sympathomimetics (see p. 35).

Parasympatholytic drugs

One of the earliest known drugs of this type is **atropine**, which is the active principle in the poisonous berry of the deadly nightshade plant. Its mydriatic properties have been known for centuries and in the Middle Ages it was used as a cosmetic, hence the name belladonna. Today one of its main uses is to dilate the pupil in patients with iritis, where the inflamed iris goes into spasm and adheres to the lens of the eye causing blindness. Because the ciliary muscle has the same nerve supply as the sphincter muscle of the iris, atropine can be used to paralyse the focusing of the eye (accommodation) for sight testing young children.

It is commonly used as eye drops of 1% or 0.5% strength and in the form of ointment. The action of this drug lasts for 18 days and it is not reversible by means of miotics. It is, therefore, unsuitable for dilating the pupil for fundal examination.

It is also dangerous as, in patients with narrow anterior chamber angles, acute angle closure glaucoma can result which will not respond to miotic treatment and will almost certainly require an emergency operation.

For most purposes a mydriatic with a shorter duration of action is appropriate. **Homatropine**, which is a homologue of atropine, can be used in 1% or 2% strengths. This has a rapid action, producing pupillary enlargement in 5–10 minutes and its effect rarely lasts for more than 24 hours and can be reversed with miotics.

A synthetic drug **cyclopentolate** is now commonly used as a mydriatic and also as a cycloplegic for sight tests in young children, in whom it is necessary to abolish their accommodation. It has a very short duration of action (about 4 hours). Its action is reversed by physostigmine eye drops.

Another short-acting mydriatic is **tropicamide** which, although it is a rapid pupillary dilator, is a weak cycloplegic and causes less blurring of vision. It is therefore useful for clinical fundal examination as it has only a slight effect on the patient's ability to read afterwards.

Sympathomimetic drugs

A typical drug is **phenylephrine**, which is used as eye drops in 10% strength. *Ephedrine* is another and also *cocaine*, which can be combined with *homatropine* to make up 'guttae H and C'. The cocaine is used at a concentration of 2% which is sufficient for it to be a controlled drug.

Sympathomimetic drugs can be used synergically to assist those of the parasympatholytic group in cases where dilatation is difficult. A particularly useful preparation named Mydricaine is available in two strengths. It contains atropine, epinephrine and procaine and is given by sub-conjunctival injection.

Miotics

Miotic drugs all act on the sphincter muscle of the iris, either directly or indirectly constricting the pupil.

Pilocarpine is used to treat chronic glaucoma. It is available in strengths of 1–4% in the form of eye drops.

A synthetic miotic called **ecothiopate** has been widely used when strong pupillary constriction is required. Unfortunately, with prolonged use it produces cysts of the iris epithelium which may largely occlude the small, miotic pupil, thereby severely reducing vision. It can now only be used under expert supervision.

During intra-ocular surgery such as cataract extraction, a rapid miosis may be required and can be achieved by the injection of *acetylcholine* directly into the anterior chamber. It is marketed as 'Miochol', a dry powder in a sterile ampoule containing its own diluent fluid. Mixing is done by breaking an inner seal but as the preparation has limited stability, it should be made up just before use. Its effect is dramatic but short-lived. After the insertion of an iris-supported acrylic lens replacement, a longer-acting miotic is often advisable.

DRUGS USED IN THE TREATMENT OF GLAUCOMA

Primary glaucoma is of two types, the *chronic open angle type* and that due to *acute angle closure*. These are two entirely different diseases, but the one common factor is that the eye pressure is raised above normal by the failure of the aqueous humour to pass through the outflow channels. The continuous secretion of aqueous by the ciliary body causes a build-up of pressure within the eye.

Drugs used in the treatment of glaucoma can be divided into two groups. Those which facilitate the outflow of the aqueous and those which reduce its production by the ciliary body. In angle closure the draining of aqueous into the canal of Schlemm through the trabecular meshwork is obstructed by the root of the iris. To treat this disorder miotics are used to constrict the iris sphincter muscle and pull the root of the iris centrally, thus relieving the obstruction. In patients with shallow anterior chambers and therefore narrow angles, both mydriatics and strong miotics can precipitate acute glaucoma. These are termed either mydriatic glaucoma or, in the case of miotics, paradoxical glaucoma. In such subjects both groups of drugs should be used with extreme caution.

Drugs modifying the autonomic nervous system

In acute angle closure glaucoma, intensive administration of 4% pilocarpine eye drops is often the first part of the treatment. This means giving one drop a minute for 5 minutes, one every 5 minutes for half an hour and quarter-hourly thereafter. If this is successful in re-opening the angle, the pupil will become small and the corneal oedema will clear in an hour or so.

It is easy to see why miotics are effective in angle closure glaucoma as they help outflow by relieving the obstruction of the drainage angle. It is more difficult to understand why they should work in glaucoma of the open angle type. It has, however, been shown that they act by speeding up the passage of aqueous humour through the trabecular meshwork, which is the band of specialized tissue which separates the anterior chamber from the canal of Schlemm, thus increasing the facility of outflow. In chronic open angle glaucoma pilocarpine is frequently used in strengths of between 1% and 4% applied four times a day as it is only effective for 6 hours.

Neutral epinephrine 1% (Eppy) has proved effective in controlling the intra-ocular pressure in cases of open angle glaucoma. It is, however, contraindicated in eyes with narrow angles where the pupillary dilatation could cause angle closure and precipitate an acute attack. It has two actions: that mediated by α receptors brings about an increase in the facility of aqueous outflow and that mediated by the β receptors causes a reduction in aqueous secretion. These two actions thus combine to lower the intra-ocular pressure.

It is usually enough for the drops to be administered twice daily. They are normally clear and are best kept at 4°C as in a domestic refrigerator. They should be discarded if they turn amber or brown in colour as they are then inactive. As side-effects they can cause ocular irritation and reactive hyperaemia. This is annoying to the patient, but not often dangerous.

A useful innovation to improve absorption is known as a *prodrug* in which the drug is modified chemically so that it passes more readily into the eye. After absorption it is split, releasing the active constituent, an example being **dipivefrin hydrochloride**, which is converted by intra-ocular enzymes to epinephrine.

Guanethidine has also been used in open angle glaucoma. Its effect in lowering the pressure is often disappointing when used by itself. However, it has been found that when combined with neutral epinephrine there is a striking reduction of ocular pressure and a much weaker concentration of epinephrine can then be used. This helps to avoid the unwanted side-effects of the epinephrine. A preparation consisting of a mixture of guanethidine and epinephrine is now available and known as '*Ganda 305*'. This contains 3% guanethidine and 0.5% epinephrine. Other concentrations are also available.

Another drug which, acting as a β blocker, causes a reduction in aqueous secretion is **timolol**. This is marketed under the name of *Timoptol* in 0.25 and 0.5% strengths. It reduces the amount of aqueous humour that is formed and thereby lowers intra-ocular pressure. It has the advantage that it does not cause unwanted changes in pupillary size and is, therefore, a very useful drug in the treatment of open angle glaucoma. For this reason, however, it is not suitable for glaucoma of the closed angle type unless a miotic is used simultaneously. Another advantage of timolol is that, so far, it has been found not to have any irritative effects on the eye in strengths of 0.5% or less. It can, however, be absorbed systemically to an extent that it may produce an unwanted fall in blood pressure in some subjects, resulting in dizziness or even collapse. It is also contraindicated in patients with known asthma and care is needed in those with chronic obstructive airways disease. **Betaxolol** is similar, but is less likely to produce systemic effects. It seems to be less effective than timolol in lowering the intra-ocular pressure. There is, however, some evidence that its absorption via the conjunctiva results in a systemic effect which may increase the blood supply to the optic nerve.

Brimonidine tartrate (Alphagan) is available as 0.2% eye drops. It is an α_2 stimulant and can be used when β blockers are contraindicated; for example, in patients with asthma.

Latanoprost (Xalatin), another pressure-reducing agent, is a prostaglandin analogue whose action is to increase the aqueous outflow. It is used in patients whose glaucoma is resistant to other drugs or who are allergic to them.

Acetazolamide (see p. 218)

(see p. 218)

This has the action of inhibiting the enzyme carbonic anhydrase which is necessary for the secretion of aqueous humour. In acute glaucoma the drug is very useful, as by reducing the aqueous production the intra-ocular pressure can be at least temporarily lowered, and this may have the effect of allowing better penetration of locally applied anti-glaucoma treatment.

Acetazolamide may also be used to avoid having to operate on a hard and inflamed eye. It does, unfortunately, have some unwanted side-effects and its diuretic action may be inconvenient. It almost always causes paraesthesia of the extremities. Neither of these effects is permanent. Gastric irritation, nausea and depression are, however, more serious and if they occur the drug should be discontinued.

Acetazolamide is available in tablets of 250 mg and a full dose is 1 g daily in divided doses. The drug is also available as a sustained-release capsule of 250 mg and is prescribed as acetazolamide SR. The recommended dose is one or two capsules daily. It produces a more even action and, as it is absorbed in the intestine, avoids the gastric side-effects.

Dorzolamide (Trusopt) is a carbonic anhydrase inhibitor which can be administered locally in the form of eye drops. This is of value in view of the great reduction in side-effects. It can also be given in combination with other antiglaucoma drugs, and is best used in this way.

Dehydrating agents

Another method of reducing the pressure in acute glaucoma before surgery involves the intravenous infusion of certain hypertonic solutions which include such substances as *urea* and *mannitol*. These have the effect of producing a vigorous diuresis and cause dehydration of the bodily tissues including the eye and at the same time produce an inhibition in the secretion of aqueous. As an alternative to the use of intravenous infusion a similar, although less marked effect, can be produced by the ingestion of a strong *glycerine solution*.

ANAESTHETICS

Because the eye is a surface organ and covered with mucous membrane it is particularly amenable to topically applied anaesthetics which produce good operative conditions.

Cocaine has been in use for over a century, its application to ophthalmic surgery being first described in 1884. Although still one of the most effective drugs of its kind, it is no longer widely used owing to the advent of highly successful synthetic homologues. Also, as an unfortunate result of its frequent abuse, the stringent regulations which, of necessity, apply to all its legitimate clinical applications have reduced its popularity. In addition, it causes clouding of the corneal epithelium. Nevertheless, the impact it had on ophthalmic surgery when first introduced, will be appreciated if a moment's thought is given to the experience of an eye operation without anaesthesia of any kind!

For surface anaesthesia—that is, of the cornea and the conjunctival sac—*amethocaine* in a 1% solution produces rapid anaesthesia which lasts for up to 20 minutes. It does, however, cause stinging when first instilled and for this reason *oxybuprocaine* (Benoxinate) may be preferred, especially in children. The action of this drug is rapid, but less well sustained, which makes it very useful for accident and emergency work as corneal sensitivity is regained relatively soon.

For the performance of eye operations under local anaesthesia, an injection is often given behind the eyeball and within the cone of muscles that surround the optic nerve. This is known as *retrobulbar injection* and may only be given by someone who is medically qualified and trained to do so. For this purpose *lidocaine* 1% can be used, up to a total volume of 2–4 ml. When a prolonged period of analgesia is required, a mixture of *lidocaine* and *bupivacaine* is effective. All these anaesthetic agents can be combined with epinephrine, but these combinations are usually avoided by ophthalmic surgeons in view of the danger of injecting directly into an orbital vein.

A more recent technique involves the injection of local anaesthetic into the tissue space surrounding the globe and extra-ocular muscles of the eye, rather than directly into the muscle cone. This is known as peribulbar anaesthesia and is less likely to cause the embarrassing and highly inconvenient, if rarely dangerous, complication of a retrobulbar haemorrhage.

For this procedure a larger volume injection is given amounting to 8 or 10 ml. As a preliminary, the conjunctiva is anaesthetized using a few drops of amethocaine. A mixture of lidocaine and bupivacaine is used and a diluted fraction is injected into the medial and lateral angles and, after a minute or so, the remainder of the main injection is given into the peribulbar space, half medially and half laterally. Such a volume does cause an excessive pressure on the outside of the eye for intra-ocular surgery to be safely performed. A balloon is therefore secured onto the front of the closed eyelids with a Velcro strap and is inflated to a pressure of 40 mmHg. After 5 minutes all the excess fluid will have been dispersed from the orbit and the effect of the anaesthesia and akinesia (absence of movement) will be complete.

To ensure rapid spread of the local anaesthetic agent, a proteolytic enzyme called hyaluronidase ('Hyalase') is often included in the injection.

In cases in which an eye is both blind and painful, a retrobulbar injection of 95% ethyl alcohol can be given. This substance destroys the branches of the fifth (trigeminal) nerve in the orbit and renders the eye permanently anaesthetized. If the first injection does not produce the desired effect, a second is generally successful. This is always an extremely painful procedure which necessitates some form of anaesthesia and can be helped greatly by the prior injection of a local anaesthetic.

STAINS USED IN OPHTHALMOLOGY

Fluorescein

Fluorescein is applied locally to the eye to stain ulcers and abrasions of the cornea and thus allow them to be easily seen. It is usually dispensed dry in the form of impregnated paper strips, as in solution it tends to form a culture medium for infecting bacteria, especially *Pseudomonas*.

It can also be used in photographic investigations of patients with retinal diseases. Here it is injected rapidly intravenously using 5 ml of a 5% or 10% solution. As it passes through the retinal blood vessels it causes them to fluoresce and any leakage through blood vessel walls as, for instance, may occur in diabetic retinopathy, can be vividly demonstrated.

Rose bengal

This is a stain of carmine hue which is taken up actively by injured or infected cells. It is thus very useful detecting an active virus infection of the corneal epithelium; for example, in *herpes simplex*.

MISCELLANEOUS PREPARATIONS

There are many different eye drops designed to replace moisture when the tear film is deficient,

as in Sjögren's syndrome. These all contain a water-binding substance, often a higher molecular weight organic sugar such as hydroxymethylcellulose, **hypromellose eye drops** being a typical product. As this preparation drips leaving a white deposit, one containing polyvinyl alcohol may be preferred.

Another highly effective preparation to treat the 'dry eye' is an ophthalmic gel, marketed as *Viscotears*. Its main constituent is polyacrylic acid.

Fluorouracil. The use of this cytotoxic drug has found a place in eye surgery as it exerts a delaying effect on the healing of scleral wounds. This is useful after drainage operations for glaucoma. The drug is given as a subconjunctival injection into the lower fornix, taking care that the bleb does not abut on the cornea. A 0.2-ml volume containing 5 mg is injected daily for 5 days. This dose is so small that serious side-effects are avoided.

DRUGS WITH ADVERSE EFFECTS ON THE EYE

Many drugs in general use have an unwanted and often disastrous effect on the eye. *Nurses in charge of patients receiving these drugs should be aware of the likely problems as their early recognition may help to avoid permanent ocular damage and possibly total blindness.* It should be remembered that where a drug is being administered systemically both eyes may be at risk. Some of the more important drugs are now described.

Chloroquine was first used as an antimalarial drug and now plays a part in the management of rheumatoid disorders and tropical diseases. It can cause opacities in the cornea and a toxic effect in the retinae. The corneal disorder is reversible when the treatment is stopped, but that in the retina is permanent and visual loss can be severe. The maximum safe dose is in the region of 250 mg a day over a period of 1 year and toxicity is very unlikely to occur if the dose of chloroquine phosphate does not exceed 4 mg/kg per day. All patients receiving this drug should be under regular ophthalmic supervision.

Drugs affecting the autonomic nervous system. A variety of drugs have a sympathomimetic or anticholinergic action as their primary or secondary effects. These include bronchodilators such as ephedrine and others used in asthma and bronchitis, antidepressants of the tricyclic group and drugs used for Parkinsonism such as benzhexol or levodopa.

All these drugs have dangers when used in patients with glaucoma, but here a distinction must be made between the open and the closed angle types of disease. A patient with open angle glaucoma may merely show a relative increase in the resistance to aqueous outflow, with the result that the ocular pressure becomes more difficult to control. One with narrow filtration angles, however, may suffer an acute attack which can be bilateral, resulting in rapid and perhaps complete blindness. In the open angle type the use of such drugs may be justified provided the risk is recognized and the glaucoma treatment suitably adjusted. In patients with narrow angle filtration these drugs should be avoided unless they are essential. When in doubt an ophthalmic opinion should be sought.

Corticosteroids which are widely used to suppress the inflammatory response, can have serious side-effects on the eye. They are also used as immunosuppressants in the longer term following organ transplantation. Such patients are subject to three major side-effects on the eye.

Steroids can, as previously mentioned, precipitate a corneal infection with herpes simplex, but with prolonged administration they can induce glaucoma of the open angle variety and can cause cataracts. The two latter effects can be produced by either local or systemic administration.

Ethambutol. This antituberculous agent can cause inflammation of the optic nerve with some visual disturbance. Fortunately, these effects regress spontaneously when treatment is discontinued and are less common if the dose of the drug does not exceed 15 mg/kg daily.

Amiodarone is very effective in treating some types of cardiac arrhythmias. It does, however, produce corneal deposits similar in appearance to those caused by chloroquine. Fortunately, retinal side-effects are absent and the corneal changes do not affect vision.

Tamoxifen. This drug, used in carcinoma of the breast, has been reported to cause blurring of vision as the result of changes in the cornea, lens and retina. This occurs mainly after high doses.

Chemical toxicity. Ocular irritation may result from substances contained in ophthalmic preparations: either the active principle, the preservative or greasy base of ointments. Prolonged use can cause chronic and sometimes permanent pathological changes in the conjunctiva. This effect can also be seen with the proprietary cleaning and sterilizing fluids used in the care of hydrophilic contact lenses.

FURTHER READING

Alward W L M 1998 Medical management of glaucoma. New England Journal of Medicine 339: 1298

Coleman Anne L 1999 Glaucoma. Lancet 354: 1803

Fraunfelder F T, Hampton R F 1980 Current ocular therapy. Saunders, Philadelphia.

Fraunfelder F T 1996 Drug-induced ocular side-effects.

Williams & Wilkins, Media, Pennsylvania.

Wilholm B-E et al 1998 Relation of aplastic anaemia to use of chloramphenicol eye drops in two international case-control studies. British Medical Journal 316: 666

26

The local application of drugs

THE SKIN

When drugs are applied to the skin the term *topical treatment* is often used. A topical application generally consists of an active application, the drug, in a base or vehicle. The type of topical application that is used depends on the type and stage of the skin disease and it is just as important to use the correct base as it is to use the correct active agent. The base consists of one or more of the following: powder, water and grease.

The most commonly used bases or vehicles are as described in the following sections.

Ointments

The distinction between modern ointments and creams is no longer so obvious because of the wide range of bases that are used for both. Ointments are generally more 'greasy' and creams are thinner and consist of emulsions of various types. Ointments are of three types:

1. *Water soluble ointments*. These bases have the advantage that they do not stain.
2. *Emulsifying ointments*—that is, those which emulsify with water. An example is *lanolin (hydrous wool fat)*, which is still very commonly used, but prolonged use in some patients can lead to sensitization to the lanolin. These bases are useful for retaining active agents in contact with the skin for as long as possible.
3. *Non-emulsifying ointments*—that is, those which do not mix with water. The paraffins form the basis of most of the very greasy ointments.

With the addition of a suitable active agent they are a good treatment of chronic, dry skin disorders, such as chronic atopic eczema, psoriasis, ichthyosis (dry skin with fish-like scales) and for common disorders such as chapping of the hands.

Creams

Creams are emulsions which are either water dispersed in oil (i.e. oily cream) or an oil dispersed in water (i.e. aqueous cream). The latter are generally very acceptable to patients cosmetically and are used to moisten and soften the skin surface. Appropriate active agents can be added. Barrier creams protect the skin against physical agents such as water or sunlight.

Pastes

Pastes can be greasy or drying and they contain a large amount of powder. They are particularly useful for localized lesions—for example, in psoriasis. In this disorder it is particularly important that the active agent should not be applied to the normal skin and therefore a paste is used for the abnormal areas. Pastes can also be used to protect inflamed or excoriated skin and can be applied very freely. A good example is *compound zinc paste*.

Lotions

Water lotions are used to cool acutely inflamed skin and may have to be frequently reapplied. *Potassium permanganate lotion* is very helpful for acute exuding lesions of the hands and feet. Lotions should generally not be used when the acute phase has subsided.

Shake lotions cool by evaporation and leave an inert powder on the skin surface. They are useful and safe for subacute lesions. *Calamine lotion* is a good example.

Dusting powders

These are drying agents and increase the effective evaporating surface. They are particularly useful in the folds of the skin. Talc, starch and zinc oxide are commonly used powders. Active agents can be added as needed—for example, antiseptics for bacterial infections and antifungal agents for athlete's foot (tinea pedis).

ACTIVE INGREDIENTS IN PREPARATIONS

From this it will be seen that the first decision is the type of base that will be used, which will depend on the acuteness of the lesion. Many lesions in fact often derive more benefit from the base than from the active agent. A decision on the active ingredient to be added generally implies a diagnosis of the skin disorder. It is no longer useful to remember detailed prescriptions because the common ones can be found in the *British National Formulary* or equivalent publications. Ointments prepared by pharmaceutical companies have complicated formulae, but it is very important to know the active ingredients and their strength in these preparations.

It is also important to check for additives in topical preparations which may be associated with sensitization (Table 26.1).

Table 26.1 Potential skin sensitizers in topical preparations

Preparations	Sensitizer
Beeswax	Isopropyl palmitate
Benzyl alcohol	Polysorbates
Butylated hydroxyanisole	Propylene glycol
Chlorocresol	Sorbic acid
Edetic acid (EDTA)	Wool fat and related
Ethylenediamine	substances including lanolin
Fragrances	(development of purified
Hydroxybenzoates (parabens)	versions of wool fat have
	reduced the problem)

Local corticosteroids

These are probably the most widely prescribed and useful ingredients to be added to the various bases. For this reason they are often over-prescribed and in particular *they should not be used alone where the cause of the skin disease is a bacterial, fungal or viral infection as they may cause spread of the infection by lowering local resistance.* They are very useful for acute and subacute disorders such as the eczemas and they are excellent for itching (pruritus).

Table 26.2 Topical corticosteroid potencies

Potency	Examples
Mild	Hydrocortisone 1%
Moderately potent	Clobetasone butyrate 0.05%
Potent	Betamethasone valerate 0.1%,
	Mometasone fuorate 0.1%
Very potent	Clobetasol propionate 0.05%

Topical corticosteroids are classified according to their potency (Table 26.2).

The choice of a topical corticosteroid should be the least-potent preparation at the lowest strength which is effective.

1. *Hydrocortisone ointment* (0.5–1%) is the most useful, standard preparation. Nothing stronger than this should ever be used in infants or on the face. (In certain cases a short course of a more potent preparation may be prescribed under strict supervision of the dermatologist.) These ointments need not be applied more than twice a day.

2. *More potent corticosteroids (e.g. betamethasone valerate)*. These can achieve a much more intense effect than hydrocortisone, but this may not be an advantage and can lead to atrophy of the skin. They are valuable for thick, dry skin disorders, such as the chronic eczemas, or with some special disorders such as lupus erythematosus. The absorption of these preparations is enhanced by occlusive dressings—for example, if they are covered with polythene. However, there is great danger of secondary infection with this method.

Sometimes corticosteroids are combined with an antibacterial or antifungal agent and used to treat dermatoses with superimposed bacterial or fungal infections.

Coal tar

Coal tar applied to the skin is an antimitotic and anti-inflammatory agent. A tar is the product of the destructive distillation of organic substances and coal tar is in many valuable preparations, although their use has been superseded by the corticosteroid preparations. For disorders such as psoriasis and chronic eczema they are preferred because there are fewer side-effects. Cosmetically acceptable preparations are now available and a liquid form can be added to the bath for the treatment of some patients with psoriasis. The *British National Formulary* calamine and coal tar ointment contains the equivalent of 0.5%–1.0% of tar. Coal tar pastes are also often used in eczemas. A useful preparation for psoriasis is betamethasone valerate ointment with liquor picis carb (tar) in yellow soft paraffin.

Dithranol is widely used to treat *psoriasis*. It is an irritant and application must be limited to the psoriatic areas as it burns normal skin, particularly if the skin is fair or has previously been treated with steroids. It should not be used if there is evidence of infection.

Antibacterial agents

If a bacterial infection is suspected it is better to send a swab to the laboratory for culture and sensitivity tests first. In addition, many infections of the skin are best treated with systemic rather than topical antibacterial agents. The prolonged use of most antibacterial agents (e.g. neomycin) on the skin carries a very high risk of sensitization to the agent so that a bacterial infection may be replaced by a contact dermatitis! Chlortetracycline is probably the best to add to an ointment. If topical antibacterial agents are used the treatment should be determined by the sensitivity of the organism. Sulfonamides and penicillin should *never* be used on the skin owing to the high risk of sensitization.

Antifungal agents

Skin scrapings to identify the fungus are best taken before commencing treatment.

Systemic treatment is used for widespread, unresponding fungal infections and nail (*tinea unguium*) and scalp ringworm. *Griseofulvin* is the drug of choice for widespread or intractable fungal infections of the skin. It is more effective in the skin than in the nails and needs to be continued for some months.

Topical treatments are usually adequate for most localized infections.

An acute fungal infection may need to be treated by *potassium permanganate* lotion 0.01% for the first few days. An ointment with salicyclic acid and benzoic acid is known as *Whitfield's ointment* and is widely used, but tends to be cosmetically unacceptable. Effective preparations which are commonly used are the imidazoles (*clotrimazole, econazole, miconazole*). The *undecoanates* and *tolnaftate* are less effective in the treatment of ringworm infections. *Terbinafine* is now also available in the form of a cream. *Amorolfine* is a newly introduced antifungal which is available as a cream for fungal skin infections and as a lacquer for fungal nail infections.

Lotions and creams are usually the vehicle of choice. As ointments have occlusive properties they should be avoided on moist areas. Dusting powders are therapeutically ineffective in the treatment of fungal infections and liable to cause skin irritation and should be avoided except for toiletry purposes.

Infections with *Candida albicans* are common in patients with diabetes mellitus and those who have been treated with antibiotics and immunosuppressive drugs. Treatment may be with the broad spectrum antifungal imidazoles. *Nystatin* is also equally effective and must be applied to the affected area, either as an ointment or a lotion.

Antiviral agents

Aciclovir cream is the treatment of choice for herpes simplex of the skin. It is extremely important that the cream should be applied as early as possible, five times a day, for 5 days.

Emollients

These are used for dry skin (xeroderma) and especially for dry, scaly skin (e.g. ichthyosis, when the scale can be removed). They soothe and smooth the skin and a simple preparation such as aqueous cream is often a good treatment. Zinc cream is a traditional remedy and E45 a more recent one. With hyperkeratotic (i.e. thickened) and scaly conditions it is important to hydrate the skin first—that is, with a bath or shower. The emollient should be applied immediately afterwards to keep the skin hydrated.

Miscellaneous

Many other agents can be applied to the skin for different, but sometimes very common, disorders. For example:

1. *Permethrin* or *malathion* is used for the treatment of scabies.

2. *Sunscreen preparations* containing substances such as aminobenzoic acid to protect the skin against UVB and sunburn. The sun protection factor (SPF) provides guidance on the degree of UVB protection offered by the preparation (e.g. using one with an SPF of 15 should enable a person to remain in the sun 15 times longer without burning).

Protection against UVA and the associated effects of long-term skin damage is offered by preparations containing reflective substances such as titanium dioxide.

3. *Cleansing agents* such as *cetrimide* are useful for removing adherent crusts or ointments.

4. *Metronidazole* is used in rosacea.

5. Preparations containing *benzoyl peroxide* or *azelaic acid* are used in the treatment of acne with comedones and inflamed lesions.

6. *Salicylic acid* may be used to soften callosities, such as corns in the feet. These agents are called keratolytics.

7. *Aluminium chloride* (20% lotion) is an antiperspirant, often effective in the treatment of hyperidrosis, at any site. It is also used in many commercially available deodorants.

8. *Barrier creams* contain water-repellent substances such as dimethicone and may be used to protect the skin in such areas as around the stomata. Barrier creams are also sometimes used in industry to try and prevent damage to the skin; however, most have been shown to be ineffective.

9. *Calcipotriol* and *tacalcitol* are vitamin D derivatives used in the treatment of mild-to-moderate psoriasis. Calcipotriol is available as a cream or ointment and in a scalp solution; it is applied twice daily to the affected areas.

10. *Tazarotene* is the first topical retinoid (vitamin A derivative) available to treat mild-to-moderate plaque psoriasis. *Tazarotene gel* should be applied thinly, once daily to the affected skin only, avoiding healthy skin and the skin folds.

11. *Tretinoin*, a vitamin A derivative, and its isomer, *isotretinoin*, may be used to treat acne.

APPLICATION OF SKIN PREPARATIONS

1. It must be remembered that drugs can be absorbed through the intact skin. It is therefore very important that the nurse wears gloves when applying any preparation to the skin, particularly one containing active ingredients.

2. Many patients will be required to apply their skin preparations over long periods so that it will be necessary that they are taught the correct technique. Adverse effects, such as redness and soreness and relapse, may require a change of treatment.

3. *Wet wraps* are warm, wet occlusive dressings made up from elasticated viscose stockinette. They are used for children in the treatment of atopic eczema to rehydrate the skin using emollients, treat inflammation with appropriate corticosteroids, cool the skin and promote skin healing. The dressings are usually applied daily for about a week.

- Lengths of the tubular bandage are used to make two body suits. They are measured and cut to fit the patient.
- The prescribed medication is applied to the skin.
- The first layer is soaked in warm water, squeezed out and applied to the body while still warm and wet.
- The second dry layer is applied over the wet layer.
- The child then can put on normal clothing.
- The process is repeated after 24 hours.

4. *Medicated baths:*

- The bath water should be approx. 36°C.
- Stir in the medication and mix well to ensure an even concentration.

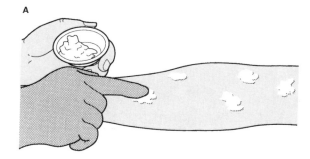

A

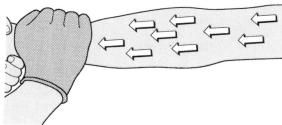

B

Figure 26.1   Application of creams and ointments: smooth on in the direction of the hair fall.

- The patient should soak for about 10 minutes.

5. *Creams and ointments:*

- Apply sparingly.
- Do not rub unless specifically prescribed.
- Smooth the preparation on gently in the direction of the hair fall (see Fig. 26.1).
- A 10 cm strip of cream or ointment from a standard nozzle of a tube of medication is the equivalent of 2 g (see Fig. 26.2).

6. *Steroid application:*

- Steroids are best applied to hydrated skin.
- Apply an emollient 20 minutes before the steroid to increase its effectiveness.
- Care should be taken to apply only the prescribed amount of corticosteroid to avoid potential side-effects. The *rule of nines* is a recognized method for

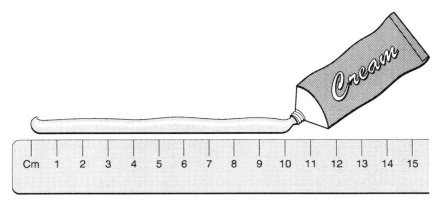

Figure 26.2 Measuring ointment/cream.

Rule of Nines

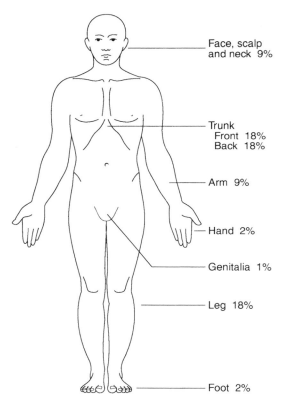

Face, scalp
and neck 9%

Trunk
Front 18%
Back 18%

Arm 9%

Hand 2%

Genitalia 1%

Leg 18%

Foot 2%

Figure 26.3 This shows the percentage of the total body surface area made up of the various parts of the body. It can be seen that the percentages are usually 9% or a multiple of 9%. In general, no more than 2 g of steroid ointment per 9% of body surface should be applied at any one time, i.e. 4 fingertip units per 9% of body surface (measured by the male finger) or 5 fingertip units per 9% of body surface (measured by the female finger).

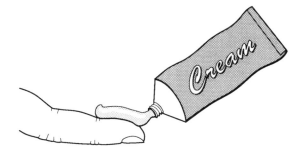

1 g ointment/cream = 2 fingertip units (males)

2.5 fingertip units (females)

Figure 26.4 Fingertip unit.

assessing the quantity of the preparation to be applied (see Fig. 26.3).

- Patients may also be advised on how to use the *'fingertip method'* to apply their topical preparations in safe quantities (see Fig. 26.4).

7. *Dithranol application:*

- Apply to affected areas only.
- Palpate skin lesions (psoriatic plaques) to identify the edges of the lesion before applying dithranol.
- Dithranol in Lassar's paste is applied to the lesions with a spatula.
- Starch powder or talc is patted on to dithranol in Lassar's paste to prevent spread of medication onto normal skin.

The medication is removed with vegetable oil.

- Dithranol in cream or ointment base is rubbed into the skin lesion with a gloved hand (powder is not used).
- Dithranol in cream in a lipid-stabilized base is removed with plenty of lukewarm water only.
- *Short contact treatment*—dithranol is left on the skin for 20 minutes or the prescribed time and then removed.

DRUG ERUPTIONS

A skin eruption due to drug treatment is now so commonly seen that this cause must always be considered whenever a patient is seen with an unusual rash. In addition, patients are often receiving more than one drug so that it is difficult or impossible to determine which one is responsible. All that can be done is to give an assessment of the possibilities.

The skin can only react in a certain number of ways, which are known as reaction patterns. A good example is *urticaria*, which can be provoked by a number of different drugs. If, however, the patient is taking aspirin or its derivatives, this is by far the most likely drug to provoke this reaction pattern. However, in practice, some drugs so commonly cause a particular eruption that this drug can be strongly suspected to be the cause if the patient is seen with a specific rash. For example, *furosemide* can cause a purpuric rash, *glutethimide* a generalized erythema and *sulfonamides* a measles-like rash.

Some drugs can cause many different types of skin eruption. *Gold* can provoke a generalized exfoliative erythroderma, which may be fatal, or a rash resembling pityriasis rosea or just a nondescript erythema associated with a stomatitis. *Penicillin* usually causes a severe erythema, and this may be so marked that a diagnosis of erythema multiforme may be considered.

In a few cases, adverse drug reactions including Stevens–Johnson syndrome and toxic epidermal necrosis (TEN) may be so severe that they become life-threatening (Table 26.3).

Table 26.3 Drugs most frequently associated with Stevens–Johnson syndrome and TEN

Sulfadoxine	Barbiturates
Sulphadiazine	Phenylbutazone
Sulfasalazine	Piroxicam
Co-trimoxazole	Allopurinol
Phenytoin	Aminopenicillins
Carbamazepine	

Table 26.4 Common allergens in contact dermatitis

Allergen	Sources
Balsam of Peru	Perfumes, citrus fruit
Colophony	Sticking plaster, collodion
Neomycin	Topical medicaments
Benzocaine	Topical anaesthetics
Parabens	Preservatives in creams and cosmetics
Wool alcohols	Lanolin, creams and cosmetics
Imidazolidinyl urea	Preservatives in creams and cosmetics
Formaldehyde (aqueous)	Cosmetics, clothing, glues, paper

Nursing point

With the advent of nurse prescribing, care should be taken to ensure that any preparation being prescribed for or recommended to a patient does not include any ingredients to which that patient is sensitive.

Contact dermatitis is an eczematous eruption produced by external agents, including some drugs (Table 26.4). Some emollients and paste bandages contain preservatives and many preparations have fragrance additives, both of which are known sensitizers. The *British National Formulary* and pharmaceutical company data sheets list additives in preparations.

Some drugs sensitize the skin to ultraviolet light. A skin eruption occurs when the photosensitive person has taken or applied the medication and then been exposed to sunlight. Two subtypes of reactions occur, phototoxic and photoallergic (Table 26.5).

Phototoxic reactions develop a few hours after exposure to sun and often resemble severe sunburn. In photoallergic reactions the onset is delayed and the rash is eczematous in nature. Table 26.6 lists other agents causing photosensitivity.

Table 26.5 Drugs causing photosensitivity reactions

Phototoxic	Photoallergic
Topical	
Coal tar preparations, e.g. dithranol	Halogenated salicylamides
Psoralens	
Furocoumarins, e.g. bergamot oil	
Systemic	
Demeclocycline	Sulfonamides
Doxycycline	Phenothiazines
Chlorpromazine	Griseofulvin

Table 26.6 Other agents causing photosensitivity

Agent type	Examples
Drug reactions	
Antibiotics	Sulfonamides, tetracycline
NSAIDs	Azapropazone
Hypoglycaemics	Chlorpropamide, glibenclamide
Sedatives	Chlorpromazine
Diuretics	Amiloride, thiazides
Contact sensitivity	
Drugs	Chlorpromazine
Sunscreens	Para-aminobenzoic acid (PABA)
Cosmetics	Perfumes, especially musk ambrette
Plants	Chrysanthemum and other compositae

Treatment is generally simple in that all drugs which are the likely cause should be withdrawn. Symptomatic treatment for symptoms may be called for, with calamine cream for pruritus or systemic antihistamines to make the patient more comfortable. It should be noted that the *topical* application of antibiotics, antihistamines and local anaesthetics should be avoided as they often cause sensitization rashes.

Nursing point

Photosensitive patients, including those with disorders such as systemic lupus erythematosus, porphyria and chronic actinic dermatitis, must be advised to wear sunscreens and protective clothing when outdoors.

CONCLUSION

From this brief review it will be seen that practically anything can be applied to the skin and often is! Patients may have used a variety of unsuitable remedies before they see a doctor or nurse and your first duty is to apply a remedy that will not do any harm. This is why many dermatologists are very conservative in the treatment that they prescribe. Like any other part of the body, when it is inflamed the skin must be allowed to rest. If there is an external cause for the trouble then this must be removed and it is as well to remember that this may be an ointment which has been prescribed. If there is an infection it must be treated. The topical application of a suitable base may be all that the skin requires. The active agents, or drugs, should only be added if there is a definite indication for their use.

SKIN CARE

There is no doubt that good skin care needs soap and water, probably almost daily. Some individuals may prefer to use a soap substitute, such as an emulsifying ointment. Make-up should always be removed at night and aqueous cream can be used to prevent drying, and as a cleansing agent to remove make-up. The skin should always be protected from excessive exposure to the sun and, if possible, excessive use of perfumes, hair dyes and so on. When it is said someone looks healthy, this means the skin is in good condition and looks normal.

FURTHER READING

Cerio R, Jackson W F 1992 Photosensitivity and photoallergy. A colour atlas of allergic skin disorders. Wolfe Publishing, London.
Dawkes K 1997 How to ... treat scalp psoriasis. British Journal of Dermatology Nursing 1(1): 8–9
Ersser S J 1998 Annotated bibliography of the dermatology nursing literature. Oxford Centre for Health Care Research and Development, Oxford.
Fincham-Gee C 1988 Safe use of topical steroids. Nursing 29(3): 1043–1045
Findlay A Y, Edwards P H, Harding K G 1989 The fingertip unit: a new practical measure. The Lancet 2: 155
Greaves M W, Weinstein G D 1995 Treatment of psoriasis. New England Journal of Medicine 332: 581
Greenhow M M 1983 Topical treatments—a simple guide. Nursing 2(10): 281–284
McClelland P B 1997 New treatment options for psoriasis. Dermatology Nursing 9(5): 295–304

Roujeau J C, Stern R S 1994 Severe adverse cutaneous reactions to drugs. New England Journal of Medicine 331: 1272

Stone L A, Lindfield E M, Robertson S 1989 A colour atlas of nursing procedures in skin disorders. Wolfe Medical, London.

Turnbull R 1994 Use of wet wrap dressing in atopic eczema. Paediatric Nursing 6(2): 22–26

THE NOSE

Drugs may be instilled into the nose. It must be remembered, however, that their effect is very transient; the cilia lining the nasal cavities completely remove them in about 20 minutes. Furthermore, medication with strong solutions of antibiotics or vasoconstrictors will paralyse the cilia and thus impede rather than help the clearance of infected material from the nasal cavities.

Nose drops are best given as follows. The patient should lie back on a couch or bed with his or her head extended over the end. About 5 ml of the appropriate drops are instilled into each nostril, the patient being instructed to breathe through the mouth, thus closing the back of the nose and holding the nose drops in the nasal cavities. This position should be maintained for 3 minutes. This method of administration may be too strenuous for elderly patients. There are a number of nose drops in use; among the most useful are:

Ephedrine nose drops 0.5%

Ephedrine	500 mg
Sodium chloride	500 mg
Chlorbutol	500 mg
Water to 100 ml	

Ephedrine nose drops are useful in sinus infection because the ephedrine causes shrinkage of the swollen and inflamed mucosa and thus clears the nasal airway and allows proper drainage from the nasal sinuses. Over-use, however, may damage the delicate ciliated epithelium lining the nasal passages and the drops should not be used for more than a week.

Interaction. Ephedrine nose drops should not be given to patients taking MAO inhibitors or within 2 weeks of stopping these drugs, owing to the risk of a hypertensive crisis. *Corticosteroids* (betamethasone 0.1%) can be given as nose drops two or three times daily or *beclomethasone* is available as a nasal spray, the dose being two sprays into each nostril twice daily. *Sodium cromoglicate* (see p. 251) can be given as a nasal spray, as drops or as an insufflation.

Allergic rhinitis can be treated locally with preparations which relieve congestion or by oral antihistamines. Local steroids appear to be the most effective.

Azelastine which is an antihistamine, can also be given as a nasal spray.

Local antibiotics have little place in the treatment of nasal infections, but a cream containing *chlorhexidine* and *neomycin* (Naseptin) can be applied locally in patients who are carriers of staphylococcus.

Mupirocin or **polyfax** ointments are used for the eradication of MRSA.

THE EAR

Although the instilling of drops into the ear may be useful in relieving symptoms, it is often done without any consideration of the underlying disease and thus proves fruitless and sometimes even dangerous.

The use of ear drops will be considered under individual disorders of the ear which can be helped by this method of treatment.

Instillation of drops

1. Warm ear drops to approximately blood heat.
2. The head is turned so that the affected ear is uppermost.
3. Discharge is gently mopped away.
4. Two or three drops are instilled and the head is held in position for a minute or two.

Wax in the ear

Wax may become hard and impacted in the ear and may resist efforts to move it by syringing. A 5.0% solution of sodium bicarbonate or warm almond or olive oil instilled for a few days will usually soften it satisfactorily.

Otitis externa

Severe infection is best managed with expert guidance as regular aural cleansing and medication are required.

Ear drops will only be effective if the meatus is cleared of debris. The following agents may be used three times daily if bacterial infection is suspected. Clioquinol 1% with flumetasone 0.02% (Locorten-Vioform) has a mild antibacterial and antifungal action, but stains the skin and clothes. Gentamicin 0.3% with hydrocortisone 1% is anti-inflammatory and antibacterial.

Other combinations of antibacterial drugs with steroids are available.

The following precautions should be observed:

1. Treatment with antibiotic ear drops should not be continued for longer than 1 week owing to the risks of drug sensitization and the development of fungal infection.

2. Gentamicin or neomycin ear drops should not be used if the eardrum is perforated as deafness may result.

In eczema of the ear, local steroids should be used to reduce irritation and inflammation. Prednisolone 0.5% or betamethasone 0.1% are satisfactory.

Otitis media

If the drum is not perforated the instillation of antibiotics into the external ear is useless as it will not reach the site of infection. Many infections are viral and require only an analgesic. Bacterial infections, which are usually due to *S. pneumoniae* or *H. influenzae*, should be treated by systemic antibiotics. Amoxicillin is usually effective and erythromycin can be used for those who are sensitive to penicillin.

FURTHER READING

Editorial 1995 Management of acute otitis media and glue ear. Drug and Therapeutics Bulletin 33: 12
Symposium 1990 Ear, nose and throat disease. Prescribers Journal 30: 191

Weiner J M 1998 Intranasal corticosteroids versus oral H antagonists in allergic rhinitis. British Medical Journal 317: 1624

27

Disinfectants and insecticides

DISINFECTANTS

Disinfection is the destruction of vegetative bacteria, but not necessarily their spores. Sterilization processes (e.g. autoclaving, gamma irradiation) destroy both vegetative bacteria and spores. However, in most circumstances (e.g. standard ward cleaning procedures, cleaning of bedpans and urinals), a reduction in the total number of bacteria is sufficient to remove the threat of infection to the average patient and disinfection is the appropriate procedure. An exception to this rule is the severely immuno-compromised patient nursed in protective isolation. Hospitals have their own protocols for the care of these very vulnerable patients. A good disinfectant is not necessarily a good cleaning agent and the two should not be interchanged.

There are two main types of disinfectant:

1. Environmental disinfectants which are used on equipment such as bedpans, urinal bottles and thermometers.
2. Those used on living surfaces such as skin and mucous membranes—sometimes called antiseptics.

These two groups are not substitutes for one another. Environmental disinfectants are often potent chemicals which damage tissue, whereas antiseptics, which have been developed to prevent such damage, are not only too expensive for environmental use, but also tend to destroy a narrower range of bacteria.

ENVIRONMENTAL DISINFECTANTS

Phenolic derivatives. Phenol was one of the first disinfectants used and it killed bacteria by combining with their proteins. It has now been replaced because it is not very effective, rapidly losing efficiency with dilution. It is very toxic, causing local corrosion of the mouth, throat and stomach if swallowed, followed by kidney damage.

Commercially available derivatives include Hycolin, which is used as a 2% or 1.5% solution, and Clearsol, which is supplied in sachets to be diluted before use. They are active against a wide range of bacteria, but are unable to destroy most spores and are inactive against some viruses. Phenolics can damage the skin and should be used with protective gloves. They should not be used on food preparation surfaces.

Hypochlorite disinfectants. These disinfectants act by releasing chlorine, the amount released being measured in parts per million of available chlorine. They can be used as environmental disinfectants.

Sodium hypochlorite solution is available in sachet form (Chlorasol) and diluted as required.

- A 1% solution (10 000 parts per million) is used as an environmental disinfectant.
- Hypochlorite disinfectants destroy hepatitis B and HIV in a 1% solution.

Diluted solutions decay rapidly and must be made up freshly before use.

Gluteraldehyde solution is used for sterilizing certain heat-sensitive instruments. It is allergenic, toxic and irritant and its use should be controlled by a code of practice.

A freshly prepared 2% solution destroys HIV, but is much more expensive than hypochlorites.

Nursing point

Wear gloves when using environmental disinfectants.

DISINFECTANTS USED ON THE SKIN AND MUCOUS MEMBRANES

Iodine is an effective disinfectant, but is rapidly inactivated by the tissues. It can also cause skin sensitization. It is now used mainly in the form of *povidone-iodine*, a non-staining and less irritant complex available as:

- Povidone-iodine 10% alcoholic solution
- Povidone-iodine 10% (aqueous) antiseptic solution, used for preoperative skin preparation
- 7.5% surgical scrub as a hand disinfectant.

Chlorhexidine is an expensive skin disinfectant and is most unsuitable for environmental use because it is effective mainly against Gram-positive bacteria (e.g. *staphylococci* and *streptococci*). It has little action against Gram-negative rods (e.g. *Pseudomonas*, *Klebsiella*, *E. coli*) and will destroy few spores or viruses.

It is used as:

- A 0.5% alcohol solution as a skin disinfectant
- A 0.2% solution of chlorhexidine gluconate as a mouthwash
- A 4% solution as a preoperative scrub
- A 0.015% solution with cetrimide (Tisept, see below) for wound cleaning.

Hexachlorophane is similar and is available in several forms including:

- 3% cream used for surface disinfecting.

It can penetrate the skin, particularly if it is excoriated and the application is not followed by rinsing. It should therefore be used with special care in newborn infants.

Hydrogen peroxide is used for irrigating infected wounds. It is not a very powerful disinfectant, but when it comes into contact with damaged tissues, enzymes which are present release oxygen which bubbles up from the wound and helps to loosen debris, thus cleaning the infected area.

Surface-acting agents lower surface tension and allow fats to be more easily emulsified. They are also bacteriocidal. This combined action is useful in that it cleans the infected area and allows the disinfectant to penetrate widely, thus extending its range of antibacterial activity. One of the most widely used is *cetrimide*, which is available as a cream or as a solution and may be combined with another disinfectant such as chlorhexidine (Tisept).

Isopropyl alcohol is used as a skin disinfectant and is most effective as a 70% solution, but it may also be used as a vehicle for other disinfectants such as chlorhexidine, marketed as '*Hibisol*', used as a hand disinfectant.

Hand decontamination

Hands can be decontaminated with soap from a wall container, a medical agent or alcoholic hand-rub. Trials have repeatedly shown the superiority of agents such as chlorhexidine over ordinary soap, but such trials have not reproduced ward conditions where nurses hurry between patients and from clean to dirty tasks. Any hand hygiene agent will only be efficient if it is used frequently and appropriately, even between such manoeuvres as mouth care and patient feeding. Hands should also be washed when plastic gloves are removed as bacteria multiply in the warm, moist environment inside them.

Whichever agent is used, all hand and inter-digital surfaces must be decontaminated and dried thoroughly as damp hands transfer bacteria more readily than dry ones. Although a thorough hand-washing technique may take longer, this is of value, particularly with medicated agents which need a minimum contact time with bacteria to be effective. When soap is used, evidence shows that the bacterial count is adequately reduced by the mechanical action of washing and thorough drying. The soreness which medicated agents are said to induce can be reduced by wetting the hands before application and rinsing and drying thoroughly.

Use of disinfectants in various circumstances

The following recommendations are necessarily incomplete and most hospitals will have their own procedures.

Ampoules	Swab neck with 70% alcohol or use a Mediswab.
Bed pans	Washer Disinfector—NB these do not sterilize.
Bladder washouts	1. Normal saline or 2. Chlorhexidine 1: 5000 aqueous solution.
Wound cleaning	0.9% Sodium chloride
Cleaning cuts and abrasion	Chlorhexidine 0.015% with cetrimide (Tisept).
Hand-washing (ward staff)	Liquid soap and water from a wall dispenser. In special circumstances, povidone-iodine surgical scrub.
Surgical scrubbing (surgeon)	Povidone-iodine surgical scrub or chlorhexidine scrub if iodine-sensitive.
Operating theatres (walls, floors, etc.)	1. Neutral detergent. 2. Infected material–Hycolin 1.5% or hypochlorite (0.1%) with detergent.
Skin preparation (injection)	70% isopropyl alcohol or 0.5% chlorhexidine in 70% alcohol.
Skin preparation (preoperative)	Povidone-iodine 10% in alcohol solution or chlorhexidine 0.5% in alcohol solution. Care is necessary if diathermy is used with alcoholic solutions. Surgeons have their preferences and may require a coloured solution to delineate the disinfected area.
Thermometers (clinical)	Individual—wipe with 70% alcohol swab after each use and store dry. After discharge—wash with detergent and soak in fresh 70% alcohol for 10 minutes and store dry.

HIV, Hepatitis B and C

These virus-carried diseases now present a special

problem and local guidelines will be available in most districts and are also available from the Royal College of Nursing, 20 Cavendish Square, London. All blood and body fluids should be regarded as potentially infectious.

Contamination should be immediately treated with 1% hypochlorite solution or, in the community, 1 part of bleach in 10 parts of water, freshly made. Gloves should be worn whenever handling blood or body fluids and the hands washed afterwards.

Nursing point

Patients often ask the nurse about the use of topical preparations such as skin disinfectants and medical insecticides. With the advent of nurse-prescribing the nurse will not only be expected to provide practical help and reassurance but to assess the circumstances in which such preparations are needed.

INSECTICIDES

Some knowledge of insecticides is important to the nurse for these substances are widely used in the disinfection of patients' bedding and houses, and some of them are highly poisonous substances which produce side-effects unless used properly.

Anticholinesterases

Malathion is commonly used. It paralyses the nervous system of the parasite. If correctly used it is not toxic, but the alcoholic solution should be avoided in patients with asthma and very young children.

Carbamates

Carbaryl is similar to the above. There is slight evidence that it may be carcinogenic and is now only available on prescription. It has been in use for many years and, so far, it has never been known to cause cancer in humans when applied locally.

Pyrethroids

This group of insecticides is obtained from the pyrethrum flowers which belong to the chrysanthemum family. They are quick-acting insecticides used in many insecticidal sprays. They are effective and, if used properly, are safe, although sensitization can occur.

MEDICAL USES OF INSECTICIDES

The two most common uses for insecticides in medical treatment are for scabies and pediculosis (lice).

Scabies

Scabies is due to a mite, the female of which burrows into the skin at certain sites, namely between the fingers, wrists, hands, buttocks and skin folds.

Therapeutics. A number of substances have been used in the treatment of scabies.

Malathion 0.5% aqueous solution (Derbac) is very effective. The solution is applied to the entire body from the neck downwards. It is very rare for the face or hair to be affected in adults. If the solution is applied to the face, avoid the eyes and around the mouth. It is left on for 24 hours. All close contacts are treated whether they have symptoms or not. The mite dies very quickly away from the skin, but it is worth laundering sheets and clothes. Itching takes about a month to subside and calamine lotion or 1% hydrocortisone ointment are useful for symptomatic treatment.

Permethrin (a pyrethroid) is available as a cream (Lyclear) which is applied over the whole body except the head. The body should be washed 12 hours later. It appears to be effective, but occasionally causes itching and erythema.

Benzyl benzoate has now been largely superseded.

Pediculosis (lice)

It is necessary to prevent the development of strains of lice which are resistant to treatment; therefore the preparations used should be rotated every 3 years. Effective preparations include:

- *Carbaryl 0.5% in alcohol (Carylderm).*
- *Malathion 0.5% in alcohol (Prioderm)* for head pediculosis.
- *Malathion 0.5% in aqueous solution (Derbac)* for pubic pediculosis or for those with abrasions or sensitive skin.
- *The pyrethroids, permethrin cream* and *phenothrin 0.2%* lotion in alcohol are used for head lice. In patients with asthma and very young children alcoholic solutions should not be used.

There is no clearly preferred preparation. Shampoos containing insecticides are not very effective and should not be used. Preparations are rubbed into dry hair, scalp or other affected areas. They are allowed to dry naturally; direct sunlight or heating should be avoided as they break down the drug and could ignite the alcohol. After 12 hours the hair is washed in the normal way using soap. Special medicated shampoos are unnecessary as the lice are already dead. The hair can be combed with a Secker comb to remove nits and treatment should be repeated after 1 week to kill lice emerging from the eggs.

Only those contacts who are infected need to be treated.

FURTHER READING

Butler M 1998 A guide to nurse prescribing of insecticides and anthelmintics. Nursing Times 94(22): 55
Editorial 1998 Treating head louse infections. Drug and Therapeutics Bulletin 36(6): 45
Elliot R, Torrance C 1998 Zoo-otic diseases. Nursing Times 94(12): 52
Gould D 1991 Hygienic hand decontamination. Nursing Standard 6(32): 33–36

Gould D 1991 Skin bacteria. What is normal? Nursing Standard 5(52): 26–29
Lowbury E J *et al* 1992 Control of hospital infection. A practical handbook, 3rd edn. Chapman and Hall, London.
Smith F, Ross F 1992 Prescribing topical agents. Community Outlook 2(7): 29–32

28

Poisoning and its treatment

The treatment of acute poisoning has of recent years become increasingly important. About 10% of acute medical admissions to hospital are due to an overdose, but 80% of these only require observation until the effects of the poison wear off. Most of the section on general treatment in this chapter applies to the more severely poisoned patient. This may be due to attempted suicide, less often to accidental poisoning and very rarely to homicide. Perhaps the commonest cause of overdosage is an attempt by the patient to draw attention to or modify some intolerable situation. In these circumstances he or she is not seeking death, but merely trying to shock relatives or friends into realization of his or her problems.

In children poisoning occurs most commonly in the 1 to 5 year age group as the child becomes mobile and is inclined to put everything in his or her mouth. Drugs and other harmful substances must be kept not only out of reach, but also out of sight as children are adept at reaching 'impossible' places. Occasionally poisoning may be due to accidental overdose of a drug.

The most frequently used suicide agents are centrally acting drugs including sedatives, hypnotics and antidepressants, analgesics including aspirin, paracetamol and opioids and a mixed bag which includes cardiovascular drugs. Coal gas, although still used, is less common than formerly as methane has replaced it for domestic use. It is, however, the most common cause of a *fatal* suicide attempt. In addition, poisoning can occur, particularly in children, from various chemicals used domestically or in the garden and from a number of berries.

GENERAL MANAGEMENT

When a patient is admitted to hospital suffering from poisoning the first step is to decide if life is at immediate risk from airway obstruction or respiratory arrest. If so, the appropriate measures should be taken at once.

The next steps are to assess the severity of the poisoning, the nature of the poison used (overdose by more than one drug is common) and to institute appropriate treatment.

Severity of poisoning

The severity of the poisoning will be based largely on three criteria.

1. Level of consciousness. This is usually classified in four grades:

- Grade I. Drowsy, but responds to light stimulation
- Grade II. Unconscious, but responds to light stimulation
- Grade III. Unconscious, but responds to severe stimulation
- Grade IV. Unconscious, with no response to stimulation.

2. Circulation. Many drugs cause circulatory failure. The nurse is frequently asked to measure the blood pressure at intervals and a low blood pressure is indicative of failing circulation. However, it must be realized that what really matters is the perfusion of vital organs such as the brain and kidney. It is possible to have a reasonable blood pressure maintained by intense constriction of blood vessels, but organ perfusion will be poor. In such a situation the hands and feet will be cold and blue and this may be a useful sign. In addition, certain drugs (particularly antidepressants) can cause cardiac arrhythmias so that ECG monitoring is necessary.

3. Respiration. Depression of respiration so that less oxygen reaches the lungs is a common cause of death in overdosage. Respiratory rate should be charted at regular intervals. Cyanosis is a useful sign of under-ventilation of the lungs, and if facilities are available the respiratory minute volume and blood gases must be measured.

Nature of poison used

The identification of the poison used will depend on history and circumstantial evidence, on clinical signs and on analysis of gastric aspirate, blood and urine. Samples should be collected, carefully labelled and analysed as soon as possible. The results may not only be useful in the management of the patient, but they may have medico-legal implications.

TREATMENT

The treatment of poisoning can be divided into:

1. Non-specific measures
2. Specific measures which are considered under individual poisons.

Non-specific measures

1. Maintenance of ventilation. In the unconscious patient the reflexes which protect the airways may be lost so there is a danger of respiratory obstruction by the tongue and the aspiration of vomit. These patients should be nursed in the coma position with an airway in place until it is possible to insert a cuffed endotracheal tube which can be kept in place for up to 72 hours. Secretions should be aspirated regularly.

With severe respiratory depression, oxygen and/or assisted ventilation will be required.

2. Reducing absorption of poisons. It is obviously desirable to minimize the absorption of poison from the gut and this can be achieved in two ways:

1. Emptying the stomach by emesis or washouts.
2. Giving substances which bind to the poison in the gut and thus prevent its absorption.

Emptying the stomach. If the patient is conscious, vomiting can be induced by stimulation of the posterior pharyngeal wall.

In the unconscious patient lavage may be used:

1. When dangerous amounts of poison have been taken within the previous hour. A longer period is reasonable with certain drugs, e.g.

Salicylates	4 h
Tricyclic antidepressants	4 h
Opioids	4 h

2. After a cuffed endotracheal tube has been inserted as there is considerable risk of inhalation of vomit in these patients.

Lavage is carried out via a 30 English gauge Jaques catheter lubricated with Vaseline, and a 50 cm length should be adequate. Great care is needed to ensure that the tube is in the stomach and not the trachea. A 300–500 ml volume of warm water should be used for each wash, which is repeated three or four times. At the end the stomach should be empty. Although gastric lavage and emetics have been used for many years in the treatment of poisoning they do not empty the stomach completely and their efficacy is under critical review. It seems probable that, except when very large amounts have been taken, they have little effect on the prognosis unless carried out within an hour of ingestion.

Absorption can also be reduced by giving *activated charcoal* by mouth. The dose is 50 g and it is usually given via a nasogastric tube. It prevents the absorption of many poisons throughout the gut and often is more effective than gastric lavage, which in many circumstances it should replace.

3. Maintenance of blood pressure. Some patients will have a low blood pressure and failing circulation. Adequate ventilation (see earlier) will often improve matters. Raising the foot of the bed is simple and is usually successful in mild poisoning. With severe hypotension the infusion of volume expanders such as dextran may be required.

4. Increasing elimination of poisons. This can be achieved by increasing elimination via the kidneys or by haemoperfusion. *Renal elimination* of some drugs can be increased by altering the pH of the urine and an example is in the treatment of salicylate poisoning (see p. 348).

In *haemoperfusion* the blood is passed through a column of charcoal or some other substance which removes the poison. This method undoubtedly removes poisons, but there is a risk of damaging platelets and blood cells so it is rarely used.

A similar effect can be more easily achieved by giving repeated oral doses of *activated charcoal*; the poison passes from the gut wall and binds to the charcoal in the lumen.

5. Nutrition, hydration and electrolyte disturbances. In comatose patients the problems of *nutrition, hydration* and *electrolyte disturbances* will require consideration, although intravenous infusion will not usually be necessary unless the coma is prolonged.

6. Follow-up. When the patient has recovered it is important that the social and psychiatric background to a suicide attempt is investigated and most of these patients will require continued supportive treatment.

INDIVIDUAL POISONS (Table 28.1)

Benzodiazepines

These drugs are widely used so it is not surprising that overdose is common. They produce coma without any specific features and cardio-respiratory depression is usually minimal. However, death can occur from respiratory depression and/or the aspiration of stomach contents, particularly if they have been combined with other more sinister agents. There is some evidence

Table 28.1 Individual poisons

	Plasma concentration producing severe overdose	Upper limit of therapeutic plasma level
Hypnotics		
Barbiturates	50 mg/l	5 mg/l
Diazepam	5 mg/l	1 mg/l
Anticonvulsants		
Phenobarbital	100 mg/l	30 mg/l
Phenytoin	35 mg/l	20 mg/l
Analgesics		
Salicylates	600 mg/l	250 mg/l
Paracetamol	200 mg/l (4 h after ingestion) 30 mg/l (15 h after ingestion)	20 mg/l
Miscellaneous		
Amitriptyline	1 mg/l	0.2 mg/l
Ethanol	3 g/l	0.8 g/l is the legal limit for driving

that death from temazepam overdose is more frequent. Some of this group of drugs have long half-lives and/or active metabolites and full recovery may take several days.

Treatment. It is usually sufficient to maintain a clear airway and give general nursing care. *Flumazenil* is a specific antidote which reverses the actions of this group of drugs, but it is only rarely required in severe overdose.

Salicylates (aspirin)

Aspirin has long been a common cause of poisoning, although in recent years its place has been partially taken by paracetamol. In addition to suicide attempts, it is particularly dangerous as a cause of accidental overdosage in children who are more sensitive to its toxic effects than adults.

Symptoms. Nausea, vomiting, tinnitus, increased respiration and with severe overdose confusion, convulsions and coma.

Aspirin also produces complicated changes in the acid-base state of the body. Early on it causes increased respiration and thus washes carbon dioxide out through the lungs and causes an alkalosis. The aspirin itself is an acid and tends to produce an acidosis after some hours.

Treatment:

1. Wash out the stomach with water. This is worth doing up to 4 hours after ingestion of the drug.
2. If the patient is conscious, give 5% sodium bicarbonate solution by mouth together with a high fluid intake.
3. In severely ill and unconscious patients (serum salicylate >500 mg/litre for adults and >300 mg/litre for children) intravenous fluid and electrolyte replacement is essential. Elimination of salicylate by the kidneys can be enhanced by infusing sodium bicarbonate solution to make the urine alkaline (forced alkaline diuresis) or haemodialysis should be considered. Equally effective is oral charcoal 50 g followed by 50 g every 4 hours, although vomiting may make this difficult. It not only prevents absorption but enhances elimination.

Paracetamol

Overdosage with paracetamol produces liver damage which may be fatal. This is due to abnormal breakdown products which do not occur with normal dosage, but only when excess has been taken. As little as 7.5 g (15 of the usual tablets) can be dangerous. Early symptoms, usually nausea and vomiting, are minimal and it is only after 2 or 3 days that jaundice with hepatic failure and/or, more rarely, renal failure develop. Patients in whom the blood level of paracetamol is above 200 mg/litre 4 hours after ingestion, or 30 mg/litre 15 hours after ingestion of the drug, are likely to develop severe liver damage.

Treatment. Activated charcoal (50 g) should be given if a large dose of paracetamol has been taken in the previous hour. There are several drugs available which alter metabolism of the drug and prevent liver damage.

- Methionine 2.5 g every 4 hours orally for 4 doses, *or*
- N-acetylcysteine 150 mg/kg in 200 ml of 5% dextrose over 15 minutes followed by 50 mg/kg infused over 4 hours, and finally 100 mg/kg infused over the next 16 hours.

Methionine is effective, but absorption is slower and may be nullified by vomiting, so N-acetylcysteine is preferred.

This treatment is very effective if given within 10 hours of ingestion of paracetamol; after this its efficacy declines. It should therefore be given *immediately* to all patients in whom there is good evidence of overdose without waiting for the results of a blood level estimation. When this becomes available treatment can be modified if necessary.

Otherwise, treatment is symptomatic.

Opioids

Morphine and related substances are common causes of poisoning. This may occur as a suicide attempt or because an addict has misjudged his or her 'fix'. Although morphine and heroin are the best known of this group, serious overdosage can occur with so-called weak narcotics such as codeine, dihydrocodeine and dextro-propoxyphene (see later), provided a large enough dose is taken.

Symptoms. The classic symptoms are coma, depressed respiration and pin-point pupils. The patient sweats and is liable to develop hypo-thermia. The pulse is slow. Pulmonary oedema may develop rapidly and is often fatal.

Treatment. Respiratory depression is reversed by naloxone (p. 118) 800 micrograms–2.0 mg given intravenously. It is, however, short-acting and repeated doses may be required. Respiratory arrest will require full resuscitation with assisted ventilation. Hypothermia should be treated in the usual way.

Dextropropoxyphene requires special mention. In the UK it is usually taken combined with paracetamol as *co-proxamol (Distalgesic)* tablets and this combination is one of the commonest causes of fatal poisoning. In relatively small doses, i.e. more than 20 tablets, it can produce marked respiratory depression and circulatory collapse. If the patient survives this there is a danger of paracetamol liver damage. The effects of dextropropoxyphene, but not paracetamol, are reversed by naloxone.

The central effects of all opioids are increased by concurrent consumption of alcohol.

Tricyclic antidepressants (imipramine, amytriptyline)

The older tricyclic antidepressants are very dangerous in overdose, largely because of their effects on the heart. Some of the more recently introduced drugs, however, are less toxic.

Symptoms. With small overdosage the patient is flushed, agitated with some blunting of con-sciousness and has a rapid pulse. The pupils are dilated and accommodation paralysed. The QRS interval on the ECG becomes progressively longer with increasing severity of poisoning. Larger doses cause fits, coma, depression of respiration and blood pressure and various cardiac arrhythmias.

Treatment. There is no specific remedy and diuresis and dialysis are no help. Wash out the stomach up to 4 hours after ingestion and leave

50 g of activated charcoal in the stomach. Further doses of charcoal, 50 g every 4 hours, should be given orally to minimize absorption. Cardiac arrhythmias are treated along the usual lines. Hypotension can be reversed by raising the cardiac output with dopamine and fits controlled by diazepam. Systemic acidosis may require cor-rection by infusion of sodium bicarbonate.

Alcohol

The patient may be conscious but mentally dis-orientated or may be unconscious. There is a smell of alcohol on the breath.

Treatment. Most patients will recover if kept warm and allowed to sleep it off. In severe cases the stomach should be washed out if the alcohol has been taken recently and treatment continued as in barbiturate poisoning. *It is very important to remember that patients who are drunk may have received injuries of which they are not aware. It should also be remembered that patients may have taken other drugs in addition to alcohol.*

Barbiturates

These are no longer the commonest cause of fatal poisoning in Great Britain.

Symptoms. The patient is confused or in a coma. The respirations are depressed and the blood pressure is low. Skin blistering is a fairly common feature.

Treatment. In barbiturate poisoning death is usually due to respiratory depression, circulatory failure, or pneumonia at a later date.

1. The airway must be kept clear and if the cough reflex is absent an endotracheal tube should be inserted, particularly for gastric lavage in the unconscious patient.
2. Gastric lavage is only justified if the drug has been taken within the previous 2 hours.
3. Ventilation is important and if there is respiratory depression some form of mechanical ventilation is required.
4. Fluid and calories must be given intravenously.

The appropriate antibiotic should be given if pulmonary infection develops.

Carbon monoxide

Carbon monoxide is the most frequent cause of fatal poisoning. It may be accidental or a suicide attempt, although the increasing use of North Sea gas (which does not contain carbon monoxide) makes this less common. It may be due to the escape of gas from faulty heating or lighting installations, to car exhaust fumes or to combustion stoves in poorly ventilated rooms.

Symptoms. Confusion or coma usually combined with cyanosis or pallor. The classical bright red colour of the skin and mucous membranes due to carboxyhaemoglobin is rare. After recovery a few subjects may develop symptoms similar to Parkinson's disease.

Treatment:

1. Get the patient out of the poisonous atmosphere.
2. Ensure a clear airway.
3. Give 100% oxygen (not oxygen and CO_2).
4. Artificial respiration may be necessary.

Phenothiazines (chlorpromazine, etc.)

Symptoms. These drugs produce coma, with hypotension and sometimes hypothermia. Chronic intoxication causes a Parkinson-like state.

Treatment is largely symptomatic, although it is worth trying gastric lavage up to 6 hours after ingestion. Parkinson-like states and other forms of dystonia respond to orphenadrine (see p. 172).

Iron compounds

These substances, particularly ferrous sulphate, are sometimes taken by children—because of their colour and sugar coating.

Symptoms. Vomiting with haematemesis; pallor, collapse and tachycardia. Fatal collapse sometimes occurs after apparent recovery. *Iron overdose in children must always be taken very seriously.*

Treatment:

1. Wash out the stomach with 5% sodium bicarbonate solution (1 oz per pint, 50 g per litre).
2. The iron chelating agent desferrioxamine, which combines with iron and prevents absorption, should be used in severe cases. Desferrioxamine can be given intravenously to a maximum dose of 80 mg/kg of body weight in 24 hours.

Paraquat

Paraquat is a weed killer. The granules available for domestic use contain only 5% of the substance and are not lethal. However, the pure substance used in agriculture is very dangerous—30 mg may be fatal. Death usually occurs after 1–2 weeks and is due to progressive lung failure, sometimes combined with kidney and liver damage. Treatment is nearly always ineffective, although, if administered soon after ingestion, an oral suspension of *Fuller's earth* has proved valuable in preventing the absorption of paraquat.

CHELATING AGENTS

These substances combine with metals and thus render them inactive. They are used in treating heavy metal poisoning.

Dimercaprol (BAL). Some heavy metals produce their toxic effects by combining with a chemical grouping found in living tissues and called SH groups. Their toxic effects can be prevented by giving dimercaprol, which also contains SH groups and thus combines with and inactivates heavy metals.

Therapeutic use. Dimercaprol is useful in poisoning by arsenic, mercury and gold.

Penicillamine is used in treating Wilson's disease, which is due to the excessive deposition of copper in the brain and liver. It chelates the copper which is then excreted. It can be given orally daily. It is also used in treating rheumatoid arthritis (see p. 128).

Information. There are six Poisons Information Centres in the UK and one in the Republic of Ireland. They can be contacted by day or night by telephone and will give information about poisoning and its treatment. Telephone numbers of these centres can be found in the *British National Formulary*.

FURTHER READING

Buckley N A et al 1995 Relative toxicity of benzodiazepines in overdose. British Medical Journal 310: 219

Davis J E 1991 Activated charcoal in acute drug overdosage. Professional Nurse 6(12): 710

Editorial 1998 Paracetamol (acetaminophen) poisoning. British Medical Journal 317: 1609

Perry J 1994 Nurse care following overdose. Nursing Times 90(38): 33

Thorsby S 1997 Methods of gastric decontamination. Nursing Times 93(21): 49

Vale J A, Proudfoot A T 1995 Paracetamol (acetaminophen) poisoning. Lancet 346: 547

29

Herbal medicines (phytotherapy). Homeopathy

Nurses, particularly if working in the community, will realize that many people use various types of alternative or complementary medicines. This chapter is not intended to deal with the underlying principles of herbal medicine or to discuss its merits or demerits—for this nurses are referred to specialist publications. However, some knowledge of this type of treatment is important for several reasons:

1. Herbal medicines may have pharmacological actions which affect the patient.

2. Not all herbal medicines are free from adverse effects.

3. Herbal medicines may interact with orthodox medicines if they are taken concurrently.

4. Patients may be more likely to tell a nurse rather than a doctor that they are taking herbal remedies, therefore a good drug history is essential.

HISTORY OF HERBAL MEDICINE

Medicines derived from plants have been used for centuries. The pragmatic and most definitive classics on Oriental medicine are *Shang Han Lung (Treatise on Febrile Disease)* and *Chin Kuei Yao Lueh (Summaries of Household Treatments)* described in southern China by Chang Chung-ching in the eastern Han dynasty (AD 25–220). This empirical system has been followed for the past 2000 years and many of the formulae in these two books are still used today.

The use of natural (herbal) medicines is a persistent aspect of present day health care and market research has estimated that in the UK the total market for complementary remedies (defined as licensed herbal medicines, homeopathic remedies and essential oils used for aromatherapy) was £72 million in 1996.

Many herbs have found their way into the pharmacopoeias of orthodox medicine, sometimes as the isolated and chemically standardized active ingredient. Such drugs as cocaine, coumarin, anticoagulants, curare, digoxin, ephedrine, morphine, quinine and quinidine, reserpine, senna and the ergot and vinca alkaloids entered orthodox medicinal use by this route.

Many other herbal substances are freely available to the public and in the UK only a small proportion comes under the direct control of the Medicines Act. Individual unprocessed traditional herbs are not considered as medicines and, therefore, do not require product licences in the UK. In Britain alone it has been estimated that 6000–7000 tons of herbs are extracted annually for use as ingredients of herbal remedies. Traditional herbs (including Chinese herbs) can be divided into three categories:

1. Licensed herbal products which are sold or supplied with claims for use as medicines (currently over 500 products are licensed). Almost all the licensed herbal medicines on the UK market have been available for some time and most originally held a Product Licence of Right (PLR). The Medicines Control Agency (MCA) has, since 1995, applied new regulations as a result of EC legislation and the Medicines Act of 1968, and, prior to marketing, all new licensed herbal products are assessed for quality, safety and efficacy.

2. Dried herbs which are exempt from licensing requirements under Section 12 of the Medicines Act and are not sold or supplied with medicinal claims on the labelling. These products, often sold as 'teas', are prepared from dried, crushed or comminuted plants, and sold under their botanical names. A survey in 1987 found that more than 100 varieties of herbal teas were on sale from pharmacies in central London and involved 117 different herbs. The exemptions under the Act give herbal practitioners the flexibility to prepare their own remedies for individual patients and will not have to prove quality, safety and efficacy.

3. Herbal products sold as food supplements with no medical claims, though some therapeutic value may be implied.

THE PRACTICE OF HERBAL MEDICINE

Medical practitioners rarely prescribe herbal remedies and medical herbalists, who constitute only a small professional body, are not consulted by most people who purchase herbal products. Consequently, the principal outlets are health food stores or mail order firms advertising in health magazines and brochures. Now they are available at community pharmacies and will probably be stocked by supermarkets.

In some areas of the UK certain immigrant races have brought their own medical traditions. Oriental medicine in particular has remained the most widely used traditional medicine. Oriental drugs are alleged to have specific characters such as the 'four properties' ('chill' and 'cool' of yin and 'lukewarm' and 'heat' of yang with 'intermediate') and the 'five flavours' ('acrid', 'sour', 'sweet', 'bitter' and 'salty'). Drugs are dispensed according to their character (e.g. diseases with fever are treated with chill and cool drugs). Over 500 herbal remedies are used in Chinese medicine and there are about 600 or more varieties of crude drugs.

Asian medicine has also been brought to the UK with the traditional practices of *Unani* and *Ayurvedic* medicine. The traditional healer is termed *hakim* if he practices the *Unani* system or *vaid* if he practices the *Ayurvedic*. Unlike Oriental medicine which follows traditional formulae, the philosophy behind the Asian system is that preparations are not uniform from country to country, i.e. a preparation sold in India under a certain name will differ from the nominally identical product prepared for sale in Britain. The addition or omission of certain herbs is usually explained by reference to different climates or temperaments of the person being treated.

In general, herbal medicines aim to use the patient's natural resistance and to restore the balance of health. They are commonly used in treating chronic disorders which respond poorly to orthodox remedies, such as arthritis, back pain, mental and stress problems and, sometimes, malignant disease.

SAFETY AND EFFICACY

Many of the plants used in herbal medicine contain principles whose effects can be demonstrated pharmacologically and the action of the whole plant extract can usually be related to that of the isolated constituents. However, for some herbal remedies it is not possible to demonstrate or evaluate their pharmacological activity and the situation is further complicated by the concurrent use of a number of drugs, the supposed active ingredients of which have not been identified. It seems to be a commonly held belief that, by and large, herbal remedies, being natural products, are inherently safer than the potent synthetic drugs of orthodox medicine which sometimes produce undesirable side-effects. However, toxicity from herbal medicines does occur, though it is rarely an acute episode due to accidental consumption of an overdose. Herbal remedies are often taken over long periods and the appearance of toxicity may be considerably delayed and may even appear after the remedy has been discontinued. The quality of the product can be affected by environmental factors, such as climate and growing conditions before harvesting, and toxicity may vary with the part of the plant used, time of harvesting, post-harvest factors and method of preparation.

Concern over the uncontrolled supply and administration of these products has led the CSM (p. 301) to remind doctors that the yellow card scheme applies as much to these products as it does to conventional medicines. However, the CSM can take little action as these medicines do not have a product licence.

HERBAL EXTRACTS OF PROVED OR SUSPECTED TOXICITY

Herbal teas

Traditionally, *comfrey* has been used as a demulcent in chronic catarrhs, as a treatment for gastrointestinal disorders and less specifically as a tonic. In the UK it is used by herbalists as a demulcent, an antihaemorrhagic and anti-rheumatic agent and as an anti-inflammatory agent. Safety concerns over comfrey centre on its content of pyrrolizidine alkaloids; their toxic effects are due to activation in the liver, leading to liver cell necrosis. Human hepatotoxicity of comfrey has been illustrated by characteristic veno-occlusive lesions with hepatomegaly and inhibition of mitosis. Hepatotoxicity has also occurred with other herbal teas containing pyrrolizidine.

A *'babchi'* herbal tea has been associated with photosensitivity. The seeds of this plant contain psoralen, isopsoralen and psoralidin, known to cause photosensitivity reactions.

Herbs used for psychotic effects

Intoxication has been noted with herbs such as *kavakava, khat, thornapple, valerian* and *skullcap*. In the UK hepatotoxicity has been reported as occurring in patients taking *'Kalms'* or *'Neurelax'* for relieving stress. Valerian was thought to be the most likely hepatotoxic component, but the report has been vigourously disputed.

Other herbal preparations

Table 29.1 summarizes some reported adverse effects of herbal medicines.

There are also problems with the apparently widespread use of *khat* or *ghat* and *betel nut*. Concern has been expressed about the incidence of carcinoma of the oral cavity when these are chewed for their stimulant properties.

Aconitine, the poisonous alkaloid in the plant acotine is cardiotoxic and can induce life-threatening arrhythmia. *Aconitum* sp is used predominantly in Chinese medicine and is well reported in Chinese literature.

Contamination

Herbal medicines may be contaminated with pesticides, mycotoxins (fungi) or substituted herbs, e.g. herbs containing podophyllum or substances with anticholinergic effects. Sometimes

Table 29.1 Possible adverse effects of herbal medicines

Herbal preparation	Indication	Adverse effect
Alfalfa seeds	Lowers cholesterol	Pancytopenia, reactivation of systemic lupus erythematosus
Aristolochic acid (tincture/infusion)	Anti-inflammatory	Carcinogenic, renal damage
Coffee enemas	Anti-cancer	Hypokalaemia
Ginseng	Anti-fatigue, anti-stress	Estrogen-like effects, hypertension
Honey (rhododendron)	Food supplement	Intoxication, nausea, vomiting, hypotension, bradycardia, reduced consciousness
Margosa oil (Neem tree extract)	Insecticide, spermicide	Hepatotoxicity
Mistletoe	Antispasmodic, diuretic, hypotensive	Hepatotoxicity (hepatitis), diarrhoea
Zemaphyte (Chinese herbs)	Eczema	Hepatotoxicity (hepatitis)

Adapted from D'Arcy (1991) Adverse reactions and interactions with herbal medicines. Part I. Adverse Drug Reactions Toxicological Review 10(4): 189–208. Published by permission of the Oxford University Press.

an orthodox drug such as aspirin or paracetamol may be added to enhance efficacy. The MCA has detected micro-organisms in some solid dosage forms.

Metals in herbal mixtures

Metals may be added to Asian and Oriental medicines in varying amounts, but in sufficient quantities to cause toxicity. Asian and East African preparations called *'Kushtay'*, used as tonics and aphrodisiacs, contain oxidized heavy metals such as arsenic, mercury, tin, zinc and lead. A typical Kushtay may contain 10–12% of each of several of these metals.

Interactions between herbal medicines and drugs used in orthodox treatment

In view of the large amounts of medicine consumed, both prescribed and over the counter, it is not surprising that interactions (some dangerous) are possible. As well as interactions between orthodox drugs (see p. 298) interactions may also occur with herbal remedies, some of which are shown in Table 29.2.

USE OF SOME COMMON HERBAL REMEDIES

There are numerous herbal drugs and just a few of those most commonly used, together with their suggested therapeutic effects, are described

here. There is no doubt that many people obtain benefits from herbal remedies and they should not be disregarded. However, some contain active substances and their use should be attended with some caution. There is a body of opinion that believes that some licensing agency is required for herbal medicine to ensure quality and to monitor any adverse effects. The scheme which is now operated in Australia would serve as a good model.

Valerian contains volatile oils and alkaloids. Its main use is as a tranquillizer, but it is also recommended for a variety of other disorders. The dose for an adult is 0.3–1.0 g of the dried root.

Ginseng (Asiatic) contains saponins, glycosides and sterols. It is claimed to have a wide variety of actions, including improvement in adrenal, muscular and cerebral function. It is used for debility and as an antidote to stress. There are constraints applied to its use which may result in increased tension and sleeplessness. In healthy adults it is advised not to take ginseng for long periods.

Echinacea. The root contains a mixture of high molecular weight branched polysaccharide and caffeic acid derivatives. It produces a non-specific stimulation to the immune system and may be useful both as a prophylactic and a treatment in common infectious diseases. It is available as an alcoholic extract in a liquid form or in the dry state as capsules or tablets. The tincture is now licensed and will be marketed for the relief of colds, influenza and other respiratory infections.

Table 29.2 Possible interactions between herbal medicines and drugs used in orthodox medicine

Herbal preparation	Orthodox medicine	Interaction
Cardiovascular		
Cardiac glycoside containing prep.	Digoxin	Potentiation, digitalis toxicity
Diuretic	Digoxin/digitoxin anti-hypertensives	Increased loss of K⁺, loss of hypertensive control
Kyushin	Digoxin	Interferes with plasma digoxin assay, false high levels
Linn prep. (ayurvedic medicine)	Amiloride + hydrochlorothiazide	Haemolysis, hypertension, fever
Liquorice	Antihypertensives	Hypokalaemia, hypernatraemia, oedema
Sedatives		
Sedative preps.	Alcohol/antihistamines, hypnotics	Potentiation
Tropane alkaloids	Alcohol/antihistamines, hypnotics	Potentiation
Anticoagulants		
Vitamin K containing preps.	Anticoagulants	Antagonism, loss of anticoagulant control
Endocrine		
Antidiabetic preps. e.g. Damsissa, Karela	Antidiabetic agents, insulin	Loss of diabetic control
Guar gum	Penicillin	Reduced bioavailability of antibiotic
Rauwolfia, ginseng	Drugs causing gynaecomastia, phenothiazines	Potentiation of gynaecomastia, galactorrhoea
Antidepressant		
Ginseng	Phenelzine	Headaches, insomnia, visual hallucinations
Hallucinogens		
Cassia bark (cinnamon)	Tetracycline	Reduced bioavailability of antibiotic (theoretical)
Hallucinogenic preps. 'magic mushroom' (*Psilocybe semilanceata*)	Propranolol, alcohol	Enhanced hallucinogenic effect, schizophrenic states
Miscellaneous		
Ispagula husk	Lithium	Reduced bioavailability of lithium
Kelp	Thyroid hormones/anti-thyroid agents/iodine preps.	Reduced thyroid control (hyper/hypothyroid)
Germander	Hepatotoxic agents	Hepatitis
Ink cap	Alcohol	Disulfiram-like reaction
Eucalyptus oil	Drugs metabolized via liver	Hepatic microsomal enzyme induction
Shankhapushpi (ayurvedic origin)	Phenytoin	Reduced seizure control

Adapted from D'Arcy (1993) Adverse reactions and interactions with herbal medicines. Part 2. Adverse Drug Reactions Toxicological Review 12(3): 147–162. Published by permission of the Oxford University Press.

Dosage of 50 drops twice daily for 5 days a week, to examine its use in the prevention of upper respiratory tract infections, has not proved effective.

Agnus castus contains volatile oils, castine and alkaloids. It is used to treat the symptoms of hormonal imbalance associated with menstruation and the menopause and is said to improve the function of the corpus luteum. The powdered fruit can be incorporated into tablets or used as a liquid extract or tincture.

Feverfew. The active ingredients are sesquiterpene lactones from the aerial parts of the plant. It is recommended for the prophylaxis of migraine in daily doses of 50 mg of the dried feverfew leaf, containing at least 0.2% parthenolide. The sesquiterpene lactones are spasmolytic and render smooth muscle less responsive to norepinephrine, acetylcholine, bradykinin, histamine, prostaglandins and serotonin. Feverfew's activity in migraine is thought to be due to its inhibition of (a) the production of the inflammatory, platelet-aggregating prostaglandins and (b) serotonin release from the platelets.

The chamomiles contain aliphatic esters of angelic and tiglic acids and other oils extracted from the flowers.

Roman chamomile promotes digestion, increases

appetite and is anti-emetic, antispasmodic and mildly sedative when taken orally.

German chamomile or *matricaria* is used most extensively as a panacea.

Preparations of warm and cold infusions of both chamomile and matricaria serve as medicinal agents and as health-related drinks. Teas, made by steeping loose fresh or dried flowers in water or teabags, are used both orally and externally.

Herbal diuretics: bearberry, celery and dandelion. These herbal diuretics are used traditionally by herbalists in the treatment of microbial infections and chronic inflammatory disorders. In more recent years they have been incorporated in over-the-counter products used for other applications, such as the symptomatic relief of premenstrual syndrome, and as slimming aids. Dandelion is probably the preferred diuretic as it is unlikely to result in toxicity and the roots and leaves contain high quantities of potassium, which reduces the likelihood of hypokalaemia. Bearberry is primarily of use as a urinary antiseptic and is effective only if the urine is alkaline. Celery may cause allergic reactions or photodermatitis in some subjects.

Garlic contains various volatile oils including alliin which is believed to form other sulphur-containing compounds responsible for its cholesterol-lowering effects. Studies have used doses of 600–900 mg of garlic powder a day or one half to one garlic clove a day to produce reductions in cholesterol of 9–12% compared with placebo in patients with hyperlipidaemia. Interest has been shown in using garlic as an antihypertensive, but clinical trials have not shown significant results. Traditionally, it has been used to treat a wide range of conditions, including chronic bronchitis, coughs, colds and influenza, and it is believed to have expectorant, antiviral, bacteriostatic and anthelmintic properties.

St John's Wort (*Hypericum perforatum*) is used extensively in both homeopathic and herbal preparations traditionally as a sedative and for wound healing. However, more recently, clinical trials have been conducted with extracts of St John's wort using doses of 350–900 mg daily for 4–8 weeks to treat mild or moderately severe depressive disorders. Similar responses have been noted when compared with drugs such as amitriptyline in mild-to-moderate depression and with imipramine in severe depression. The greater tolerability demonstrated by hypericum recommends further study. A known side-effect of St John's wort is photosensitivity and so patients should be advised of this when taking it. Most extracts of hypericum are standardized on their hypericin content although it is considered that the effects of hypericum may be due to a variety of constituents. Hypericon induces enzymes which increase the breakdown of some drugs including the combined contraceptive pill and warfarin, and therefore reducing their efficacy.

Ginkgo biloba (maidenhair tree) has been used medicinally for thousands of years. Traditionally, as a tea for the treatment of asthma and bronchitis. It is widely used in France and Germany in licensed herbal remedies for the treatment of circulatory insufficiencies (peripheral and cerebral). Many clinical studies of varying quality have examined its use in cerebral insufficiency employing doses of 120 mg daily for 4–6 weeks or 50 mg three times a day for up to 52 weeks. Further study is required but clinically significant effects have been found for improving cognitive impairment and daily living/social behaviour.

Coltsfoot (*Tussilago farfara*). The leaves and flowers from this common wild plant have been used in the form of tea as a popular remedy for coughs and bronchial congestion. The mucilage produced from the leaves is thought to produce a throat soothing effect. The preparations available often contain complex mixtures of different medicinal plants. Safety concerns have been expressed about its long-term use and use in pregnancy due to its content of pyrrolizidine alkaloids which could be potentially tumour-inducing.

Essential oils

Essential oil constituents are found in conventional medicinal products, e.g. peppermint oil for the relief of abdominal colic and distension.

However, the practice of aromatherapy for the palliative care of patients with cancer and for hospice patients has brought the use of essential oils into a different area for the nurse. Some midwives are using aromatherapy for pregnancy and childbirth and for both the mother and infant after birth.

Essential oils are obtained from plant material, e.g. root, leaves, flowers, seeds, usually by distillation, although physical expression is used to obtain some essential oils, mainly those from citrus fruit. It should be noted that there are no controls on the quality of the product sold to the consumer. The concentration of constituents can vary between plant sources and adulteration and contamination is known to occur with pesticides, synthetic oils and other oils. The chemistry of essential oils is complex. A typical essential oil will contain about 100 or more chemical constituents, but most will be present in concentrations below 1%. In aromatherapy it is the constituents of the oils that are thought to provide the 'relaxant' or 'stimulant' effect. Examples of constituents found in some essential oils:

Constituent	Source
Limonene	Citrus oils, e.g. bergamot
Thymol	Thyme oil
Cineole	Eucalyptus oil
Citral	Lemongrass
Linalyl acetate	Lavender oil

Essential oils are believed to act in two ways: by exerting pharmacological effects following absorption into the circulation and via the effects of their odour on the olfactory system. Topical application (i.e. massage) and inhalation have been shown to result in constituents absorbed into the circulation. However, some oils can cause skin irritation or contact dermatitis even when highly diluted in a bath, and some, particularly citrus fruit (with the exception of mandarin), have resulted in photosensitvity. Tea tree oil has been used for the treatment of certain skin infections and clinical trials have shown its potential for use in treating acne.

Patients wishing to consult an aromatherapist should be advised to choose one who has undertaken relevant training, is registered with an appropriate professional body and who has adequate professional indemnity.

FURTHER READING

British Medical Association Report 1986 Alternative therapy. British Medical Association, London
Chan T Y K et al 1995 Poisoning due to Chinese proprietary medicines. Human and Experimental Toxicology 14: 434
D'Arcy P E 1991 Adverse reactions and interactions with herbal medicines. Adverse drug reactions, Toxicological Reviews 10(4): 189
De Smet P 1992 Adverse effects of herbal drugs. Springer-Verlag, Berlin
Editorial 1994 Herbal medicines. Pharmaceutical Journal 253
Editorial 1995 Should herbal medicine-like products be licensed as medicines? British Medical Journal 310: 1023
Editorial 1998 Alternative medicine—the risks of untested and unregulated remedies. New England Journal of Medicine 339: 839
Ernst E 1998 Health food shops, risks of complementary medicine and ethical standards of research. Journal of the Royal College of Physicians London 32: 399
Fulder S 1989 The handbook of complementary medicine, 2nd edn. Coronet Books, London
MacGregor F B 1989 Hepatotoxicity of herbal remedies. British Medical Journal 299: 1156
Mills S 1989 The complete guide to modern herbalism. Thorsons, London
Ministry of Agriculture, Fisheries and Food, Department of Health 1991 Dietary Supplements and Health Foods
Newall C A, Anderson L A, Phillipson J D 1996 Herbal medicines. A guide for health care professionals. Pharmaceutical Press, London
Penn R G 1983 Adverse Reactions Bulletin No. 102

FURTHER INFORMATION

It would further research if any suspected adverse effects which are thought to be due to herbal remedies were reported to the National Poisons Information Service, Medical Toxicology Unit, Avonley Road, London SE14 5EP. Telephone: 0171 635 1062.

HOMEOPATHY

Homeopathy is perhaps one of the most controversial complementary therapies, but at the same time appears to be one of the most popular in the UK. There is a lack of conclusive evidence that the clinical effects of homeopathy are completely due to placebo, but at the same time there is insufficient evidence that homeopathy is clearly efficacious for any single clinical condition.

Classical homeopathy has the following characteristics:

1. Medicines are chosen on the basis of the similarity between the symptoms they produce in healthy people and the symptoms from which the patient is suffering
2. The medicines are given singly
3. The medicines are given in small doses
4. Medicines are not repeated routinely, but only when the patient's symptoms demand it.

In practice there are wide variations in how these principles are applied; a good deal depends on the orientation of the particular homeopath with respect to the symptoms they consider important (physical and psychological), the type of illness and whether the illness is acute or chronic. Many homeopaths ignore the 'single remedy' rule, preferring to adopt a multiple prescribing approach, e.g. remedies for hay-fever.

History and philosophy

The basic principle of homeopathy has been known since the time of the Ancient Greeks. Devised from the Greek word '*homios*' meaning 'like', homeopathy is the medical practice of treating like with like.

In the eighteenth century Dr Samuel Hahnemann (1755–1843), a German-born physician, appalled by the medical practices of the day sought a method of healing which would be safe, gentle and effective. He believed that human beings have a capacity for healing themselves and that the symptoms of disease reflect the individual's struggle to overcome their illness. He reasoned that instead of suppressing symptoms he could seek to stimulate them and so encourage and assist the body's natural healing process.

Hahnemann discovered that when he self-administered an infusion of cinchona bark (quinine) it produced the symptoms of malaria. When given to a patient suffering from the disease it alleviated the symptoms. He used this procedure with numerous active substances from animal, vegetable and mineral sources in healthy volunteers to determine the 'symptom

picture' of each substance. This approach came to be known as 'proving'. He than went on to establish the smallest effective dose to reduce the toxicity of the substance. He diluted his medicines and subjected them to vigorous shaking ('succussion') at each dilution step. He claimed that the more dilute the remedies were, the more potent they became; this process of serial dilution and succussion became known as 'potentization'.

Diagnosis and treatment

In addition to the basic principles of classical homeopathy there are other basic tenets of homeopathy. Homeopaths believe that illness results from the body's inability to cope with challenging factors, such as poor diet and environmental conditions, and that the signs and symptoms of disease represent the body's attempt to restore order. Homeopathic remedies are believed not to act directly on the disease process but to stimulate the body's own healing activity known as the 'vital force'. As homeopaths believe that the 'vital force' is expressed differently in each individual, their choice of treatment is based on each individual's unique set of symptoms. It is usual for a homeopath during a first consultation to take a very detailed history to determine the patient's physical, mental and emotional symptoms. A homeopath may then use a homeopathic repertory to choose a remedy that most closely fits a patient's symptom picture. Computerized repertories are now available which greatly facilitate this process.

Having chosen the remedy the homeopath must select the potency and the form, e.g. tablets, pills or powders. The method of preparing a homeopathic medicine usually commences with the 'mother tincture' as in the case of a herbal medicine, an alcoholic extract. One drop of this is mixed with 99 (or sometimes 9) drops of water and shaken hard to give the first potency, i.e. 1c the first centesimal dilution. One drop of this preparation is then mixed with 99 drops of water and shaken to give the second potency (2c), and this process is repeated for as many times as required. Insoluble substances, such as metals, are ground up in a mortar and mixed with lactose. Some commonly used potencies are the 6c, 12c and 30c. Modern molecular theory suggests that the 12th centesimal potency is the limit beyond which no molecules of the original substance would be present. This is therefore taken as the boundary between 'low' and 'high' potencies. In practice the high potencies are considered more powerful than the low ones despite the absence of any of the original substance as it is said they have been 'dynamized' to a greater extent. The 'seriousness' of the symptoms determine how frequently the remedy is administered and the number of total doses.

Mechanism of action

The lack of a plausible mechanism of action continues to be one of the arguments against homeopathy. Probably the most known work in this area is that of Benventiste and colleagues who believed that they had shown that ultra-high dilutions of immunoglobulin E (IgE) anti-serum could trigger degranulation in human basophils *in vitro*. This has subsequently been disputed when attempts have been made to replicate the experiments and the original experiments discredited as flawed. (See further reading for a summary of Benventiste's results: Schiff M).

Numerous hypotheses of the mechanism of action of homeopathic potencies exist. How the solution 'remembers' information from the original substance is speculative. Results from rigorous placebo-controlled trials do not support the hypothesis that it is a placebo effect and further studies are required to investigate any positive benefit these remedies may have.

Safety

Homeopathic remedies are often claimed to be entirely free from adverse effects. However, there are isolated reports in the literature of suspected adverse effects, usually allergic reactions, following the use of homeopathic remedies. Also, it is often stated that a patient may experience an 'aggravation' (a temporary worsening of symptoms) within a few days of starting treatment. Homeopaths claim that this is a sign that the correct remedy has been chosen and that it is working.

There have been reports of homeopathic remedies adulterated with corticosteroids and of homeopathic preparations that contain unusually high levels of arsenic. The Committee on the Safety of Medicines (CSM) accepts yellow card reports for any licensed homeopathic medicines.

Certain homeopaths (usually lay practitioners) have been criticized in the past for advocating the use of homeopathic remedies as an alternative for immunization in childhood. Under UK law anyone can set themselves as a homeopath, regardless of whether or not they have had any training. Patients seeking a consultation should be advised to check that the homeopath has recognized qualifications, is registered with a relevant professional body, e.g. Faculty of Homeopathy, Society of Homeopaths of UK Homeopathic Medical Association, and has adequate professional indemnity. There is also a plethora of remedies available for self-administration. Choosing the right remedy is not always easy.

It is often claimed that the use of caffeine, aromatic substances (e.g. peppermint, essential oils) or certain orthodox drugs (e.g. corticosteroids) can inactivate homeopathic remedies if used concurrently. However, there does not appear to be any reliable evidence to support this and there is no evidence that homeopathic remedies interact with conventional medicines, although homeopaths may claim that a patient's symptoms may be 'masked' by conventional medicines, therefore making an accurate choice of homeopathic remedy more difficult.

Homeopathic remedies

In the UK, the majority of homeopathic remedies can be bought in pharmacies, health stores and other retail outlets. Some low-potency (i.e. high-concentration) homeopathic remedies are however classified as prescription-only medicines. About 65% of homeopathic remedies are prepared from extracts of plant materials. The remainder may be of animal, insect, biological, chemical or other origin with over 1600 substances routinely in use today. For example:

Arsenicum album	chemical
Arnica (*Arnica montana*)	plant (all parts)
Apis mellifica (honey bee)	insect (bee sting)
Calcarea fluorica	chemical
Hamamelis virginia (witch hazel)	plant (bark)
Nux vomica	plant (seeds)
Sulphur	chemical

The British Homeopathic Pharmacopoeia was first published in 1870; a new edition, published by the British Homeopathic Manufacturers Association, became available in 1993 and is designed to be used in conjunction with the German Homeopathic Pharmacopoeia.

The remedies are usually prescribed as tablets or pills with the following advice:

- Do not take remedies within 30 minutes of eating, drinking, smoking or using toothpaste
- Avoid touching the remedies (tip tablets and pills onto the bottle cap and then onto the tongue)

- Hold remedies in your mouth for a few seconds before swallowing
- Store remedies away from strong smelling substances
- Do not stop taking conventional medicines unless told to do so by the doctor who prescribed them.

Each remedy is thought to be of benefit for a range of symptoms, for example:

Arnica

Use after any injury
Bruises
Sprains
Physical exhaustion following sustained exercise, e.g. a day's gardening or a long walk
Insomnia due to over-tiredness
Muscle-ache all over
Bed feels too hard—constant desire to move to a soft part
Cannot bear to be touched
Great sensitivity to pain
Gout, rheumatism, with a fear of being touched
Use when symptoms are worse: from touch; from motion; in damp, cold conditions
Use when symptoms are better: when lying down; with head low.

FURTHER READING

Castro M 1990 The complete homeopathy handbook. A guide to everyday health care. Macmillan, London
Ernst E and Hahn E 1998 Homeopathy. A critical appraisal. Butterworth-Heinemann, Oxford
Kayne S B 1997 Homeopathic pharmacy. An introduction

and handbook. Churchill Livingstone, Edinburgh
Linde K et al 1997 Are the clinical effects of homeopathy placebo effects? A meta-analysis of placebo controlled trials. Lancet 350: 834–843
Schiff M 1994 The memory of water. Thorsons, London

Weights and measures

WEIGHTS AND MEASURES

Weight

1 kilogram (kg)	=	1000 grams (g)
1 gram (g)	=	1000 milligrams (mg)
1 milligram (mg)	=	1000 micrograms (mcg)
1 microgram (mcg)	=	1000 nanograms (ng)

Capacity

1 litre (l)	=	1000 millitres (ml)
1 decilitre (dl)	=	100 millilitres (ml)

1 litre of water at 4°C weighs 1 kilogram.

Quantity

1 mole (mol)	=	1000 millimoles (mmol)
1 millimole (mmol)	=	1000 micromoles (mcmol)

Percentage solutions

0.1% solution	=	100 mg in 100 ml (1 mg/ml)
1% solution	=	1 g in 100 ml (10 mg/ml)
10% solution	=	10 g in 100 ml (100 mg/ml)

Domestic measures

1 teaspoonful	=	about 5 ml
1 dessertspoonful	=	about 7.5 ml
1 tablespoonful	=	about 15 ml
1 tumblerful	=	about 250 ml

Infusion sets

Standard giving set

20 drops (15 for blood) deliver 1 ml

Microdrop set

60 drops deliver 1 ml

Appendix 2

Glossary of terms used

TYPES OF DRUGS REFERRING TO MODE OF ACTION

General anaesthetics depress cerebral function, induce unconsciousness and prevent all sensation.

Local anaesthetics interfere with the function of a nerve or nerve ending and prevent all sensation from a localized area without loss of consciousness.

Analgesics relieve pain without interfering with consciousness.

Anthelmintics kill or aid the removal of worms from the intestines.

Antiepileptics prevent fits.

Antipyretics reduce body temperature when it is raised above normal.

Antibiotics are prepared from living organisms and kill or prevent multiplication of bacteria in the body. Many antibiotics are now prepared synthetically.

Aperients loosen the bowels.

Carminatives promote belching.

Chemotherapeutic agents are prepared synthetically to kill or prevent the multiplication of bacteria within the body.

Contraceptives prevent conception.

Cytotoxic agents are drugs which damage or kill malignant cells and are used in treating cancers.

Diaphoretics induce sweating.

Disinfectants kill bacteria.

Diuretics increase the secretion of urine by the kidneys.

Emetics produce vomiting.

Expectorants make the bronchial secretion more liquid and therefore more easily expelled.

Hypnotics produce sleep.

Hypotensive drugs lower blood pressure.

Mydriatics dilate the pupil.

Myotics constrict the pupil.

Neuroleptics are anti-psychotic drugs.

Opioids have a similar action to opium.

Prodrug a substance which is inactive, but is converted into an active drug in the body.

Sedatives soothe, but may also cause drowsiness.

Styptics stop local bleeding.

Tonics are said to restore general well-being, but are of doubtful value.

Tranquillizers promote mental relaxation without drowsiness.

Terminology referring to administration

Although many hospitals now have special prescription forms which have eliminated the use of many of the following terms, they are still widely used when prescribing in outpatients departments and general practice. It would be better if most of them were eliminated from prescription writing as they are a potential source of error.

a.c.	— before meals
ad lib	— as much as required
b.d.	— twice daily
b.i.d.	— twice daily
gutt.	— drops
i.m.	— intramuscular
inj.	— injection
I.U.	— International Units
i.v.	— intravenous
o.h.	— every hour
o.m.	— every morning
o.n.	— every night
p.c.	— after meals
p.o.	— orally
p.r.	— per rectum
p.v.	— per vaginam
q.d.s.	— four times daily
q.i.d.	— four times daily
rep	— repeat
s.o.s.	— if necessary
stat	— at once
t.d.s.	— three times daily
t.i.d.	— three times daily

Proprietary and other drug names

The following list of proprietary names of drugs with the non-proprietary equivalent or similar preparation is not intended to be complete, but merely to include drugs which are often prescribed under their proprietary names.

Proprietary or trade name	rINN of drug or similar preparation
Acepril	Captopril
Achromycin	Tetracycline
Actilyse	Alteplase
Actinomycin D	Dactinomycin
Acupan	Nefopam
Adalat	Nifedipine
Adcortyl	Triamcinolone
Adenocor	Adenosine
Adriamycin	Doxorubicin
Alcobon	Flucytosine
Aldactone	Spironolactone
Aldomet	Methyldopa
Alexan	Cytarabine
Alimix	Cisapride
Alkeran	Melphalan
Aludrox	Aluminium hydroxide
Alupent	Orciprenaline
AmBisone	Amphotericin liposomal
Amikin	Amikacin
Amoxil	Amoxicillin
Anafranil	Clomipramine
Antabuse	Disulfiram
Antepsin	Sucralfate
Anturan	Sulphinypyrazone
APD	Disodium pamidronate

Proprietary or trade name	rINN of drug or similar preparation	Proprietary or trade name	rINN of drug or similar preparation
Apresoline	Hydralazine	Cedocard Retard	Isosorbide dinitrate
Aprinox	Flumethiazide	Celevac	Methylcellulose
Apsifen	Ibuprofen	Ceporex	Cefalexin
Aricept	Donepezil	Cervagem	Gemeprost
Arret	Loperamide	Chloromycetin	Chloramphenicol
Artane	Benzhexol	Choledyl	Choline theophyllinate
Asacol	Mesalazine	Ciproxin	Ciprofloxacin
Ativan	Lorazepam	Cidex	Glutaraldehyde
Atrovent	Ipratropium	Claforan	Cefotaxime
Augmentin	Amoxicillin + potassium clavenulate	Clarityn	Loratadine
		Clinoral	Sulindac
Aureomycin	Chlortetracycline	Clozaril	Clozapine
Avomine	Promethazine theoclate	Colofac	Mebeverine
Azactam	Aztreonam	Cordarone X	Amiodarone
AZT	Zidovudine	Cordilox	Verapamil
Bactrim	Co-trimoxazole	Corlan	Hydrocortisone pellets
Becosym	Vit B compound	Corsodyl	Chlorhexidine mouthwash
Becotide	Beclomethasone		
Benemid	Probenecid	Coversyl	Perindopril
Benerva	Thiamine	Cozaar	Losartan
Beta-Cardone	Sotalol	Crystapen	Benzylpenicillin
Betadine	Povidone iodine	Cyklokapron	Tranexamic acid
Betaloc	Metoprolol	Cytamen Injection	Cyanocobalamin injection
Betnesol	Betamethasone		
Betnovate	Betamethasone topical	Cytosar Injection	Cytarabine injection
Bioral gel	Carbenoxolone gel	Cytotec	Misoprostol
Blocadren	Timolol	Daktarin	Miconazole
Bricanyl	Terbutaline	Dalacin C	Clindamycin
Brocadopa	Levodopa	Dalmane	Flurazepam
Brufen	Ibuprofen	Danol	Danazol
Burinex	Bumetanide	Daraprim	Pyrimethamine
Buscopan	Hyoscine butylbromide	Deltacortril	Prednisolone
Buspar	Buspirone	De-Nol	Bismuth chelate
Cafergot	Ergotamine + caffeine	Depixol	Flupenthixol
Calpol	Paracetamol paediatric elixir	Depo-Medrone	Methylprednisolone
		Depo-Provera	Medroxyprogesterone
Calsynar	Calcitonin (salmon)	Deseril	Methysergide
Camcolit	Lithium carbonate	Dexedrine	Dexamfetamine
Camsilon	Edrophonium	DF118	Dihydrocodeine
Canesten	Clotrimazole	Diamox	Acetazolamide
Capoten	Captopril	Diazemuls	Diazepam injection
Cardura	Doxazosin	Diconal	Dipipanone + cyclizine
Catapres	Clonidine	Difflam	Benzydamine
CCNU	Lomustine	Diflucan	Fluconazole

Proprietary or trade name	rINN of drug or similar preparation
Dioctyl	Docusate sodium
Diprivan	Propofol
Disipal	Orphenadrine
Disprin	Dispersible aspirin
Distalgesic	Paracetamol + dextroproproxyphene (co-proxamol)
Dixarit	Clonidine
Dolobid	Diflunisal
Dramamine	Dimenhydrinate
Droleptan	Droperidol
D.T.I.C.-Dome	Dacarbazine
Dulco-Lax	Bisacodyl
Duphalac	Lactulose
Durabolin	Nandrolone phenylpropionate
Durogesic patch	Fentanyl patch
Dytac	Triamterene
Elantan	Isosorbide mononitrate
Eldepryl	Selegiline
Emblon	Tamoxifen
Eminase	Anistreplase (Apsac)
Endoxana	Cyclophosphamide
Entero-vioform	Clioquinol
Entocort	Budesonide capsules
Epanutin	Phenytoin
Epilim	Sodium valproate
Eppy	Epinephrine eye-drops
Erythrocin	Erythromycin
Esidrex	Hydrochlorothiazide
Euglucon	Glibenclamide
Fansidar	Sulfadoxine + pyrimethamine
Feldene	Piroxicam
Fentazin	Perphenazine
Flagyl	Metronidazole
Fluothane	Halothane
Fortral	Pentazocine
Fortum	Ceftazidime
Fosamax	Alendronic acid
Frumil	Co-amilofruse
Fucidin	Sodium fusidate
Fungilin Lozenges	Amphotericin lozenges
Furadantin	Nitrofurantoin

Proprietary or trade name	rINN of drug or similar preparation
Genticin	Gentamicin
Glibenese	Glipizide
GlucaGen	Glucagon
Glucobay	Acarbose
Glucophage	Metformin
Heminevrin	Chlormethiazole
Hibiscrub	Chlorhexidine
Hibitane Gluconate	Chlorhexidine gluconate
HRF	Gonadorelin
Humalog	Insulin lispro
Hypnovel	Midazolam
Hypovase	Prazosin
Hytrin	Terazosin
Ikorel	Nicorandil
Ilosone	Erythromycin
Imigran	Sumatriptan
Imodium	Loperamide
Imuran	Azathioprine
Inderal	Propranolol
Indocid	Indomethacin
Innovace	Enalapril
Intal	Sodium cromoglicate
Isoket	Isosorbide dinitrate
Isordil	Isosorbide dinitrate
Istin	Amlodipine
Jectofer	Iron sorbitol
Kabikinase	Streptokinase
Keflex	Cephalexin
Kemadrin	Procyclidine
Klaricid	Clarithromycin
Kloref Tablets	Potassium chloride effervescent tablets
Konakion	Phytomenadione (vitamin K)
Lamictal	Lamotrigine
Lanoxin	Digoxin
Largactil	Chlorpromazine
Lariam	Mefloquine
Larodopa	Levodopa
Lasix	Furosemide
Ledermycin	Demeclocycline
Lentizol	Amitriptyline (sustained release)

Proprietary or trade name	rINN of drug or similar preparation	Proprietary or trade name	rINN of drug or similar preparation
Leukeran	Chlorambucil	Nivaquine	Chloroquine sulphate
Librium	Chlordiazepoxide	Nizoral	Ketoconazole
Lindane	γ Benzene hexachloride	Nolvadex	Tamoxifen
Lioresal	Baclofen	Nuelin	Theophylline Liquid
Lipostat	Pravastatin	Nurofen	Ibuprofen
Livial	Tibilone	Omnopon	Papaveretum
Lomotil	Co-phenotrope	Oncovin	Vincristine
Lopresor	Metoprolol	One alpha	Alfacalcidol
Losec	Omeprazole	Oramorph	Morphine solution
Madopar Capsules	Co-beneldopa	Pabrinex	Vitamin B and C injection
Malarone	Atovaquone + Proguanil	Palfium	Dextromoramide
Maloprim	Dapsone + pyrimethamine	Paludrine	Proguanil
Manerix	Moclobemide	Panadol	Paracetamol
Marcain	Bupivacaine	Paramol	Paracetamol + dihydrocodeine
Maxolon	Metoclopramide		
Melleril	Thioridazine	Parlodel	Bromocriptine
Meptid	Meptazinol	Penbritin	Ampicillin
Metopirone	Metyrapone	Pepcid	Famotidine
Midamor	Amiloride	Persantin	Dipyridamole
Minocin	Minocycline	Phenergan	Promethazine
Mithramycin	Plicamycin	Phyllocontin	Aminophylline slow release
Mitoxana	Ifosfamide		
Mobic	Meloxicam	Physeptone	Methadone
Modecate Injection	Fluphenazine decanoate injection	Physiotens	Moxonidine
		Picolax	Sodium picosulphate
Moduretic	Co-amilozide	Pipril	Piperacillin
Mogadon	Nitrazepam	Piriton	Chlorphenamine
Molipaxin	Trazodone	Ponderax	Fenfluramine
Motilium	Domperidone	Ponstan	Mefenamic acid
Myleran	Busulphan	Praxilene	Naftidrofuryl
Mysoline	Primidone	Prednesol	Prednisolone soluble
Naprosyn	Naproxen	Premarin	Conjugated estrogens
Narcan	Naloxone	Prepidil	Dinoprost
Nardil	Phenelzine	Prepulsid	Cisapride
Natrilix	Indapamide	Primaxin	Imipenem + cilastatin
Natulan	Procarbazine	Pripsen	Piperazine
Navidrex	Cyclopenthiazide	Pro-Banthine	Propantheline
Negram	Nalidixic acid	Propaderm	Beclomethasone topical
Neo-Cytamen	Hydroxycobalamin	Proscar	Finasteride
Neo-NaClex	Bendroflumethiazide	Prostigmin	Neostigmine
Nephril	Polythiazide	Prothiaden	Dosulepin
Netillin	Netilmicin	Provera	Medroxyprogesterone tablets
Neurontin	Gabapentin		

Proprietary or trade name	rINN of drug or similar preparation	Proprietary or trade name	rINN of drug or similar preparation
Prozac	Fluoxetine	Sustenon	Testosterone propionate injection
Pulmicort	Budenoside inhaler		
Questran	Colestyramine	Symmetrel	Amantadine
Rastinon	Tolbutamide	Synacthen	Tetracosactide
Redoxon	Ascorbic acid	Syntometrine	Oxytoxin + ergometrine
Retrovir	Zidovudine		
Rifinah	Rifampicin + Isoniazid	Synalar	Fluocinolone
Risperdal	Risperidone	Tagamet	Cimetidine
Rivotril	Clonazepam	Tambocor	Flecainide
Rogitine	Phentolamine	Targocid	Teicoplanin
Rynacrom	Sodium cromoglicate nasal spray	Taxol	Paclitaxel
		Tegretol	Carbamazepine
Rythmodan	Disopyramide	Temgesic	Buprenorphine
Sabril	Vigabatrin	Tenormin	Atenolol
Salazopyrin	Sulfasalazine	Terramycin	Oxytetracycline
Saluric	Chlorothiazide	Theo-Dur	Theophylline slow release
Sando K Tablets	Potassium chloride effervescent tablets		
		Tildiem	Diltiazem
Sandostatin	Octreotide	Tofranil	Imipramine
Sanomigran	Pizotifen	Trandate	Labetalol
Saventrine Tablets	Isoprenaline slow release	Transiderm-Nitro	Glyceryl trinitrate patch
Scoline	Suxamethonium	Trasicor	Oxprenolol
Scopolamine	Hyoscine	Tridil	Glyceryl trinitrate injection
Securopen	Azlocillin		
Senokot	Senna	Triludan	Terfenadine
Septrin	Co-trimoxazole	Tritace	Ramipril
Serc	Betahistine	Tryptizol	Amitriptyline
Serenace	Haloperidol	Tylex	Co-codamol (30/500)
Serevent	Salmeterol	Uniphyllin Continus	Theophylline slow release
Sinemet Tablets	Co-careldopa		
Sinequan	Doxepin	Utinor	Norfloxacin
Slow K Tablets	Potassium chloride slow release	Valium	Diazepam
		Vallergan	Alimemazine
Sotacor	Sotalol	Vancocin	Vancomycin
Staril	Fosinopril	Velbe	Vinblastine
Stelazine	Trifluoperazine	Ventolin	Salbutamol
Stemetil	Prochlorperazine	Vepisid	Etoposide
Stilnoct	Zolpidem	Vermox	Mebendazole
Streptase	Streptokinase	Viagra	Sildenafil
Stugeron	Cinnarizine	Vibramycin	Doxycycline
Surmontil	Trimipramine	Visken	Pindolol
Sustac	Glyceryl trinitrate sustained release	Voltarol	Diclofenac
		Welldorm	Chloral betaine

Proprietary or trade name	rINN of drug or similar preparation	Proprietary or trade name	rINN of drug or similar preparation
Xylocaine	Lidocaine	Zirtek	Cetirizine
Yomesan	Niclosamide	Zithromax	Azithromycin
Zamadol	Tramadol	Zocor	Simvastatin
Zantac	Ranitidine	Zofran	Ondansetron
Zarontin	Ethosuximide	Zoladex	Goserelin
Zestril	Lisinopril	Zovirax	Aciclovir
Zimovane	Zopiclone	Zydol	Tramadol
Zinacef	Cefuroxime	Zyloric	Allopurinol
Zinamide	Pyrazinamide	Zyprexa	Olanzapine

Information about drugs

There are now many books and articles about drugs. Three important publications which should be available in every School of Nursing library give clear and up-to-date information about drugs and treatment:

Prescribers Journal (published quarterly)
Enquiries to: HMSO
           PO Box 276
           London SW8 5DT

Drug and Therapeutics Bulletin (published monthly)
Enquiries to: Dept. DTB
            Consumers Association
            Castlemead
            Gascoyne Way
            Hertford X, SG14 ILH

The *British National Formulary* (BNF), which is published twice a year, is a very useful book of reference. It contains essential details of all drugs currently available in the UK with brief sections on treatment. A copy should be kept on every ward.

Pharmaceutical companies provide a data sheet for each of their products. These sheets contain information about the nature and action of the drug, its dose and therapeutic use, adverse effects and contraindications. They are also published annually as a compendium and are a useful source of information.

There are several good textbooks of clinical pharmacology. The most prestigious and arguably the best is *The Pharmacological Basis of Therapeutics*

(9th edn) by A.G. Goodman and L.S.T. Gilman, Pergamon Press, New York, 1996. It is, however, extensive and expensive; it is also orientated to the USA.

Considerably more readable and shorter are *A Textbook of Clinical Pharmacology* (4th edn) by J.M. Ritter, L.D. Lewis and T.G.K. Mant, Edward Arnold, London, 1999 and *Clinical Pharmacology* by D.R. Laurence, P.N. Bennet and M.J. Brown, Churchill Livingstone, Edinburgh, 1997.

A book containing multiple choice questions for study and self-examination, based on *Clinical Pharmacology for Nurses*, is now available: *Test Yourself in Clinical Pharmacology for Nurses* by J. Trounce and D. Gould, Churchill Livingstone, Edinburgh, 1997.

Index